Craig's Care of the Newly Born Infant

Craig's Care of the Newly Born Infant

T. L. Turner MB ChB FRCP(Edin) FRCP(Glas)
Consultant Paediatrician,
Royal Hospital for Sick Children and
Queen Mother's Maternity Hospital, Yorkhill, Glasgow
Honorary Clinical Lecturer, University of Glasgow

Jean Douglas RGN SCM
Sister,
Department of Neonatal Medicine and Surgery,
City Hospital, Hucknall Road, Nottingham

F. Cockburn MD FRCP(Edin) FRCP(Glas) DCH
Samson Gemmell Professor of Child Health, University of Glasgow
Honorary Consultant Paediatrician, Royal Hospital for Sick Children
and Queen Mother's Maternity Hospital, Yorkhill, Glasgow

EIGHTH EDITION

CHURCHILL LIVINGSTONE
EDINBURGH LONDON MELBOURNE AND NEW YORK 1988

CHURCHILL LIVINGSTONE
Medical Division of Longman Group UK Limited

Distributed in the United States of America by
Churchill Livingstone Inc., 19 West 44th Street, New
York, N.Y. 10036, and by associated companies,
branches and representatives throughout the world.

First edition 1956
Second edition 1962
Third edition 1966
Fourth edition 1969
Fifth edition 1974
  Reprinted 1975
Spanish edition 1977
Italian edition 1978
Sixth edition 1978
Seventh edition 1982
Eighth edition 1988

ISBN 0-443-03342-0

British Library Cataloguing in Publication Data
Craig, W. S.
    Craig's care of the newly born infant. —
    8th ed.
    1. Infants (Newborn) — Diseases
    I. Title II. Turner, T. L. III. Douglas,
    Jean IV. Cockburn, Forrester
    618.92'01   RJ254

Library of Congress Cataloging-in-Publication Data
Craig, W. S. (William Stuart), 1903–1975.
    Craig's care of the newly born infant.

    Includes bibliographies and index.
    1. Infants (Newborn) — Care. 2. Pediatric nursing.
I. Turner, T. L. II. Douglas, Jean. III. Cockburn,
Forrester. IV. Title. V. Title: Care of the
newly born infant. [DNLM: 1. Infant Care. 2. Infant,
Newborn, Diseases — nursing.   WY 159 C886n]
RJ253.C7   1988   618.92'01   87-26824

Produced by Longman Singapore Publishers (Pte) Ltd.
Printed in Singapore

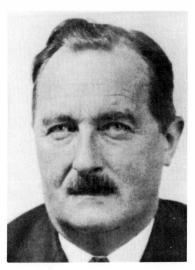

William Stuart McRae Craig
B.Sc., M.D., F.R.C.P. (Edin.), F.R.C.P. (Lond.), F.R.S.E.
1903–1975

Stuart Craig who prepared the first four editions of this, his book, died in Edinburgh after a short illness on 21st June, 1975.

The son of a Scottish family doctor he was educated at Bingley Grammar School, Yorkshire, George Watson's College, Edinburgh and the Universities of Glasgow and Edinburgh at the last of which he was awarded the Buchanan Scholarship and the James Thomson Medal.

His initial paediatric training was gained when working at the Royal Hospital for Sick Children, Edinburgh, under the guidance of Professor Charles McNeil to whom he became first assistant in the newly formed Department of Child Life and Health in the University of Edinburgh.

From 1946 to 1968 he was the first full time Professor of Paediatrics and Child Health in the University of Leeds. In 1969 he gave the first Charles McNeil Memorial Lecture at the Royal College of Physicians of Edinburgh. In addition to many contributions to the medical literature his major publications included: *Child and Adolescent Life in Health and Disease*, 1946; *Care of the Newly Born Infant*, 1956; *John Thomson, Pioneer and Father of Scottish Paediatrics*, 1968; *History of the Royal College of Physicians of Edinburgh*, 1976.

Preface

This Eighth Edition builds on the firm foundations laid by Professor W S Craig in the first four editions published between 1956 and 1969. Dr A J Keay, Dr D M Morgan and Nora H J Stephen, in the three editions published in 1974, 1978 and 1982, have with great skill kept to the original format while keeping up-to-date with a very rapid increase in knowledge. *Craig's Care of the Newly Born Infant* has provided for more than 30 years a view of current thinking about the provision of care for the newly born infant.

The present authors have endeavoured to maintain the basic structure and to keep the information given up-to-date and relevant to present day practice. Changes in the provision of care for the newborn human infant during this past 30 years came about through improved understanding of the normal and abnormal birth processes and the early requirements, adaptations and behaviour of the mother, father and baby. Improved knowledge and understanding has resulted in a much greater chance of undamaged survival for the infant and for the subsequent growth of a healthy child.

When first approached by the publishers and Dr Alex Keay about the task of up-dating 'Craig', we were conscious of the considerable part the book has played in medical and nursing education and of the continuing need for the book. We were also conscious of the considerable responsibility placed upon us. It is our hope that we have managed to maintain the continuity and standards achieved during the past three decades whilst making extensive revision of the text. If we have succeeded, thanks must go to those readers of previous editions who have given generously of their time and expertise to make constructive criticisms. In particular, we would wish to acknowledge the help of Mrs Bess Waddington, Queen Victoria Hospital, Adelaide, South Australia.

The authors are most grateful to Miss Jean Hyslop and

Mr Alastair W M Irwin of the Department of Medical Illustration of the Royal Hospital for Sick Children, Yorkhill, Glasgow for the preparation of new illustrations, and to Dr Susan Cole of the Information Services Division of the Scottish Home and Health Department for providing the up-dated statistical information used in Chapter 2. We thank the staff of Churchill Livingstone for their courtesy and understanding. We are most grateful to Mrs Jean Barr for her considerable secretarial assistance and good humour.

As with our predecessors we are happy to acknowledge the love and support of our families during the preparation of this edition.

Glasgow, 1987   T. L. T
                                                        J. D
                                                        F. C

Contents

1

The challenge

Our health and happiness in later childhood and adult life depend to a large extent on our well-being before, during and after birth. This formative period of our lives therefore presents all those concerned with the management of mother and infant with a formidable challenge. Although recent years have seen great advances in our understanding of the physiology and pathology of this all-important period of our lives, new discoveries often only serve to reveal our ignorance in other respects.

Changing emphasis

Inevitably the development of care of the newborn has been subject to the same influences which have conditioned progress in medicine as a whole. The influence of the anatomist was followed by that of the pathologist. A new but complementary approach resulted from the growth of bacteriology, later to be extended with the advent of virology. Most recently we have seen the advent of genetic techniques in chromosomal and gene analysis, in which DNA probes are used to unravel the causes of inherited congenital malformations and metabolic disorders, and of some tumours. This is opening up the exciting prospect of early detection and treatment or prevention of these genetically determined disorders. Research in biochemistry, biophysics and immunology have added greatly to our knowledge of the manner in which the newborn infant reacts to his environment. Behavioural studies are demonstrating that these reactions are not just physical but involve degrees of awareness and social responsiveness of which we have not previously been aware. It has become increasingly evident that many of the factors affecting the health of the newborn infant act before birth, during the pregnancy or in the parents before conception has taken place.

1

Development of perinatal health services

Until the beginning of the century pregnancy and delivery were associated with a major risk to the life and health of the mother and an even greater risk to the newborn infant. Concern at this state of affairs led to the establishment in the UK of the Central Midwives Board, which was formed to regulate the professional practice of midwives and to supervise their training. Continuing high rates of maternal deaths in the 1920s promoted a national drive towards safer maternity by encouraging higher professional standards among doctors, midwives and nurses. The Royal College of Obstetricians and Gynaecologists was founded in 1929 and promoted improved standards of medical management and training. Local health authorities by the late 1930s were obliged by law to provide a comprehensive midwifery service. The introduction of antibiotics and of compatible blood transfusion reduced the risk from infection and haemorrhage. Confidential enquiries into every maternal death began in the 1950s and are now being followed by similar enquiries into infant deaths in the perinatal period. By such methods of medical audit the perinatal health services are able to keep themselves under ongoing review. The present perinatal health services will be considered in more detail in Chapter 2. At this point it is of interest to consider how each of the professions engaged in perinatal care has evolved.

The midwife

Until the end of the eighteenth century no specific hospital provision was made for mothers in labour or for their infants. Foundling hospitals were formed mainly for the care of unwanted infants but indirectly they were instrumental in stimulating a new interest in care of the newborn. In the eighteenth century the family doctor acted as man-midwife to those families able to afford his services. Deliveries of mothers in poor circumstances were attended by 'handy women'. The University of Edinburgh in 1726 appointed a Professor of Midwifery with the instruction of midwives as his primary commitment. In 1739 Manningham opened a small school for midwives and medical students in a workhouse infirmary in Westminster. William Smellie in 1741 organized a scheme combining free domiciliary attendance on women in labour with instruction of students in midwifery.

Registration of midwives. The Midwives Institute was founded in 1881, the Obstetric Society having previously established a voluntary examination for the award of a certificate of proficiency which had become the hallmark of trained midwives. Responsibility for the awarding of this certificate was assumed in 1905 by the Central Midwives Board which had been established in accordance with the terms of the Act of 1902. The name of the Midwives Institute was changed to that of College of Midwives in 1941 and six years later was designated by Charter the Royal College of Midwives.

Subsequent regulations pertaining to legal entitlement to practise reduced the number of midwives on the Roll of the Central Midwives Board. Despite this the combined effect of a fall in the birth rate and of the official policy to expand institutional midwifery resulted in there being a surplus of domiciliary midwives. The Midwives Act 1936 established the municipal midwife, employed by the local supervising authority or by a voluntary organization acting for the local supervising authority. She was available to act as maternity nurse in a doctor's case but frequently took complete responsibility for the confinement and worked in close co-operation with the local health authority antenatal clinic. In many parts of the country municipal midwives requiring a medical opinion tended to refer to general practitioners with a particular interest in midwifery and subsequent regulations relating to the National Health Service encouraged the custom. One result was the development of a body of general practitioner obstetricians, many of whom held the Diploma of the Royal College of Obstetricians and Gynaecologists.

The obstetrician

Obstetrics was a recognized special interest among consultants prior to the beginning of the nineteenth century and was practised in the larger cities by a limited number, some of whom were primarily physicians and others primarily surgeons. With the association of gynaecology with obstetrics those practising obstetrics became more closely linked with surgery. The College of Obstetricians and Gynaecologists was founded in 1929 and granted a Royal Charter in 1946.

Of successive advances in obstetrics many have had some bearing on perinatal care. J W Ballantyne in Edinburgh and P C Budin in France at the end of the nineteenth century laid the basis for the study of perinatal care. Ballantyne, an enthusiastic advocate of antenatal care, established the first clinic in this country for expectant mothers.

Since the 1950s obstetricians have been increasingly involved in the study of normal pregnancy and delivery and in finding means to prevent the complications which may occur. This has involved them in closer contact with paediatricians who over the same period have been developing an interest in the newborn infant and his problems.

The paediatrician

Study of disease and health in the newborn was slow to begin and slow to develop despite the fact that the first book on paediatrics written in English, *The Boke of Chyldren* by a general physician, Thomas Phaire (1544), referred to the newborn and gave advice on breast feeding.

Prior to the 1914–18 world war Henry Ashby of Manchester, John Thomson of Edinburgh and George Frederick Still of London were the only physicians who confined their practice to children. At the same time many general physicians dealt with sick children in the course of their routine consultant activities. In this they were continuing the practice of their predecessors. Their work among the newborn was limited and to a considerable extent shared with their obstetric colleagues.

What may be termed concentrated paediatric study of the newborn dates back no further than 1930, although St Thomas's Hospital, London was unique in establishing a paediatric unit in 1919 which incorporated the work of a mothercraft centre and supervision of healthy and ailing babies in the maternity department of the hospital.

As with the obstetricians the advances made in medicine generally since the 1950s have stimulated paediatricians to study in much greater detail the physiology of the adaptations which the infant has to make at birth and to apply this knowledge to clinical management. Many of the factors involved act before delivery and both the obstetrician and paediatrician are keenly interested in the development of the fetus. Perinatal medicine is therefore of concern to both, and we are beginning to see the evolution of the perinatologist. In the UK there are now joint committees of the Royal College of Obstetricians and British Paediatric Association (BPA) on perinatal definitions and working arrangements, and there is a British Association for Perinatal Medicine affiliated with the BPA. Nurses involved in perinatal care have formed The Neonatal Nurses Group.

Throughout most of the developed and some parts of the developing countries there are groups of trained professionals promoting improved care for the fetus and newborn infant. The International Paediatric Association has recently formed a perinatal subgroup which makes recommendations for perinatal care relevant to individual country's needs.

Social legislation

The compulsory notification of births and deaths brought about an increase in public awareness of the high mortality in the very young and was an important factor in stimulating medical and other professionals to improve the care of mothers and infants. Legislation has made further major contributions to the welfare of the newborn by providing assistance for families in need, and for such contingencies as unemployment and sickness. Other important provisions include family allowances, maternity grants and maternity allowances. The trend of modern advances in curative and, more especially, preventive care of the newborn has been largely determined by administrative improvements based on social legislation, together with integration of obstetric and paediatric practice in antenatal and perinatal care.

Measures to allow working mothers maternity leave, to encourage good antenatal and intrapartum care and to allow the mothers to care for their infants during the important early months are the result of recent legislative reform in the UK. Other countries such as France have similar legislation and encourage mothers to attend antenatal clinics early in pregnancy by making such attendance a condition for receiving maternity benefits. Improved facilities for breast-feeding mothers are now found in many firms, factories and shops.

Recent advances

Improvement in the care of the fetus and newborn infant since the beginning of this century is reflected in the progressive decline in perinatal mortality rates (Chapter 2). Much of this improvement is secondary to the socioeconomic advances which have occurred with a resulting rise in the standard of living and higher standards of health and education generally. More recently the increasing volume of basic research into the physiology of pregnancy and delivery has led to a better understanding of the changes occurring.

Some of the instruments involved in this research have been adapted for clinical use.

As a result, intensive care of very low birth weight infants now permits the survival of many infants weighing less than 1000 g at birth. This in turn opens to question whether the present limit of 28 weeks in the definition of stillbirth is still justifiable. Many feel that the 'age of viability' should now be reduced to 22 or 24 weeks.

Teamwork

The complexity of the physiological problems being investigated is generally beyond the ability of a single research worker and most work is carried out by teams of workers, each with his or her own particular skill to contribute. Similarly in clinical work co-operation between several branches of the nursing, midwifery, medical and paramedical services is necessary to provide the optimum service for the fetus and the newborn. The paediatrician is as interested in the progress of the fetus as is the obstetrician in the progress of the baby in the nursery. Although much of the care of the newborn will continue to be in the hands of general paediatricians, the most highly specialized units require the full-time services of paediatricians confining their attention to the newborn period. Such neonatal paediatricians will on occasions, however, require the support of paediatric systems specialists such as paediatric cardiologists. As mentioned earlier, in some centres doctors are employed as perinatologists rather than as obstetricians or paediatricians.

Special care nurseries

The success of special care nurseries depends more on the quality of the nursing care provided than on the equipment available. Training schemes in the special care and intensive care nursing of the newborn are available at many centres. The National Board for Nursing, Midwifery and Health Visiting for Scotland and their equivalents have established standards which must be met before such schemes can be approved by these bodies. It is to be hoped that this highly specialized branch of nursing will be given the recognition which it deserves. The shortage of nursing staff generally has in this, as in other areas, led to the production of monitoring instruments designed to reduce the nursing load. The use of electronic gadgetry has greatly improved the ability to monitor the infant and his environment. In this as in other aspects of care of the newborn the distinction between nursing and medical functions becomes blurred. The concept of working as a team is clearly to the advantage of all concerned.

Intensive therapy

Intensive therapy involving a high concentration of nursing and medical skills is essential for the survival of the very low birthweight (less than 1500 g) infant and those with serious medical or surgical problems. Advances in controlled ventilation, parenteral nutrition, temperature control as well as in surgical and anaesthetic technique have greatly improved the chances of survival of the very small or very ill infant.

Supporting services

No clinical team of nurses, physicians and surgeons can work efficiently without support from the radiology and laboratory services. Most of the advances at present being made depend on the rapid provision of detailed investigation services. In many cases it has been advances in these departments that have paved the way for subsequent advances in therapy. It must also be recognized that advances in the services provided by physiotherapists, social workers, health visitors, etc. have been essential components of the general advance in the services provided for the newborn.

The mother

With such a plethora of staff and services the danger is that mother's place is forgotten and downgraded. What may prove to be the most significant recent advance is the recognition of the need of a mother to maintain contact with her baby from birth onward. Her baby belongs to her, and she has need of her baby as much as her baby will later need her continuing love and care. Separation of mother and infant makes the establishment of a permanent emotional bond more difficult. Involvement of mother in the care of her infant helps to maintain the link and prevents the feeling of detachment and uselessness which distresses some mothers whose infants are being cared for in special care nurseries.

Unsolved problems

Preterm delivery, limited intrauterine growth and abnormal intrauterine development are major factors contributing to perinatal mortality and morbidity. Improved understanding of the various aetiologies will allow us to prevent premature birth and avoid factors which damage the embryo and fetus. There will always be crises and accidents which result in the birth of damaged or abnormal infants. Education and carefully planned management should ensure that such happenings are kept to an absolute minimum. Appropriate help for families with infants born with handicapping conditions must be available without the need to pursue compensation from Health Services, doctors and nurses in the courts of law.

Promotion of good health of both parents and the concept of every child a wanted child will eventually reduce such problems to a very low level. By implementing present knowledge such as prevention of rubella and other intrauterine infections, avoidance of irradiation and drugs, especially alcohol, and the taking of a good diet from before conception and throughout pregnancy and lactation will reduce perinatal mortality and morbidity. Giving the next generation a good start is everybody's business.

Peripheral influences

The successful rearing of a child into a young adult with normal physical, intellectual and emotional development has always been subject to influences over which medical and nursing staff have had little control. Many of these are related to the social and economic circumstances of the community concerned and include such factors as nutrition, housing and education. Much of the present improvement in the health of our newborn population is related as much to the rise in the general standard of living as to advances in medical and nursing skill. Enlightened political actions based on good information can make major differences in the health of infants and young children, as demonstrated in Japan and France in recent times. In some parts of the world religion or local folklore may have a major influence on ideas about conception, pregnancy and the upbringing of children. Some aspects of management appear to be fashionable at one time but not at another. Breast feeding provides a good example of this. Fashions can be created and interest in breast feeding corresponds with the amount of effort expended in advocating its use.

The continuing challenge

Complacency is the enemy of progress and unless we can accept that there is a continuing challenge to provide the best possible care for the newborn infant further progress will not be made. As will be shown in the next chapter it is safer for infants to be delivered in some other countries than it is for them to be born in England or Scotland. Further improvement in the standard of perinatal care is therefore called for. This requires co-operative work by legislators, administrators, research scientists, doctors, midwives, teachers and parents. The training of the midwife and the doctor must strike a successful balance between instruction in clinical· observation, developing awareness of emotional aspects of birth and child rearing and the appropriate use of the technologies of modern intensive care. Much of the knowledge of normal behaviour in the newborn has followed many hours of diligent observation of individual infants. At the same time other major advances in management have only been made possible by the examination of blood or other body tissues in the laboratory. Clinical and laboratory medicine are complementary. Students must be taught the merits of each. The clinician must respect the contribution of the research scientist, and the laboratory worker must understand the problems facing the clinician. Team work is essential and further advance will not be made without full co-operation between all those working to the same end.

There is a risk that as the team caring for the infant increases in size the infant's parents feel remote from their baby and deprived of their joy in welcoming a newcomer to their family. Parents and particularly mothers must be closely involved in the care of their infants when they are very small or ill. Weeks of work in a special care nursery are of no avail if by the time an infant is ready for discharge home his mother feels that he is no longer her infant and that she cannot give him the love and care which he needs. Such aspects of the mother – infant relationship have received too little attention in the past and are a significant part of the continuing clinical challenge now presented to us.

FURTHER READING

House of Commons Social Services Committee (1980) *Perinatal and Neonatal Mortality* (The Short Report). London: HMSO.

House of Commons Social Services Committee (1985) *Perinatal and Neonatal Mortality* (Follow up). London: HMSO.

Lancet (1980) *Better Perinatal Health. A Survey*. London: *The Lancet*.

National Medical Consultative Committee (1980) *Report of the Joint Working Party on Standards of Perinatal Care in Scotland*. Edinburgh: SHHD.

2

Perinatal health services

In many countries in the western world obstetrics developed in relation to gynaecology and neonatal medicine has become a branch of paediatrics. Whereas the midwife has training in both the care of the mother during pregnancy and of her infant after delivery, there has developed a tendency for two groups of doctors, the obstetricians and the neonatal paediatricians, to be involved in the sole care of the mother on the one hand and of the infant on the other. Training schemes have evolved which are likely to perpetuate this split. Fortunately the disadvantages and even dangers of such an artificial division of interest and responsibility are being recognized and renewed attention is now being given, particularly in Australia and the USA, to the concept of perinatal medicine and the health services which are required to improve standards of care in the perinatal period.

Measurement of success

At the beginning of the twentieth century maternal mortality due to childbirth was a major cause for concern and efforts at improving maternity services were aimed at reducing the risk to the mother. In 1970 in England 109 mothers died from childbearing, a rate of 15 deaths per 100 000 deliveries. This compares with rates of the order of 500 per 100 000 deliveries at the beginning of the century. The maternal mortality rate is no longer a useful measure by which to assess the success of maternity services and attention is now focused on the infant. A successful pregnancy is one which results in an infant who is fully capable of developing his inherited powers of physical and mental development. Measurement of success is, however, not possible at birth. Our assessment still has to rely on measurement of failure as with maternal mortality. When an infant is stillborn or is alive at birth but dies within a few days the pregnancy cannot be considered to have had a successful outcome. Many infant deaths in the first year of life are due to causes directly or closely related to factors occurring during fetal life or during delivery. Stillbirths and deaths during the first seven days of life have therefore many causes in common to both and are termed perinatal deaths. Before discussing this matter further it is important to state the definitions of the terms involved.

DEFINITIONS USED IN PERINATAL STATISTICS

For the requirements of the law and for purposes of statistical analysis certain situations in relation to the birth of an infant have to be carefully defined. The definitions given below are those of the Standing Joint Committee of the BPA and RCOG as reported in *Archives of Disease in Childhood* (1986) by M L Chiswick and are based on current WHO definitions.

Commentary on current World Health Organisation definitions used in perinatal statistics

There is an urgent need for those collecting and disseminating perinatal statistics, whether at national, regional, district, or local hospital level to adhere to standard definitions. It is strongly recommended that current World Health Organisation (WHO) definitions are used in the collection of statistical data. Listed below are the relevant definitions together with short commentaries where this is felt appropriate.

It is appreciated that gestational age often cannot be determined by reference to the last menstrual period. Nonetheless, whichever method of gestational age assessment is used the definitions of various gestational age categories are still appropriate. The definitions also highlight the need for all live births and fetal deaths to be accurately weighed as soon as possible after birth. Indeed, the accurate weighing of babies at birth is a necessary part of good clinical practice.

Finally, it must be stressed that adherence to the WHO definitions are for statistical purposes only and that the existing definitions governing, for example, legal requirements to register stillbirths remain unchanged.

Definitions and recommendations

Live birth. 'Live birth is the complete expulsion or extraction from its mother of a product of conception, irrespective of the duration of the pregnancy, which, after such separation, breathes or shows any other evidence of life, such as beating of the heart, pulsation of the umbilical cord, or definite movement of voluntary muscles, whether or not the umbilical cord has been cut or the placenta is attached; each product of such a birth is considered live born.'

Fetal death. 'Fetal death is death prior to the complete expulsion or extraction from its mother of a product of conception, irrespective of the duration of the pregnancy; the death is indicated by the fact that after such separation the fetus does not breathe or show any other evidence of life, such as beating of the heart, pulsation of the umbilical cord, or definite movement of voluntary muscles.'

Birthweight. 'The first weight of the fetus or newborn obtained after birth. This weight should be measured preferably within the first hour of life before significant postnatal weight loss has occurred.'

Comment
Ideally the naked baby, alive or dead, should be weighed to the nearest gram, preferably on an electronic weighing balance. Suitable weighing machines should be stationed in delivery units close to resuscitation trolleys so that even ill babies can be rapidly weighed at a convenient time before they are attached to apparatus that may not be relinquished for days or weeks. The initial record of weight must be the one that is recorded on all birthweight documentation, ie hospital birth book, special care baby unit (SCBU) notes, maternity ward notes, discharge letters, etc. It is essential to ensure that several different measurements of 'birthweight' made on the delivery unit, SCBU etc are not simultaneously used.

Low birthweight. 'less than 2500 g (up to, and including, 2499 g).'

Gestational age. 'The duration of gestation is measured from the first day of the last normal menstrual period. Gestational age is expressed in completed days or completed weeks (eg events occurring 280 to 286 days after the onset of the last normal menstrual period are considered to have occurred at 40 weeks of gestation). Measurements of fetal growth, as they represent continuous variables, are expressed in relation to a specific week of gestational age (eg the mean birthweight for 40 weeks is that obtained at 280–286 days of gestation on a weight-for-gestational age curve).'

Comment
However gestational age is measured, a completed week is 7 days. Thus a pregnancy at 40 weeks (280 days) on 26 July is only 39 weeks (279 days) on 25th July; and not 41 weeks (287 days) until 2nd August.

Pre-term. 'Less than 37 completed weeks.'

Comment
A birth is pre-term if it occurs up to and including the 258th day of gestation. A new day commences at midnight. Thus a pregnancy at 37 weeks (259 days) on 4th July is classified as pre-term if the baby is born on 3rd July at 11.59 pm (23.59 hours).

Term. 'From 37 to less than 42 completed weeks.'

Comment
259 days up to and including 293 days.

Post-term. 'Forty-two completed weeks or more.'

Comment
294 completed days or more.

Perinatal mortality statistics. 'It is recommended that national perinatal statistics should include all fetuses and infants delivered weighing at least 500 g or, when birthweight is unavailable the corresponding gestational age (22 weeks) or body length (25 cm crown-heel), whether alive or dead. It is recognised that legal requirements in many countries may set different criteria for registration purposes, but it is hoped that countries will arrange the registration or reporting procedures in such a way that the events required for inclusion in the statistics can be identified easily. It is further recommended that less mature fetuses and infants should be excluded from perinatal statistics unless there are legal or other valid reasons to the contrary.'

Comment
In Britain, the 'fetal death' component of perinatal mortality includes only those fetuses who have completed 28 weeks (196 days) in the womb. This is convenient only because it corresponds with the legal requirement to register stillbirths who have, by definition, completed 28 weeks (196 days) in the womb. Thus, a fetus that is 28 weeks (196 days) on 1st May is not classified as stillborn if born dead on 30th April at 11.59 pm (23.59 hours) but is classified as an abortion. However, this restrictive interpretation of perinatal mortality is unsatisfactory for many reasons, not the least being the illogicality of including within the liveborn component of perinatal mortality *all* babies regardless of their gestational age.

Thus there is much sense in defining perinatal mortality as 'fetal deaths weighing 500 g or more *PLUS* deaths occurring less than 7 completed days after birth (ie 6 d 23 h 59 m or less) in babies weighing 500 g or more'. The inclusion of extremely low birthweight babies within the definition of perinatal mortality underlines the need for all fetal deaths and live births to be accurately weighed. In this way perinatal mortality can be analysed within specific birthweight groups (see below) and when comparing perinatal mortality rates, allowances can be made for differences in birthweight distributions between populations.

Statistical tables. 'The degree of detail in cross-classification by cause, sex, age, and area of territory will depend partly on the purpose and range of the statistics and partly on the practical limits as regards the size of particular tables. The following patterns, designed to promote international comparability, consist of standard ways of expressing various characteristics. Where a different classification is used (eg in age-grouping) in published tables, it should be so arranged as to be reducible to one of the recommended groupings.'
  (a) Age classification for special statistics of infant mortality
  (i) Under 24 hours, 1–6 days, 7–27 days, 28 days up to but not including 3 months, 3–5 months, 6 months but under 1 year.
  (ii) Under 7 days, 7–27 days, 28 days but under 1 year.

Comment
Early neonatal death (included in perinatal mortality): death less than 7 completed days from birth (ie up to and including 6 d 23 h 59 m).

Late neonatal death (not included in perinatal mortality): death from 7 completed days to less than 28 days from birth (ie up to and including 27 d 23 h 59 m).

Post neonatal death: death from 28 completed days to less than 1 year from birth (ie up to and including 364 days).
Early neonatal death may be further subdivided as shown below: —
(iii) Under 1 hour, 1–23 hours, 24–167 hours.

(b) Birthweight classification for perinatal mortality statistics
By weight intervals of 500 g ie 500–999 g, 1000–1499 g 1500–1999 g etc.

(c) Gestational age classification for perinatal mortality statistics
Under 28 weeks (under 196 days), 28–31 weeks (196–223 days), 32–36 weeks (224–258 days), 37–41 weeks (259–293 days), 42 weeks and over (294 days and over).

Comment
The influence of birthweight and gestational age on mortality is particularly marked in very low birthweight babies. Therefore data should be collected in a way that allows birthweight groupings to be expressed also by intervals of 250 g (ie 500–749 g, 750–999 g, 1000–1249 g etc) and by ungrouped gestational ages.

M L CHISWICK
On behalf of the Standing Joint Committee
of the British Paediatric Association and
Royal College of Obstetricians and Gynaecologists
(*Archives of Disease in Childhood* **61**: 708–710)

In the UK these definitions are used as the basis for the Registrar General's statistical analysis.
Birth rate is the number of births (live and still) registered per 1000 of the population.
Stillbirth rate is the number of stillbirths registered per 1000 live and still births.

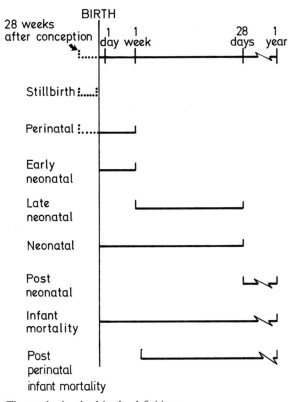

Fig. 2.1 Time scales involved in the definitions.

Neonatal mortality rate is the number of deaths registered of infants dying under the age of 28 days per 1000 registered livebirths in the same year.

Perinatal mortality rate is the number of stillbirths and early neonatal deaths per 1000 live and stillbirths.

Infant mortality rate is the number of deaths registered of infants dying under 1 year of age per 1000 registered livebirths in the same year.

Postperinatal infant mortality rate is the number of deaths between the eighth day and the end of the first year of life per 1000 livebirths.

Perinatal epidemiology

The recognition that study of the perinatal period is more

rewarding than the study of the prenatal or postnatal periods separately has led to the establishment of the National Perinatal Epidemiology Unit in Oxford, England and the Social Paediatric and Obstetric Research Unit in Glasgow, Scotland. At present the index for success or failure in promoting better perinatal health has to be the perinatal mortality rate. Although measurement of mortality rates is clearly an index of failure rather than of success it is a precise measurement of a defined event, the cause of which can generally be ascertained and recorded. Crude perinatal mortality rates vary with factors such as social background and environment which are not directly under medical or nursing control. Attempts have therefore been made to use 'adjusted perinatal mortality rates' which allow for birth weight and for major malformations which are incompatible with extended post-natal life. Such adjusted figures will give a better indication of the standard of perinatal care than crude perinatal mortality rates. The most satisfactory index of perinatal health is the subsequent growth and development of the baby into a healthy happy child who becomes a healthy adult fully able to fulfil his genetic potential. In other words we are primarily interested in the quality of survival. Measurement of such factors is, however, extremely difficult and imprecise and involves a long time delay. For the present, there-fore, we have to use the information which is most readily available to us in the form of perinatal mortality rates. In order to improve the accuracy of information available about perinatal deaths it has been proposed that a 'Certificate of Cause of Perinatal Death' should be used.

Perinatal mortality

As will be seen from Figure 2.2 there has been a steady fall in the perinatal mortality rate in the UK since these figures have been available. This is largely due to improvement in living standards and in particular to higher standards of nutrition and hygiene. The improvement began before the introduction of the sulphonamides and antibiotics which helped to increase the rate of fall by reduc-tion of mortality from non-viral infections. Notification of still-births was not required by law until 1928 in England and Wales and 1939 in Scotland. Perinatal mortality rates could not therefore be calculated on a national basis before 1928 in England and Wales

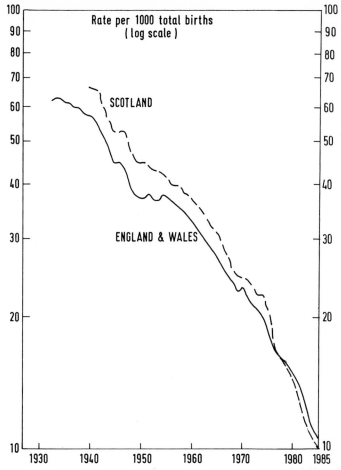

Fig. 2.2 Comparison of the fall in perinatal mortality rates in England and Wales and in Scotland.

Table 2.1   Perinatal mortality rates per 1000 total births

Year	England and Wales	Scotland
1950	37.4	42.7
1960	32.8	35.4
1970	23.5	24.8
1975	19.3	21.1
1980	13.7	13.1
1985	10.0	9.8

Table 2.2   Perinatal mortality rates in selected countries in order of rates for 1975

	1965	1970	1975
Sweden	19.7	16.4	11.1
Finland	24.5	17.0	12.5
Denmark	18.7	17.9	13.4
Netherlands	23.1	18.6	14.0
Norway	21.3	19.1	14.0
New Zealand	22.3	19.6	16.5
France	27.7	23.4	18.3
England and Wales	26.9	23.5	19.3
USA	28.1	23.6	20.7
Scotland	31.5	24.8	21.1
Northern Ireland	34.5	27.6	25.9

Table 2.3   Perinatal mortality rate per 1000 total births by Health Board of Residence, 1975–1985

Health Board of Residence	1975	1980	1985*
Argyll & Clyde	24.3	13.4	10.1
Ayrshire & Arran	23.1	18.3	9.0
Grampian	18.1	8.1	11.1
Greater Glasgow	22.5	13.8	10.5
Lanarkshire	20.0	14.0	8.8
Lothian	19.5	11.7	10.8
Tayside	16.4	13.3	7.3
SCOTLAND	21.1	13.1	9.8

* Provisional
Source: GRO (Scotland)
  By kind permission of Dr Susan Cole, Information Services Division — Scottish Health Service Common Services Agency.

or 1939 in Scotland. Comparison of the rates for these two parts of the UK is shown in Table 2.1. In each country there has been a steady fall but Scotland has until recently lagged behind England and Wales. Such comparisons between countries can be extended both by widening the net so that comparisons are made with countries outside the UK (Table 2.2) and by narrowing the net to make comparisons between regions within a country (Table 2.3). It can be seen from Table 2.3 that different regions of Scotland have perinatal mortality rates varying between 7.3 and 11.1 for the year 1985 and it can be shown that within areas such as Greater Glasgow the perinatal mortality rates in some city areas are up to five times those in more advantaged parts of the city.

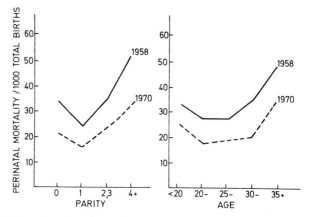

Fig. 2.3 The effect of parity and maternal age on perinatal mortality rates (*British Births 1970*).

Factors involved in perinatal mortality

Parity and maternal age. Figure 2.3 shows the effect on perinatal mortality of parity and maternal age. In each case the figures for 1970 are lower than those for 1958 but show the same pattern in relation to increasing parity and increasing age.

Birth weight. The increase in perinatal mortality with decreasing birth weight is discussed in Chapter 9.

Social factors. There is a continuing discrepancy in perinatal mortality between the social classes and between legitimate and illegitimate infants. Such differences continue to exist in spite of our egalitarian society. Taller mothers have fewer perinatal deaths. Unsupported mothers have an even higher risk of perinatal loss of their infants than mothers in social class V and a rate which is five times higher than that for married mothers in social class I.

Use of antenatal services

Studies carried out in many countries have shown that perinatal mortality is lowest amongst those who attend for antenatal care earliest and highest for those who do not attend until late in their pregnancy. Distance of home from hospital also affects the number of attendances at antenatal clinics, those nearest attending more regularly. Taking antenatal care from hospital out to the local health centre, clinic or home results in earlier identification of pregnancies at risk and referral to hospital for expert management. Improved and better organized antenatal services are likely to contribute to a reduction in perinatal mortality.

Changes in perinatal mortality

Comparison between countries shows that it is those with the highest standard of living which have the lowest perinatal, neonatal and infant mortality rates. The improvements in these figures which have occurred in individual countries during this century are in line with their rate of socioeconomic progress. The factors involved are many but include better nutrition resulting in better physique, improved hygiene and housing conditions resulting in fewer infectious illnesses, better education resulting in a better understanding of the need for antenatal care and, more recently, planned parenthood limiting the size of families and forestalling the birth of an unwanted or abnormal infant. The improvements made are largely the result of activity at national government level. This does not mean that further gains cannot be achieved by improvement of the services at the level of the maternity unit.

Hospital statistics

The use of statistical evidence can equally well be applied to the local situation. If such data is collected uniformly throughout the country by the use of a national Neonatal Discharge Form (Fig. 2.4) comparisons between hospitals are made easier. It should be the duty of every maternity unit to keep under review not only individual failures in the form of stillbirth or neonatal death but also total performance over a period of one or more years. By comparison with earlier periods in the same unit, with the same period in other similar units or with national figures the success or failure of the unit can be assessed.

Table 2.4 shows the birth weight and gestation specific perinatal mortality rates in normally formed singletons born in Scotland in 1985. By further examination of obstetric and paediatric information related to the perinatal deaths (Tables 2.5 and 2.6) one can begin to identify preventable causes of perinatal mortality.

By studying the figures for such statistics as stillbirth rate, neonatal death rate and perinatal mortality rate within a hospital department much can be learned of the success or failure of the methods of care being used. Problems such as the high mortality

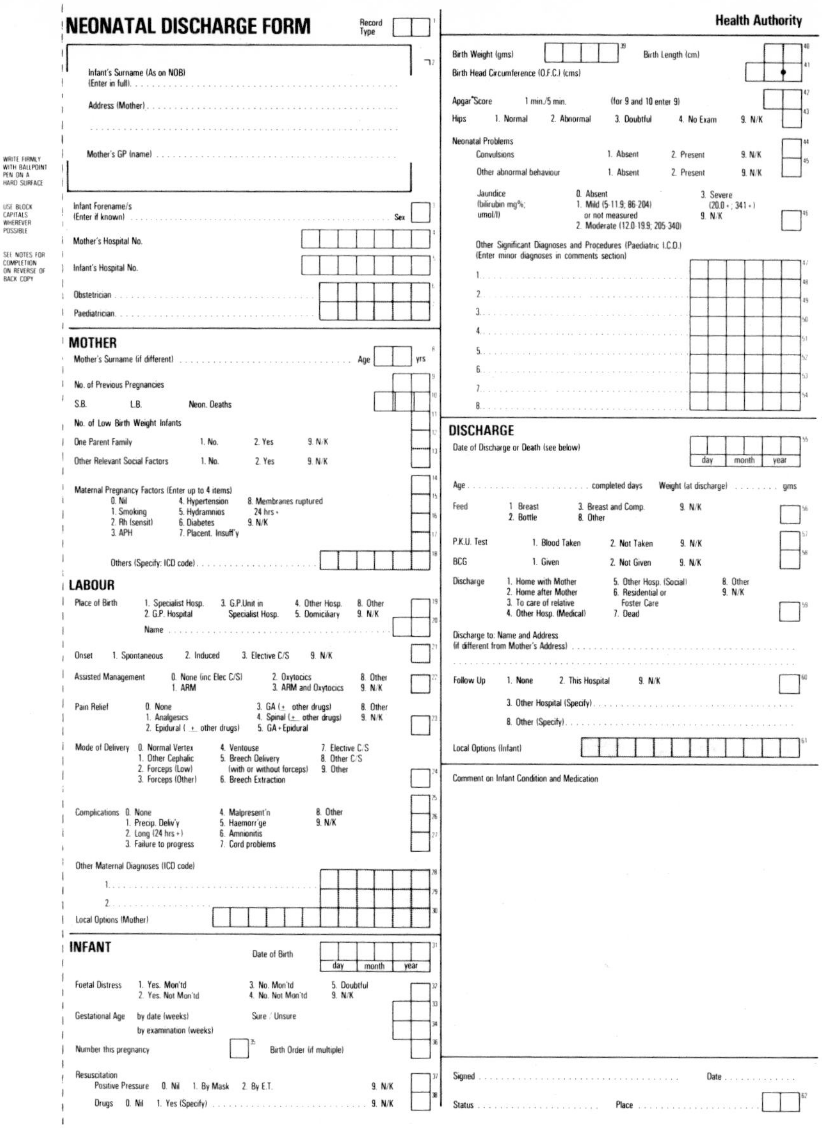

NEONATAL DISCHARGE FORM   Record Type ☐   **Health Authority**

WRITE FIRMLY WITH BALLPOINT PEN ON A HARD SURFACE

USE BLOCK CAPITALS WHEREVER POSSIBLE

SEE NOTES FOR COMPLETION ON REVERSE OF BACK COPY

Infant's Surname (As on NOB) (Enter in full) ....

Address (Mother) ....

Mother's GP (name) ....

Infant Forename/s (Enter if known) ....   Sex ☐

Mother's Hospital No. ☐

Infant's Hospital No. ☐

Obstetrician ....

Paediatrician ....

MOTHER

Mother's Surname (if different) ....   Age ☐ yrs

No. of Previous Pregnancies

S.B.   L.B.   Neon. Deaths ☐

No. of Low Birth Weight Infants

One Parent Family   1. No.   2. Yes   9. N/K

Other Relevant Social Factors   1. No.   2. Yes   9. N/K

Maternal Pregnancy Factors (Enter up to 4 items)
0. Nil   4. Hypertension   8. Membranes ruptured
1. Smoking   5. Hydramnios   24 hrs +
2. Rh (sensit)   6. Diabetes   9. N/K
3. APH   7. Placent. Insuff'y

Others (Specify: ICD code) ....

LABOUR

Place of Birth   1. Specialist Hosp.   3. G.P.Unit in   4. Other Hosp.   8. Other
2. G.P. Hospital   Specialist Hosp.   5. Domiciliary   9. N/K

Name ....

Onset   1. Spontaneous   2. Induced   3. Elective C/S   9. N/K

Assisted Management   0. None (inc Elec C/S)   2. Oxytocics   8. Other
1. ARM   3. ARM and Oxytocics   9. N/K

Pain Relief   0. None   3. GA (+ other drugs)   8. Other
1. Analgesics   4. Spinal (+ other drugs)   9. N/K
2. Epidural (+ other drugs)   5. GA + Epidural

Mode of Delivery   0. Normal Vertex   4. Ventouse   7. Elective C/S
1. Other Cephalic   5. Breech Delivery   8. Other C/S
2. Forceps (Low)   (with or without forceps)   9. Other
3. Forceps (Other)   6. Breech Extraction

Complications   0. None   4. Malpresent'n   8. Other
1. Precip. Deliv'y   5. Haemorr'ge   9. N/K
2. Long (24 hrs +)   6. Amnionitis
3. Failure to progress   7. Cord problems

Other Maternal Diagnoses (ICD code)
1. ....
2. ....

Local Options (Mother)

INFANT   Date of Birth   day month year

Foetal Distress   1. Yes. Mon'td   3. No. Mon'td   5. Doubtful
2. Yes. Not Mon'td   4. No. Not Mon'td   9. N/K

Gestational Age   by date (weeks)   Sure / Unsure
by examination (weeks)

Number this pregnancy   Birth Order (if multiple)

Resuscitation
Positive Pressure   0. Nil   1. By Mask   2. By E.T.   9. N/K
Drugs   0. Nil   1. Yes (Specify)   9. N/K

Birth Weight (gms) ☐   Birth Length (cm) ☐
Birth Head Circumference (O.F.C.) (cms) ☐

Apgar Score   1 min./5 min.   (for 9 and 10 enter 9)
Hips   1. Normal   2. Abnormal   3. Doubtful   4. No Exam   9. N/K

Neonatal Problems
Convulsions   1. Absent   2. Present   9. N/K
Other abnormal behaviour   1. Absent   2. Present   9. N/K

Jaundice   0. Absent   3. Severe
(bilirubin mg%;   1. Mild (5-11.9; 86-204)   (20.0 +; 341 +)
umol/l)   or not measured   9. N/K
2. Moderate (12.0-19.9; 205-340)

Other Significant Diagnoses and Procedures (Paediatric I.C.D.)
(Enter minor diagnoses in comments section)
1. ....
2. ....
3. ....
4. ....
5. ....
6. ....
7. ....
8. ....

DISCHARGE

Date of Discharge or Death (see below)   day month year

Age .... completed days   Weight (at discharge) .... gms

Feed   1. Breast   3. Breast and Comp.   9. N/K
2. Bottle   8. Other

P.K.U. Test   1. Blood Taken   2. Not Taken   9. N/K
BCG   1. Given   2. Not Given   9. N/K

Discharge   1. Home with Mother   5. Other Hosp. (Social)   8. Other
2. Home after Mother   6. Residential or   9. N/K
3. To care of relative   Foster Care
4. Other Hosp. (Medical)   7. Dead

Discharge to: Name and Address
(if different from Mother's Address) ....

Follow Up   1. None   2. This Hospital   9. N/K
3. Other Hospital (Specify) ....
8. Other (Specify) ....

Local Options (Infant)

Comment on Infant Condition and Medication

Signed ....   Date ....
Status ....   Place ....

Fig. 2.4 Proposed National Neonatal Discharge Form.

rate among infants of very low birth weight are underlined and an assessment can be made of efficiency in reducing low birth weight mortality.

Quality of survival. Further reduction in mortality rates presents

Table 2.4 Birth weight and gestation specific perinatal mortality rates in normally formed singletons 1985

Birth weight	<33		33–36		Gestation 37+		NK		Total	
	No.	Rate	No.	Rate	No.	Rate	No.	Rate	No.	Rate
<1000	108	744.8	3	333.3	—	—	—	—	111	720.8
1000–1499	71	245.7	15	182.9	—	—	—	—	86	221.1
1500–1999	22	79.2	32	91.2	5	36.5	—	—	59	76.7
2000–2499	3	41.1	30	31.5	22	14.6	—	—	55	21.0
2500+	2	125.0	22	15.1	123	2.1	—	—	147	2.4
NK	2	—	1	—	1	—	8	—	12	—
TOTAL	208	256.2	103	36.0	151	2.5	8	—	470	7.2

By kind permission of Dr Susan Cole, Information Services Division — Scottish Health Service Common Services Agency.

Table 2.5 Obstetric classification by birth weight and time of death 1985 (multiple births are shown in brackets)

Obstetric classification	<1000	1000–1499	1500–1999	2000–2499	2500–2999	3000–3499	3500–3999	4000–4499	4500+	NK	Total
Congenital anomaly AP	3	3	4 (2)	3	2	—	—	—	—	1	16 (2)
IP	1	2	2	3 (2)	2	2	1	—	1	—	14 (2)
Wk 1	2	10 (1)	16 (2)	18	18 (1)	14	4	1	1	—	84 (4)
Wk 2–4	—	1	3	2 (1)	8	4 (1)	6	—	—	1	25 (2)
Pregnancy Hypertension AP	7	5	8 (1)	3	2	2	—	—	—	—	27 (1)
IP	2	—	— (1)	—	1	1	—	—	—	—	4 (1)
Wk 1	7	4	1	— (1)	—	—	1	—	—	—	13 (1)
Wk 2–4	1	1	—	—	—	—	—	—	—	1	3

											Total
APH	AP	6	11	11	11	4	5	1	—	—	—	49
	IP	2	3 (1)	2	3	5	—	1	—	—	—	16 (1)
	Wk 1	21 (2)	8	1	1	—	1	—	—	1	1	34 (2)
	Wk 2–4	1	—	—	—	—	—	—	—	—	—	1
Other*	AP	2	—	6	4	6	5	3	2	1	—	27
	IP	—	(2)	1	1 (1)	2 (1)	2	2	2	—	2	10 (4)
	Wk 1	3	3 (1)	2	1	3	3	3	2	3	—	25 (1)
	Wk 2–4	1	2	2	—	1	2	1	1	—	1	11
Unexplained LBW	AP	23 (4)	23 (2)	18 (5)	28 (2)	—	—	—	—	—	—	92 (13)
	IP	2	2 (1)	2	—	—	—	—	—	1	—	6 (1)
	Wk 1	36 (24)	26 (6)	7 (2)	3	—	—	—	—	—	—	73 (32)
	Wk 2–4	10 (3)	3 (1)	4 (1)	1 (1)	—	—	—	—	—	—	18 (6)
NBW	AP	—	—	—	—	24 (1)	17	15	4	1	—	61 (1)
	IP	—	—	—	—	3 (1)	2	3	1	—	—	9 (1)
	Wk 1	—	—	—	—	5	5 (1)	4	—	—	—	14 (1)
	Wk 2–4	—	—	—	—	—	—	1	—	—	—	1
No information	AP	— (1)	1	—	—	—	—	—	—	—	2	3 (1)
	IP	—	—	—	—	—	—	—	—	—	—	—
	Wk 1	—	—	—	—	—	1	—	—	—	6	7
	Wk 2–4	—	—	—	—	—	—	—	—	—	6	6
TOTAL	AP	41 (5)	43 (2)	47 (8)	49 (2)	38 (1)	29	19	4	2	3	275 (18)
	IP	7	7 (4)	7 (1)	7 (3)	13 (2)	7	7	3	1	—	59 (10)
	Wk 1	69 (26)	51 (8)	27 (4)	23 (1)	26 (1)	24 (1)	11	4	5	10	250 (41)
	Wk 2–4	13 (3)	7 (1)	9 (1)	3 (2)	9	6 (1)	8	1	—	9	65 (8)

* Includes maternal disease, trauma, isoimmunization and other.

By kind permission of Dr Susan Cole, Information Services Division — Scottish Health Service Common Services Agency.

Table 2.6 Birthweight by paediatric cause — neonatal deaths 1985 (multiple births are shown in brackets)

Paediatric cause	Wk	Birth weight										Total
		<1000	1000–1499	1500–1999	2000–2499	2500–2999	3000–3499	3500–3999	4000–4499	4500+	NK	
Congenital anomaly	Wk 1	2	10 (1)	16 (2)	18	18 (1)	14	4	1	1	—	84 (4)
	Wk 2–4	—	1	3	2 (1)	8	4 (1)	6	—	—	1	25 (2)
Isoimmunization	Wk 1	—	—	1	—	—	—	—	—	—	—	1
	Wk 2–4	—	—	—	—	—	—	—	—	—	—	—
Anoxia	Wk 1	9 (1)	11 (1)	4 (2)	3	4	9 (1)	5	1	3	1	50 (5)
	Wk 2–4	2	1	1	1	—	—	1	—	—	—	6
Trauma	Wk 1	—	1	—	—	—	—	—	—	—	—	1
	Wk 2–4	—	—	—	—	—	—	—	—	—	—	—
Immaturity	Wk 1	37 (17)	2	—	—	—	—	—	—	—	1	40 (17)
	Wk 2–4	—	—	—	—	—	—	—	—	—	—	—
HMD	Wk 1	17 (7)	19 (5)	1	— (1)	1	—	—	—	—	1	38 (13)
	Wk 2–4	4 (1)	2	2 (1)	—	—	—	—	—	—	—	9 (2)
Haemorrhage	Wk 1	2	—	1	—	1	—	—	—	—	—	4
	Wk 2–4	1	1	—	—	—	—	—	—	—	—	2
Infection	Wk 1	1 (1)	3 (1)	3	1	1	—	—	1	—	—	10 (2)
	Wk 2–4	3 (2)	1 (1)	2	— (1)	1	—	—	—	—	1	8 (4)
Other	Wk 1	1	5	2	1	1	—	2	1	1	2	16
	Wk 2–4	3	1	—	—	—	2	1	1	—	—	8
No Information	Wk 1	—	—	—	—	—	1	—	—	—	6	7
	Wk 2–4	—	—	—	—	—	—	—	—	—	6	6
TOTAL	Wk 1	69 (26)	51 (8)	27 (4)	23 (1)	26 (1)	24 (1)	11	4	5	4	250 (41)
	Wk 2–4	13 (3)	7 (1)	9 (1)	3 (2)	9	6 (1)	8	1	—	9	65 (8)
TOTAL BIRTHS*		205	469	965	2956	11 788	25 385	18 792	5564	812	97	67 033
Singletons		154	389	768	2542	11 359	25 214	18 760	5561	812	83	65 642
Multiples		51	80	197	414	429	171	32	3	—	14	1 391

* Estimated birth weight distribution for 1985.
By kind permission of Dr Susan Cole. Information Services Division — Scottish Health Service Common Services Agency.

us with a new problem — the quality of life for those who survive. This is not easy to present in the same manner as rates for perinatal mortality. Quality of life can be estimated for an individual but national figures can only be assessed indirectly by noting changes in such factors as school performance and admission rates to schools for the physically or mentally handicapped. Should an increased number of admissions to such schools be evident five to ten years after the introduction of a new method of management of the newborn, suspicion should be aroused and the efficacy of the method reassessed. As an example one may quote the harmful effect of delay in feeding of small infants practised during the 1950s which has led to impaired school performance and cerebral palsy in many of the children so treated. This was not evident or easy to foresee at the time the practice was in vogue. The association of retrolental fibroplasia and oxygen therapy is another example. Close co-operation between all branches of the health services dealing with infants and children is essential to ensure that the long-term effects of changes in management of the newborn are communicated to those responsible for making and applying policy decisions in nurseries for the newborn.

As will be discussed in more detail in Chapter 7 it is essential to have a record prepared for individual infants in the pre and postnatal period in a form which will allow the accurate collection of the basic information about an infant's pre and postnatal condition suitable for subsequent statistical analysis. Where the facilities are available this information should be collected in a form ready for computer analysis. It is hoped that information collected in the perinatal period will eventually form the basis of an ongoing lifelong record of health for that individual.

Organization of services for the newborn

Experience in this country and elsewhere has shown that the services provided for the newborn vary in efficiency from one region to another. This can be demonstrated by comparing perinatal mortality rates for regions with similar socioeconomical and demographic patterns. Differences existing between such similar areas are frequently due to factors which are capable of correction by bringing the standard of perinatal care up to the standard practised in better areas. The most dramatic improvements are likely to occur in developing countries but in such situations it may well be more effective to use those monies available for the improvement of hygiene and nutrition before large sums are spent on services for the newborn. In countries with a high socioeconomical standard, however, services for the newborn may not reach standards available elsewhere and it is useful to consider how standards can be improved.

Administration. Within the health services of any country or region of a country there are a number of variable factors responsible for success or failure. These include efficiency of the organization of the services and its responsiveness to changing circumstances, the provision and maintenance of suitable buildings and equipment, the supply of well-trained nursing, medical and paramedical staff but above all the willingness of patients to use the facilities available and their confidence in the staff and in the methods employed. Ease of access to clinics and possible financial inducements to attend are factors to be considered. Satisfactory provision will not be identical throughout the world but in any area it is essential that the service be self-critical and be prepared to keep under frequent review its effectiveness in providing a good economic service which is acceptable to the local population.

The national health service

At the time of the introduction into the UK of a National Health Service the country had already seen the benefit of the introduction of set standards of practice for doctors, nurses and midwives but was only beginning to accept the need for organized health services on a wide basis. The service was introduced as a tripartite system based on the hospitals, the general practitioners and the local authority health services. Maternity services including those for the newborn were divided between the three branches and it took some time before satisfactory co-operation between these branches was achieved. The National Health service Act (1974) attempted to remedy some of the faults of the 1948 Act by planning for an integrated health service. Experience has not justified all the high hopes of the reformers and further changes in the structure of the service and in administration will be required before a satisfactory state is reached. The erection of some new hospitals serving a district and replacing one or more older buildings offers an opportunity of assessing how best maternity services can be organized. In most parts of the UK 95 per cent or more of deliveries take place in hospital. Changing attitudes towards contraception and abortion make it difficult to assess the number of infants likely to be delivered in the years ahead. The birth rate which was falling until 1980–1982 now shows sign of rising. The report in 1980 of Mrs Renee Short's Parliamentary Social Services Committee on Perinatal and Neonatal Mortality analyses the situation in detail and makes radical recommendations for perinatal provisions which the Government would be wise to accept.

Reports on Perinatal Health Services. In the UK the concern of the general public and of the Government with regard to perinatal health services is reflected in the number of reports which have been published on this subject. These include the Peel Report (1970), Sheldon Report (1971), Oppé Report (1974), Court Report (1976) and several other documents of a more general nature in which reference is made to the problems of the perinatal health services. These reports are referred to in the most recent and most comprehensive reports on Perinatal and Neonatal Mortality prepared by the Parliamentary Social Services Committee under the chairmanship of Mrs Renee Short MP. These reports, which were published in 1980 and 1985, will be referred to here as the Short Reports.

The Short Reports

The 1980 Short Report contained 152 recommendations and it would clearly not be possible to refer to all of them here. Many of these recommendations had been made previously in the earlier reports mentioned and the need to repeat them is an indication of the lack of action taken following earlier recommendations. Of the 152 recommendations made, the Committee considered that 98 could be carried out with little or no extra cost and should be implemented immediately. A further 40 should also be implemented immediately and the cost borne by a special financial allocation. In only 14 of the recommendations was immediate implementation not considered necessary. Both the number and urgency of the recommendations indicate the concern which the Parliamentary Committee felt about our present perinatal health services.

Recommendations. The recommendations cover all aspects of the perinatal health services, including health education, social services, financial assistance, general practitioner, obstetrics, etc., but here we will concentrate on those recommendations referring particularly to the care of the infant. The Committee support hospital delivery in large units with better selection for delivery in small consultant units. They consider that home delivery should be further phased out. There is little support for the creation of 'perinatologists' but it is recognized that there is a need for consultant obstetrician posts to be created that have more time allocated to obstetric rather than gynaecological practice and that there should be an urgent increase in the number of consultant neonatal paediatricians. The Committee do not recommend an overall increase in special care nurseries but do recommend an immediate increase in the provision of intensive care nurseries: 'Every region should have one or two referral units which are equipped and staffed to provide the best possible intensive care for mother, fetus and newborn infant.' Further, each region should designate a number of additional large maternity hospitals, perhaps three to five, as subregional perinatal centres where mothers and babies with problems that cannot be dealt with in every district general hospital could be cared for. All maternity hospitals and units not designated as regional or subregional centres should be supplied with facilities for the provision of short-term intensive care. The report makes many recommendations with regard to the staffing of such units and suggests that new guidelines are required. It is expected that the level of staffing required will be at least that recommended by the Sheldon Report. The 1985 Short Report reinforced the 1980 report and regrets the lack of government action. In 1987 there is little or no evidence that the UK government has any intention of implementing the recommendations of the Short Reports.

The Sheldon Report

Although the Report of the Expert Group on Special Care for Babies (the Sheldon Report) was issued in 1971, it was not until 1976 that it was given formal approval and many of its recommendations have still not been implemented. The Report made detailed recommendations with regard to the provision of special care and intensive care nurseries and in particular the number and training of the midwifery and nursing staff involved. This will be considered further in Chapters 6 and 10.

Transport facilities

The Short Reports and the Sheldon Report lay emphasis on the advantage to both mother and infant of delivery taking place in a unit fully equipped and staffed to deal with any emergency which may arise. As such emergencies are more likely to occur in high-risk mothers every effort should be made to ensure that they are delivered in major obstetric units with facilities for special and intensive care. It is not always possible to identify beforehand every mother who is likely to develop such a problem and some apparently low-risk mothers will still be delivered at home. Should problems develop in such a pregnancy, transfer to hospital becomes essential. Although the baby at risk travels most safely in utero it has to be recognized that a situation may arise where infants are born at a distance from special care nurseries and require to be transported to them. Arrangements for suitable ambulance equipment and staffing have to be made and kept under regular review. The ambulance must be adequately lit, ventilated and heated. It must contain all the equipment necessary to maintain continuing ventilation and temperature control with full monitoring on at least two babies. Most ambulance services have found that they cannot equip and maintain ambulances used solely for the transfer of sick newborn. Transport incubators with the appropriate ventilator and monitoring equipment are now available and suitable anchorage and service points for these incubators within 'standard' ambulances (air and land) must be provided. Regional teams of doctors and nurses equipped and trained can allow the safe transfer of even the sickest of the low birth weight infants.

Design of nurseries

The architectural design of nurseries has a very important bearing on the successful function of a unit. This is not the place for any detailed discussion of the relative merits of different architectural solutions to the problems presented but it is useful for those who work in nurseries to have some idea of the basic principles involved in the design of a special care or intensive care nursery. Adequate space must be provided to allow easy access to an infant by more than one member of staff and for positioning of any special apparatus required. At the same time cots or incubators must not be so widely spread that observation of more than one infant by one nurse is not practical. In order to use nursery staff and equipment in the most economical manner at least two rooms per unit should be capable of holding six to eight cots or incubators with an allocation of floor area of 4 m^2 per cot. In smaller rooms the floor area should be 5 m^2 per cot. In a special care unit there should be at least two single isolation cubicles. The remaining cots should be in rooms containing four to six cots each. Panelling between rooms should be glazed from a level below cot height to a sufficient height to allow ready observation between rooms and of each room from the nurse's station. The grouping of room and the circulation areas must be aimed at allowing ready access with the minimum amount of movement. Separation of clean and dirty lines of communication is an advantage. Careful planning of air movement will do much to prevent cross-infection and this may mean that artificial ventilation systems are essential. Similarly, good design, choice of material and good workmanship will eliminate unnecessary dust-traps and make cleaning easier. The temperature of each room should be controlled by the staff within the range 20–30 °C. Double glazing is advisable, and if there are large areas of window facing the sun suitable means of preventing overheating by direct radiation has to be provided. There should be ample power points. Piped oxygen, compressed air and suction prevent the rooms being cluttered with unnecessary equipment. Lighting must be of a high standard and capable of variation in intensity. Each room should have an intercommunication system linked with the nursing station. In modern obstetric units the newborn nursery is adjacent to or an integral part of the delivery suite. Whether the nursery is close to the delivery area or not it is necessary to have a good communications system between the paediatricians and nurses involved in both areas.

It is essential to provide back-up provisions to ensure continued supplies of essential services such as electrical power, gases and water in the event of mains supply failure.

Mothers' rooms. A number of ancillary rooms will be necessary and should include single rooms for mothers with day-room facilities. Since mothers will take an increasing part in the care of their infant as the time for discharge home is approached, allowance for the presence of mothers (and fathers) must be made in planning space and facilities in nurseries. One or more rooms will be required for the training of parents and for the education of staff. Other provision for staff will depend upon the relationship of the unit to the remainder of the hospital. In some situations a bedroom for medical staff on call will be necessary. Provision of a quiet area where staff can relax away from the noise and bustle of the unit is essential. In planning the layout some thought must be given to allow young siblings and grandparents to visit the new addition to their family.

Special care and intensive care

The categories of infants requiring different intensity of management will vary between hospitals. It is convenient to consider three major categories for planning neonatal care. These are normal care, special care and intensive care. A memorandum prepared by the BPA and BAPM gives these categories and their resource implications in terms of staffing and equipment.

1. **Definitions of Neonatal Care**
1.1 *Intensive Care*
    Care given in a special or intensive care nursery which provides continuous skilled supervision by nursing and medical staff.
1.2 *Special Care*
    Care given in a special care nursery or on a postnatal ward which provides observation and treatment falling short of intensive care but exceeding normal routine care.
1.3 *Normal care*
    Care given, usually, by the mother in a postnatal ward, supervised by a midwife and doctor but requiring minimal medical or nursing advice.
2. **Clinical Categories**
2.1 *Intensive Care*
2.1.1 Babies receiving assisted ventilation (Intermittent Positive Pressure Ventilation (IPPV), Intermittent Mandatory Ventilation (IMV), Constant Positive Airway Pressure (CPAP)) and in the first 24 hours following its withdrawal.
2.1.2 Babies receiving total parenteral nutrition.
(Some units may wish to record these first two categories as a special and major subdivision of intensive care).
2.1.3 Cardiorespiratory disease which is unstable, including recurrent apnoea requiring constant attention.
2.1.4 Babies who have had major surgery, particularly in the first 24 post-operative hours.
2.1.5 Babies of less than 30 weeks gestation during the first 48 hours after birth.
2.1.6 Babies who are having convulsions.
2.1.7 Babies transported by the staff of the unit concerned. This would usually be between hospitals, or for special investigations or treatment.
2.1.8 Babies undergoing major medical procedures, such as arterial catheterisation, peritoneal dialysis or exchange transfusions.
2.2 *SPECIAL CARE*
(Some units may find it useful to make a sub-division, for example into high and low dependency special care to allow more detailed audit of their workload.)
2.2.1 Babies who require continuous monitoring of respiration or heart rate, or by transcutaneous transducers.
2.2.2 Babies who are receiving additional oxygen.

2.2.3   Babies who are receiving intravenous glucose and electrolyte solutions.

2.2.4   Babies who are being tube fed.

2.2.5   Babies who have had minor surgery in the previous 24 hours

2.2.6   Babies with a tracheostomy.

2.2.7   Dying babies.

2.2.8   Babies who are being barrier nursed.

2.2.9   Babies receiving phototherapy.

2.2.10 Babies who receive special monitoring, (for example frequent glucose or bilirubin estimations).

2.2.11 Other babies receiving constant supervision (for example babies whose mothers are drug addicts).

2.2.12 Babies receiving antibiotics.

2.2.13 Babies with conditions requiring radiological examination or other methods of imaging.

3   Resources Required for Neonatal Care

3.1   These are the present recommendations of the BPA.

3.2   INTENSIVE CARE

3.2.1   *Medical Staff*
Minimum medical staff should consist of both an experienced paediatric registrar and SHO on duty and available in the intensive care area at all times with an appropriately trained consultant in charge.

3.2.2   *Nursing Staff*
There should be an establishment to allow a ratio of four *trained* nurses (with neonatal intensive care experience) to each cot. This ratio allows for 24 hour cover and leave. The optimum ratio is 5:1.

3.2.3   *Equipment*
The following equipment must be available for each baby receiving intensive care:

> 1 intensive care incubator, or unit with overhead heating
> 1 respiratory, or apnoea, monitor
> 1 heart rate monitor
> 1 intravascular blood pressure transducer or surface blood pressue recorder
> 1 transcutaneous PO_2 monitor or intravascular oxygen transducer
> 1 transcutaneous PCO_2 monitor
> 2 syringe pumps
> 2 infusion pumps
> 1 ventilator
> 1 continuous temperature monitor
> 1 phototherapy unit
> 1 ambient oxygen monitor

Facilities for frequent blood gas analysis using micromethods
Facilities for frequent biochemical analysis including glucose, bilirubin and electrolytes by micromethods.
Access to ultrasound equipment for visualisation of organs such as the brain
Access to equipment for radiological examination.

3.3   *SPECIAL CARE*

3.3.1   *Medical Staff*

Minimum medical staff for 24 hour cover: an appropriately experienced SHO should be on duty, and an experienced more senior member of staff should be on call, with a consultant paediatrician in charge.

3.3.2   *Nursing Staff*

There should be an establishment to allow a ratio of 1.25 nurses (with neonatal experience) to each cot. This ratio allows for 24 hour cover and leave. The optimum ratio is 1.5 : 1.

3.3.3   *Equipment*

The following equipment must be available for each baby:
1 incubator, or cot adequate for temperature control
1 ambient oxygen anaiyser
1 apnoea alarm
1 heart rate monitor
1 infusion pump
1 phototherapy unit
1 ventilator to be used for short-term ventilation
Access to frequent blood gas analysis using micromethods
Access to biochemical analysis (including glucose, bilirubin and electrolytes) by micromethods.
Access to equipment for radiological examination.

3.3.4   Special care may take place on a post-natal ward, particularly in an area specially set aside for the purpose.

3.4   *NORMAL CARE*

Minimal requirements are a low reading thermometer, facilities for clearing the upper airway, for cord and skin care, and for weighing the baby. Emergency resuscitation equipment must be readily available.

4   **The Use of Categories of Neonatal Care in Hospital**

4.1   The list of categories in paragraph 4 should not be regarded as exhaustive but serves as a guide. The categories allow a nursing officer to count the number of babies receiving each level of care at a particular time. It must be understood that Intensive Care includes the categories described under Special Care, and there is therefore a hierarchy of care.

4.2   Some units may find it useful to subdivide intensive and special care to allow a more detailed audit of their workload.

4.3   The babies to be counted are those using the facilities or staff of the unit. This would include babies who are in an operating theatre or being transferred between hospitals when the count is made.

4.4   In order to obtain a complete picture of the workload it will be necessary to collect returns from the postnatal wards for those babies receiving special care. Babies who clearly require a level of care which cannot be provided because of shortage of staff or facilities should be included in the category reflecting the level of care required.

4.5   It may be necessary to undertake a count several times within a 24 hour period to demonstrate that there are times, for instance during the night, when the workload is not matched by the available resources.

Follow-up

The value of improved special care services for infants can only be assessed by the long-term follow-up of infants treated in such units. Arrangement for such follow-up requires co-operation with other branches of the health services. It is important that adequate records be kept of each stage in the progress of an individual infant and also of the performance of a special care nursery as a unit. There is now in the UK a standard code for the newborn produced by the BPA, which is compatible with the International Classification of Disease (ICD) Code and which is beginning to allow collection of national data on morbidity as well as mortality. Such information will be invaluable to those engaged in research and planning of medical and educational services.

Services for the newborn are not yet uniformly well developed in all parts of the UK. It is to be hoped that improvements in organization, the provision of physical facilities and in staffing will soon allow those parts of the country with the highest perinatal mortality rates to bring their results into line with the areas which have already achieved as high a standard as appears possible in the light of present-day knowledge.

FURTHER READING

British Medical Journal (1979) Towards fewer handicapped children. **iv**, 1458.
Chiswick, M. L. (1986) Commentary on current World Health Organisation definitions used in perinatal statistics. *Archives of Disease in Childhood*, **61**, 708–710.
Davies, P. (1980) Perinatal mortality. *Archives of Disease in Childhood*, 55, 833.
Lancet (1980) *Better Perinatal Health. A Survey*. London; *The Lancet*.
House of Commons Social Services Committee (1985) *Perinatal and Neonatal Mortality* (The Short Report). London: HMSO.
House of Commons Social Services Committee (1985) *Perinatal and Neonatal Mortality* (Follow up). London: HMSO.
Office of Health Economics (1979) *Perinatal Mortality in Britain — a question of class*. London: OHE.

3

The parents

An addition to the family is always a great event to which all relatives look forward. The arrival of the newborn infant must therefore always be seen in the context of the family to which he or she will belong. That family is of interest to the obstetrician, midwife and paediatrician before their infant arrives. The parents may have come to seek advice before even embarking on a pregnancy. In some situations advice may be requested, before marriage is contemplated, about possible difficulties in producing a normal infant. Others, after marriage, may seek advice about the spacing of pregnancies. This change in attitude to planned parenthood is chiefly due to advance in our knowledge of hereditary factors and to our ability to examine the embryo and fetus in utero as well as to control fertility. Parents are mainly concerned about possible abnormal development of their child before birth. Further discussion of the significance of heredity and perinatal diagnosis will be found in Chapter 4, which is concerned with the fetus.

Planned parenthood

Apart from their concern as to possible congenital abnormality, parents are are also anxious to make sure that they are in a satisfactory position to look after a new infant properly. Problems may arise because of poor housing, an inadequate income, ill-health or the presence of previous children. Many such factors tend to deter parents from having children when they are young and newly married. Perinatal mortality, however, is at its lowest in mothers who are between 20 and 30 years of age and who have had less than four pregnancies. Close spacing of pregnancies adds to the burden on mother's health and to the calls on her energy and purse. A prolonged interval between pregnancies may cause problems to some families. Careful planning of parenthood may obviate some of these difficulties and dangers and to this end doctors and midwives should be prepared to give advice about contraception or arrange for parents to visit a family planning clinic.

Social problems

A social worker is an essential member of the team in the antenatal clinic and expectant mothers should be encouraged to discuss their social problems. This service should be extended to fathers-to-be. The prospect of the responsibility of having to look after their first infant may present some young couples with problems of management of their lives and financial resources beyond their unaided capacity. Understanding, help and education at this stage may help them to establish a happy family and prevent much unnecessary misery.

The expectant mother should be told of help available during pregnancy, for instance protection of employment and the right to time off with full pay to attend antenatal clinics.

Contraception

The failure to have children may be a cause of great distress and disappointment to some couples and conversely in others there is a need to regulate fertility. Many social and personal factors influence the methods used. There is no 'best' method of contraception, only that which is most suitable to meet the needs of that particular couple. Male and female sterilization is available under the UK NHS. Throughout the world limitation of family size is being widely encouraged in order to diminish the population explosion. Attitudes towards the use of induced abortion also vary from country to country and are dependent upon a number of religious and other factors. In general, however, there is at present a much greater understanding than hitherto of the need for limitation of family size and for planned parenthood.

Infertility

It has been estimated that in about one in seven of all marriages there are problems with infertility. The introduction of methods for investigation of endocrine and anatomical disorder has helped many previously infertile couples, for example by induction of ovulation and artificial insemination techniques.

More recently the introduction of the techniques of in vitro fertilization has, for some previously infertile couples, brought about the miracle of parenthood. There are many legal and ethical dilemmas to be faced by society in coming to terms with technologies which observe embryos in test-tubes, and which can identify inherited metabolic or other defects prior to implantation within a uterus which may or may not be that of the donor of the ovum or wife of the donor of the sperm. For a fuller consideration of the implications, read the report of the RCOG ethics committee on in vitro fertilization and embryo replacement or transfer (RCOG, 1983) and the Warnock Report (1984).

Preparation for parenthood

Radio and television programmes have broken down the 'mystique' of the past surrounding pregnancy, labour and the care of the newly born baby and have indirectly played a major part in developing male interest. The role of the expectant father has radically changed. Husband and wife face pregnancy, labour and the care of the baby together. Changes in attitudes of the midwife have occurred, and it is now accepted that the loving and comforting presence of a husband during labour and delivery is an everyday part of the labour ward scene. There must therefore be provision for both parents in an antenatal education programme.

At school

Preparation for parenthood begins in childhood when children watch and note how their own parents and relatives bring up children. More formal education starts at school. With the school leaving age now being 16 years more time could be devoted to this subject in education programmes. Education authorities and teacher training colleges should be encouraged to add instruction in parentcraft to lessons on home management and sex education and to ensure that teachers have the appropriate knowledge and understanding of its importance. Involvement of midwives, health visitors, social workers and doctors in teacher training might help to enlarge experience on both sides.

A programme for education in parenthood to be used in school could cover the following subjects.

Choosing a partner. This difficult subject might be used to open a discussion on what a boy or girl expects from a partner in marriage and how they see their own role as parents. From this they could be led to discuss the role of their partner, what attributes they would expect of each other and whether they consider that each other's demands are reasonable. An introduction should be made to the concept of family responsibility particularly with regard to children.

Home management. The importance of budgeting the family income should be stressed, showing how money can be allocated to cover the necessities of life such as food, fuel, clothing and housing. Of particular importance is the need to convey to young people the value of eating a good nutritious diet not only for their own health, but also for that of their children. Young people do begin to have some idea that a healthy body is maintained in large part by a healthy life style and good nutrition. Basic information about the dietary values of different foods and the need for a varied and balanced nutrient intake must be provided. Planning of housework and its relation to work outside the home should be discussed. The need for relaxation and leisure enjoyment should not be forgotten.

Health education. The basic concepts of positive health as opposed to treatment of disease can be used as an introduction to the higher chance of a successful pregnancy with healthy parents. Girls who have no natural immunity to rubella should be immunized before reaching reproductive age. The particular risks of smoking and drinking alcohol during pregnancy can be underlined. Avoidance of accidents and poisoning in the home should be discussed. Special attention should be paid to the effect of parental habits on children and the responsibilities of parenthood. The value of services provided by health visitors should be stressed.

Social services. An outline of the social services available and of the particular help given to parents and their children should be given. Examples of the type of problems which young parents experience can be presented. The social benefits available should be explained.

Planning parenthood. On the presumption that sex education has already been given, the concept of spacing of a family and limitation of the number of children should be introduced. This leads into a description of contraceptive methods which might be given by a doctor or nurse from the Family Planning Service.

Bringing up children. A general discussion on the pleasures and responsibilities of bringing up a family could round off this series. A couple with young children might be willing to take part or the pupils might visit a day nursery.

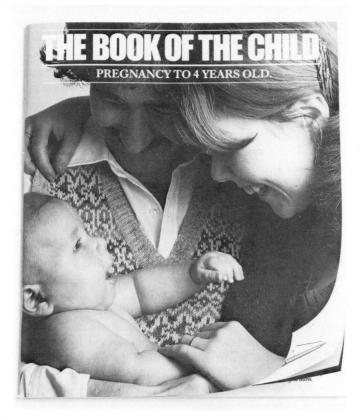

Fig. 3.1 *The Book of the Child* issued by the Scottish Health Education Group to all mothers attending antenatal clinics.

Films, slides and other visual aids may be used to make the parentcraft programme as attractive as possible. A variety of books, leaflets and magazines could be available for further study (Fig. 3.1).

Parentcraft

Although great strides have been made in the provision of classes for the expectant parents there are still a considerable number of people who are not motivated to attend and see no need for this very special kind of education even although they are totally ignorant of the subject. Many of these people are also clinic defaulters and come from poor social backgrounds and are in the high risk category. In order to encourage this very important group to attend, parentcraft classes must be taken out from the hospital into the community. The classes can be held in the local community centre, health centre or church hall with community midwives and local health visitors. Health Authorities have health education centres with excellent resources from which posters, leaflets and visual aids can be obtained. Great benefit can be derived from small classes and the chance to talk over problems with others in the same situation. Expectant parents are a delightful class to teach as they are uniquely receptive and every opportunity should be taken to exploit this willingness for health education.

Antenatal classes

Attractive environment for the classes is important with a friendly and relaxed atmosphere. The early classes directly concerned with pregnancy should be conducted by the hospital or community midwife depending on the location of the class. Later in the programme the obstetrician, paediatrician, health visitor, dentist and physiotherapist can be involved. The majority of patients are working in early pregnancy but in some countries recent legislation for pregnant women allows time off during the working day to attend classes. Special evening sessions for husband and wife should be arranged with an opportunity to visit the maternity hospital and take part, perhaps over a cup of coffee, in an informal question and answer session.

Confident parenthood

Parentcraft classes in the antenatal period must concentrate on giving young couples confidence in their ability to be good parents. Facilities for classes will vary from place to place according to the availability of staff and accommodation for this purpose. The following outline of a suggested programme may be beyond the capacity of some maternity departments but is an indication of what can be done under favourable circumstances.

General care during pregnancy. This session is an introduction to the facilities available to help a mother-to-be during her pregnancy. The value of regular attendance for antenatal examination by midwife, general practitioner or obstetrician must be stressed and the routine of antenatal clinics explained. General advice about care during pregnancy can be given together with reference to minor ailments which may arise and how these can be managed. The maternity benefits available should be explained and instructions given as to how they can be obtained.

Normal pregnancy. This will involve a simplified explanation of the course of pregnancy and the changes which take place in mother and fetus. Further explanation of the need for antenatal care can touch on some of the problems which may occur and how these can be avoided. An introduction to breast feeding can be given.

Educating both parents. Both parents are given an opportunity to meet some of the maternity department staff. Husbands can be advised about the effect of pregnancy on their wives. A film of a delivery may be shown. This is a useful opportunity for questions and answers and a discussion group.

Health education. Topics which were mentioned in the school programme must be further elaborated. Advice on diet and weight control can be given by a dietitian. The dangers of smoking and drinking alcohol or taking unnecessary medicines, particularly during pregnancy, are emphasized (Fig. 3.2). Warning is given of potential dangers in the home which might cause accidents and the risk of children taking poisonous substances is stressed. The role of the health visitor during pregnancy and after delivery is explained.

Preparing for baby's arrival. This is a practical session at which advice is given about the purchase of a layette, cot, pram and other items which will be required. Samples should be available for display.

Baby's arrival. The labour ward sister gives a simple explanation of the process of labour and demonstrates how pain is relieved. Advice is given about recognizing the onset of labour and admission procedure explained. The role of the father during labour can be discussed. This session can be concluded by a visit to the labour suite.

Arrangements in hospital. In this final session both parents are introduced to hospital routine. They are told how members of the staff can be identified and what functions they perform. Arrangements for visitors and for receiving and making telephone calls are explained. The hospital policy with regard to smoking is stated. Finally a tour of the hospital can be made pointing out where the various facilities are available.

The first five classes could be given at weekly intervals in early pregnancy and the remainder in the last month of pregnancy.

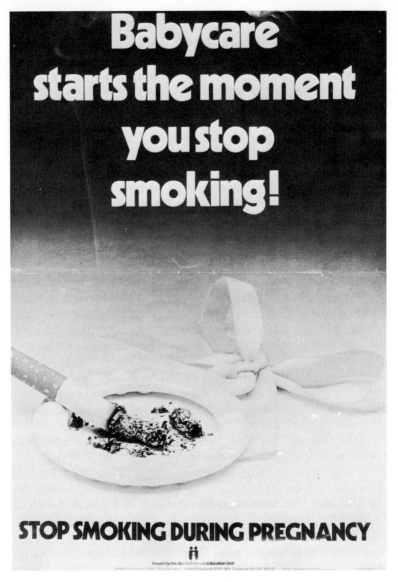

Fig. 3.2 Poster for display in antenatal clinic. (By courtesy of the Scottish Health Education Unit.)

As many visual aids as possible should be used to make the classes more attractive. Coloured slides of the unit and of the equipment used such as intravenous drips and monitors are very helpful as an introduction before a visit. Posters covering a wide range of subjects are readily available. There are excellent anatomical illustrations available which are particularly useful in the talk dealing with labour.

The requirements for bathing baby are shown using a doll. This demonstration is helpful to stress the importance of various items of equipment but the actual technique of bathing is best taught in the puerperium with mother's own baby.

A layette can be demonstrated using actual garments. Maternity fashions can be discussed including advice on suitable clothing. Samples of leaflets describing articles can be obtained from the firms supplying such articles or from local shops.

Breast feeding. Publicity for the advantages of breast feeding can readily be included in such a programme. Fashions vary with regard to the popularity of breast feeding. Interest in breast feeding should be stimulated at the antenatal clinic during the first visit. A midwife with special interest in lactation should discuss the advantages of breast feeding, examine the breasts and advise accordingly. She should arrange to see the patient at least twice again during the pregnancy in conjunction with an ordinary antenatal visit. The National Childbirth Trust hold classes to which expectant mothers may be invited. Their tutors place special emphasis on breast feeding preparation and may give individual support to new mothers in the postnatal period from members of the Trust who have successfully breast fed their own babies.

Several films about breast feeding are available and should, if possible, be shown during the antenatal period. Unless a mother has thought about breast feeding before delivery it is unlikely that she will be persuaded to give her baby the advantage of receiving human breast milk (Chapter 8).

In planning such a programme it must be remembered that the expectant mother has to travel to and from the parentcraft centre, and care must be taken not to overtax her unduly. At the same time it is essential to provide sufficient information to allay her fears and give her confidence in hospital and in the hospital team before she comes in to have her baby.

Parentcraft in the puerperium is discussed at the end of this chapter.

ANTENATAL CARE

The marked improvement in the standard of antenatal care which
has occurred during this century has been one of the greatest
factors in reducing maternal mortality, stillbirths and neonatal
deaths. Antenatal care may be shared by the consultant obstetrician, with the hospital midwife, the family doctor and domiciliary
midwife. 'At risk' patients are asked to attend the hospital clinic
for care throughout pregnancy whilst others attend the hospital
clinic at specific stages of the pregnancy. Patterns of shared care
vary. The advantage to the patient of this system is that she usually
has a family doctor near her own home and thus avoids travelling
long distances to the hospital. She continues to receive care from
her own family doctor whom she already knows in familiar
surroundings. Physiotherapists and social workers have a major
role to play and their services are available in the community as
well as in the hospital. The paediatrician and the clinical geneticist
may also on occasion be invited to join the team when particular
problems are involved (see Chapter 4).

Family history

At the first visit to the antenatal clinic the mother's history is carefully recorded, paying particular attention to her own previous
history and the history of both her own and her husband's family.
Reference may have to be made to her family doctor for details of
which the mother may not be aware. This applies particularly to
the occurrence in either parent's family of conditions which are
know to be inherited. It may be possible to reassure the mother
that conditions which have occurred in other members of the
family are not inherited. More young couples are attending pre-
pregnancy clinics and information of this nature would already
have been recorded and discussed.

Mother's medical history

Any period of admission to hospital must be carefully recorded and
enquiry made about any blood or blood product transfusion
received following, for example, a road accident or operation. It
is important to note the name and address of the hospital and the
patient's name and address at that time so that further enquiries
can be made. Specific enquiry must be made into a history of acute
rheumatism, chest infections, jaundice and urinary tract infections

as the extra burden of pregnancy may reveal diminished reserves of function which are the residual effect upon the heart, lungs, liver and renal system of such illnesses.

Obstetric history

It is essential to find out the mother's normal menstrual pattern so that the expected date of delivery can be calculated as accurately as possible from the date of the last menstrual period. This becomes of great importance if the maturity of the fetus is in doubt. A full summary of all previous pregnancies and abortions must be recorded with the following points being noted:

> Duration of pregnancy and whether labour was spontaneous or induced
> Complications of pregnancy
> Type of labour
> Delivery — spontaneous, forceps, breech, Caesarean section
> Liveborn or stillborn
> Birth weight of baby and type of feeding — breast or artificially fed
> Complications of the puerperium. Duration of hospital stay of mother and infant(s) is helpful in assessing the severity of the complication.

Social history

In order to assess the patient's social conditions it is necessary to make enquiries into her educational level and employment as well as that of her husband or partner and details of the house in which she is living.

Medical examination

A full medical examination is carried out with particular reference to the heart, blood pressure and lungs. The urine is tested for protein and sugar. If indicated a specialist physician is consulted to advise on the management of any abnormality detected. Height is recorded carefully as a woman of small stature might have a contracted pelvis (150 cm or under may be significant). Weight is recorded. An obese patient at the beginning of pregnancy will be a bad obstetric risk during the pregnancy. Dietary advice should be given and weight control achieved early in pregnancy. Blood is examined for ABO blood group, rhesus factor, VDRL slide test or Wassermann reaction and haemoglobin estimation. In some centres the immunological state with regard to such infections as rubella, cytomegalovirus, toxoplasmosis and hepatitis B is established by appropriate tests on the serum at the 15th to 16th week. At the same time blood may be examined for serum alphafetoprotein levels (Chapters 4 and 11). The rhesus-negative woman will need special monitoring during pregnancy and this will be intensified if antibodies are demonstrated (Chapter 15). The possibility of congenital syphilis in the fetus can be avoided by treating the mother in early pregnancy.

The size of the uterus must be checked with the period of amenorrhoea. This may be assessed by bimanual examination but a more accurate measurement and fetal assessment can be made by ultrasonography (Chapter 4).

Antenatal visits

Visits are arranged monthly until the 28th week of pregnancy, fortnightly till the 36th week, and weekly until delivery. At each of these visits the blood pressure and weight are recorded and the urine tested for sugar and protein. The abdomen is examined to ensure normal progress and growth of the uterus and, later, lie and presentation of the fetus. The haemoglobin estimation is repeated at the 28th, 32nd and 36th week of pregnancy, and more frequently if the readings are not satisfactory. Regular antenatal examination can detect early signs of abnormality of pregnancy and appropriate advice or treatment can be given.

The midwife helps the mother to lead a healthy life during pregnancy by advice and by encouraging her to attend the parentcraft talks which have already been detailed. These talks help to dispel the fears many women have of childbirth by enabling them to understand how the fetus develops and how the body functions during labour. The physiotherapist contributes to the confidence of the woman by teaching exercises to aid posture during the later weeks of pregnancy and to encourage relaxation when in labour. The medical social worker may be required to advise about arrangements for the care of the rest of the family while mother is in hospital. She may assist in providing for the new baby and in cases of hardship may even have to ensure that there is a suitable home for him to return to with his mother. The careful supervision of the mother during pregnancy is one of the chief factors in the reduction of maternal and perinatal mortality.

Mothers over 35 years of age. As the incidence of chromosomal abnormality, including Down's syndrome, in the fetus increases markedly in mothers over 40 years of age and to a lesser extent in mothers between 35 and 40 years of age, mothers should be encouraged to complete their families before this age. If pregnancy occurs after 35 years of age the mother can be offered screening tests to exclude such abnormalities in her fetus (Chapter 11). Should the examination confirm that the fetus has an abnormal chromosome karyotype, therapeutic termination of pregnancy can be offered.

High-risk mothers

Unfortunately many patients who come into this category are slow to seek antenatal care and frequently fail to keep antenatal clinic appointments. Studies have shown that many mothers will not travel more than a short distance to antenatal clinics and a reassessment of arrangements for providing optimal antenatal services is needed. Defaulters should be followed up by the domiciliary midwife or health visitor. In some cases antenatal care may have to be given in the patient's own home.

Older primigravidae

Patients coming into this classification are women going through their first pregnancy from the age of 30 years onwards. There may be a history of infertility. The maximum fertility in a woman is at about the age of 24 years and there is a gradual decline with increasing age. There is a greater tendency for preeclampsia and hypertension to develop in older mothers. These factors could precipitate accidental haemorrhage or the premature onset of labour. In labour such patients tend to become anxious and labour may be prolonged and the functional activity of the uterus poor. There is a higher ratio of operative deliveries in older primigravidae and consequently both mother and baby are at greater risk.

Bad obstetric history

Patients who come under this category are those who have had previous pregnancies with unsuccessful outcomes such as abortion, stillbirth, neonatal death and abnormal infants. Information regarding the previous pregnancies must be obtained from the hospital where she was previously confined including a report of any post-mortem examination carried out. Certain factors may recur such as cervical incompetence, preeclampsia, hypertension. If the size of the pelvis is in doubt previous pelvimetry results must be studied and the weight of previous babies taken into consideration. The possibility of chronic ill-health of the mother as a causative factor must be considered and such conditions as chronic pyelonephritis or diabetes mellitus excluded.

The grand multipara

This term is generally applied to women who have had five babies or more. With increasing age these patients have a greater tendency to obesity. In many cases social conditions are poor and they are overworked and tired out. Dietary deficiencies may be present as they tend to feed their children and neglect themselves. There is a greater tendency to the complications of pregnancy particularly anaemia, pre-eclampsia and hypertension with their attendant risks of antepartum haemorrhage and preterm delivery. The grand multipara has a greater chance of multiple pregnancy, of placenta praevia and of antepartum haemorrhage. Malpresentations and malpositions are more common due to the laxity of the muscles of the abdominal wall and a pendulous abdomen. In labour complications are more liable to occur for reasons already mentioned and the stillbirth and neonatal death rate is greatly increased.

The unsupported mother

The unmarried or unsupported mother is at greater risk as she may be living in poor social conditions. She may try to conceal her pregnancy and continue working and therefore will get little antenatal care. The unmarried mother requires very tactful and sympathetic consideration and the medical social worker can give her most valuable advice and support.

Check lists

Check lists can be used to ensure that all the necessary information has been collected and that no important items have been overlooked. The decision regarding specialist antenatal care in hospital or shared antenatal care with the family doctor will depend on the risk factors present.

Delivery

Delivery is the climax of a pregnancy to which parents look forward with both excitement and fear. Most maternity hospitals recognize the great significance of this event to both parents and encourage fathers to be beside their wives during labour and delivery. This can give great pleasure to both, and fathers can be a source of comfort and strength to their wives. It must be emphasized, however, that some husbands cannot deal with the stress of labour and especially delivery. They should not be allowed to feel guilty on this account. Guidance and help for the husband should be provided in the antenatal period and a firm decision made by the couple as to whether the husband wishes to be with his wife.

The puerperium

As stated earlier the puerperium is a most important learning time when teaching is more meaningful because of the presence of the newly born baby. A policy of rooming-in increases the opportunities for mother to learn about her baby.

Parentcraft in the puerperium

Informal classes can be held while mother is in the postnatal wards. With the present tendency for shorter periods in hospital after delivery the opportunity for postnatal education is limited and advantage must be taken of every opportunity offered.

The following subjects can be covered.

Care of the breasts and nipples. A simple explanation of the physiology of lactation is given stressing that lactation is a natural function which is favoured by rest, a tranquil outlook and a good diet.

Bottle feeding. For mothers who choose not to breast feed instruction is given on the sterilization of bottles and teats and the preparation of feeds. The types of milk on sale can be discussed.

Caring for baby at home. A health visitor can usefully introduce education about the management of baby at home with particular reference to maintenance of temperature. Further care can be discussed introducing the advantage of regular attendance with baby at a clinic for periodic checks and for immunization procedures.

Family planning. This is a useful time to talk to mothers about contraception. Some mothers are more willing to discuss this

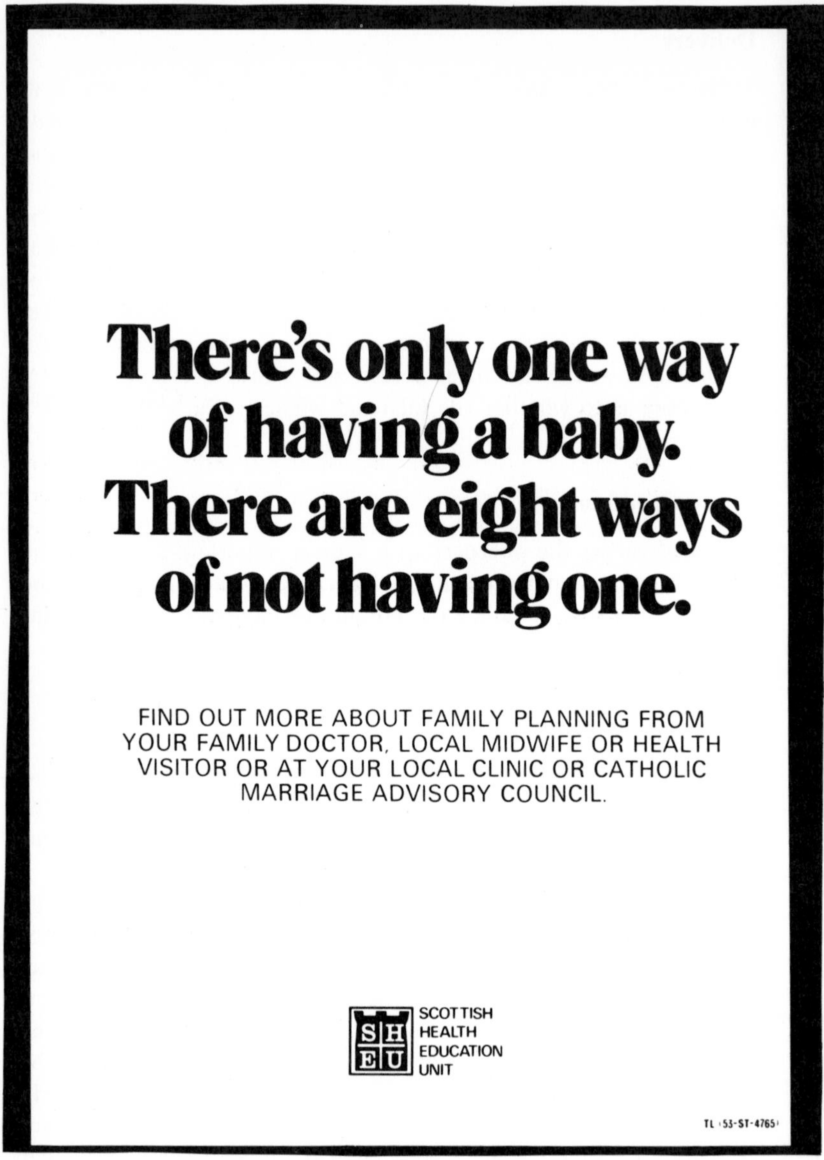

There's only one way of having a baby. There are eight ways of not having one.

FIND OUT MORE ABOUT FAMILY PLANNING FROM
YOUR FAMILY DOCTOR, LOCAL MIDWIFE OR HEALTH
VISITOR OR AT YOUR LOCAL CLINIC OR CATHOLIC
MARRIAGE ADVISORY COUNCIL.

SCOTTISH
HEALTH
EDUCATION
UNIT

TL (53-ST-4765)

Fig. 3.3 Poster for display in postnatal clinic. (By courtesy of the Scottish Health Education Unit.)

subject with their midwife after delivery. Excellent leaflets are prepared by the Family Planning Service and can be distributed to parents (Fig. 3.3).

Adoptive parents. Special parentcraft classes covering some of these subjects can be given to prospective adoptive parents.

The father

The role of the father in supporting his wife and the rest of the family during his wife's pregnancy and delivery is often overlooked not least by fathers themselves. Many of the problems which arise during pregnancy could be prevented or diminished by more sympathetic understanding of the situation by the father-to-be. Ignorance of his wife's needs is the most common cause of this apparent neglect of duty and many fathers-to-be are very upset when their lack of support for their wives is pointed out to them. They commonly reply, 'I never realized. . . .' This unawareness on the part of father is more often due to lack of education than to lack of will and underlines the importance of the comments made earlier in this chapter on education in parentcraft at school and in the antenatal clinic. It takes two parents to act in unison before a child is conceived. We must make sure that both parents understand the responsibilities which follow their action.

FURTHER READING

Bock, G. & O'Connor, M. (1986) *Human Embryo Research: Yes or No?* The Ciba Foundation, London: Tavistock Publications.

Docherty, R. C. (Ed) (1979) *The Book of the Child: Pregnancy to 4 years.* Edinburgh: Scottish Health Education Unit.

Harvey, D. (1987) Parent-Infant Relationships. *Perinatal Practice*, Vol. 4. Chichester: Wiley Medical.

Loudon, J. D. O. (Chairman) (1983) *Report of the RCOG Ethics Committee on In Vitro Fertilisation and Embryo Replacement or Transfer.* London: Royal College of Obstetricians and Gynaecologists.

Myles, M. F. (1985) *A Textbook for Midwives*, 10th edn. Edinburgh: Churchill Livingstone.

Warnock, M. (Chairman) (1984) *Report of the Committee of Inquiry into Human Fertilization and Embryology.* London: HMSO.

Williams, M. & Booth, D. (1974) *Antenatal Education — Guidelines for Teachers.* Edinburgh: Churchill Livingstone.

4

The fetus

Study of the factors involved in perinatal mortality and morbidity (Chapter 2) clearly indicates that the majority of these exert their effect before the onset of labour and many are associated with the mother's general health and upbringing before conception occurred. It is therefore appropriate that consideration of the care of the newly born infant should not ignore the antenatal period. Knowledge of embryonic and fetal development is essential to the proper understanding and management of the newborn infant. This chapter deals with subjects which are more directly the concern of the obstetrician and which are dealt with in more detail in textbooks of obstetrics and fetal medicine. Prenatal medicine is nevertheless equally of interest to all who deal with the infant following delivery, and the recent developments in knowledge about fetal medicine serve only to indicate how much more we still have to learn about this relatively short period of our lives which shapes our future.

HEREDITY

Variability and abnormality

The fertilization of the maternal ovum by the paternal sperm is the starting point of a new and eventually independent life. Before emergence as a newborn infant the fertilized ovum has to pass through an intrauterine stage of growth and development of such complexity that it is amazing how relatively alike one human being is to another.

Capacity for variability. Fortunately for us differences do exist and we are not produced as identical copies of either parent. It is this capacity for variability which allows for evolutionary forces to act over long periods of time and this has been to the advantage of the human and to other species.

Limitation of variability. The capacity for variability within an individual is limited by the genetic factors inherited equally from both parents. These may act either to his or her benefit or detriment. Where the result is sufficiently detrimental, conception may not be successful or the fertilized ovum may die at an early stage.

Abnormality. With progressively less serious forms of abnormality intrauterine growth may proceed for longer periods resulting in abortion, stillbirth or the live birth of an abnormal infant. During the first 8 weeks after conception the embryo develops to become recognizably human and to have formed most major organs. During the subsequent 30 weeks fetal growth and development takes place. The progress of development may be disturbed by genetic disorder at the time of conception or by subsequent damage to the growing embryo and fetus by external influences. These subjects are considered further in Chapter 11.

Normality. The tendency for most major abnormalities of conception to cause death before development is well advanced ensures a high degree of normality and viability in surviving fetuses. In this chapter consideration will be given to the development of the normal fetus but mention will also be made of factors which can interfere with the normal development of a fetus which begins life without inherited abnormality. The absence of abnormality does not make us all identical and it is clear that we inherit characteristic features of physique and possibly behaviour from our parents which make us different from our siblings without being abnormal.

Genes and chromosomes

Inherited characteristics are carried in deoxyribonucleic acid (DNA) as genes on chromosomes contained in the nucleus of body cells. In humans there are 22 pairs of autosomes and 2 sex chromosomes giving a total of 46 chromosomes. This is known as the diploid number. The ovum and the spermatozoon each contain half that number, 22 autosomes and 1 sex chromosome, and this is known as the haploid number. At fertilization the autosomes of the spermatozoon pair up with the autosomes of the ovum to form the 22 pairs of somatic chromosomes. A female has two X chromosomes, and a male has an X and a Y chromosome. These are known as the sex chromosomes. Every fetus receives one X chromosome from the mother and either an X or a Y chromosome from the father. The fetal sex chromosome constitution therefore

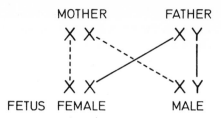

Fig. 4.1 Inheritance of sex chromosomes indicating that it is the sex chromosome received from the father which determines the sex of the fetus.

depends upon which sex chromosome is received from the father (Fig. 4.1).

Inheritance

Each chromosome carries very large numbers of genes which are the ultimate factors governing inheritance. With the pairing of autosomes at conception the fetus receives pairs of genes, one from each parent.

Dominant. Some inherited abnormalities are carried on a single gene. In some conditions the presence of abnormality in one only of the gene pair is sufficient to produce its effect on the fetus. Such conditions are termed dominant.

Recessive. In other situations both genes in the pair must have the same abnormality before the fetus is affected. This type of inheritance is termed recessive.

Zygosity. If a person has only one gene carrying such a recessively inherited condition and the other gene of the pair is normal that person is not usually affected by the single abnormal gene but is a carrier of that gene. Where only one gene of a pair is abnormal the subject is heterozygous for that gene. If both genes are the same the subject is homozygous for that gene. If both genes are normal the subject is normal for that trait. If both are abnormal so is the subject.

Risk. If a male and a female carrier (heterozygotes) of a recessively inherited gene such as phenylketonuria or cystic fibrosis marry there is a 1 in 4 chance that each infant will be a homozygote and affected. There is also a 1 in 4 chance that he will be an unaffected homozygote. The remaining 2 of the 4 chances will be heterozygotes and therefore unaffected but carriers.

Sex linked. Certain inherited traits such as haemophilia are carried on the X chromosome as a recessive character. In the male with a single X chromosome the trait will be manifest. The female with two X chromosomes will generally be heterozygous. The trait will not be manifest but the female is a carrier. Her sons have a 1 in 2 chance of being affected. Her daughters have a 1 in 2 chance of being carriers. This is called sex-linked or X-linked recessive inheritance.

Eugenics

While some inherited disorders (Chapter 11) fall into these relatively simple patterns of dominant, recessive and sex-linked inheritance originally described by Mendel, much more complicated patterns of inheritance govern the majority of normal variations which constitute our individuality. Our genetic inheritance is at present a sequel to the mutual attraction between our parents. Some scientists foresee the time when chance will be given a less free hand and artificial selection of genetic characteristics will be possible by eugenically planned mating, whether this be physiological or in the test-tube. Others look forward to the possibility of altering genes. Many authors have warned of the potential risks of such concepts. Fortunately at present the human race remains dependent on chance to select the maternal and paternal genes of a fetus. This haphazard method has served us well in the past and it is difficult to believe that more organized control would result in a benefit which outweighed the dangers inherent in such proposals. In families afflicted by severe inherited disorders, genetic techniques can be applied to remove unnecessary anxieties through DNA and other analyses.

The ovum

A detailed study of the development of the fertilized ovum is not called for in a book which is chiefly concerned with the newborn infant. It is helpful, however, to have some knowledge of intra-uterine development as a preparation for the study of the infant at birth and it is hoped that the following outline will suffice.

Before implantation

Fertilization almost invariably takes place while the ovum is in the ampulla of the Fallopian tube. After fertilization the ovum is propelled along the tube to the uterus and at the same time under-

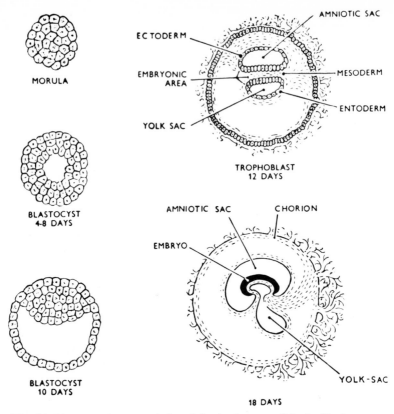

Fig. 4.2 Diagrammatic representation of the development of the fertilized ovum.

goes repeated cell division. As a result the ovum assumes the form of a ball of cells (morula) in which a cavity (blastocele) appears — at which stage the ovum is known as a blastocyst. The multiplying cells of the blastocyst undergo a patterned distribution, some cells being gathered together to form what is called the inner cell mass and others remaining on the surface as a covering layer (trophoblast). At one point the trophoblast and the inner cell mass remain connected by a stalk of cells known as the body stalk. Arriving at this stage of development the ovum comes in contact with the uterine endometrium (Fig. 4.2).

Implantation

During the secretory phase of the menstrual cycle the endometrium undergoes changes intended to prepare it for reception of a fertilized ovum. If a fertilized ovum becomes embedded in it the endometrium undergoes further development, becoming greatly increased in thickness, vascularity and softness. The ovum or blastocyst penetrates and eventually becomes completely embedded in the endometrium, which is now known as the decidua.

The embryo

Two cavities develop in the inner cell mass of the blastocyst. One is known as the amniotic sac and the other as the yolk sac. Between them there is a cellular area called the embryonic area or plate because it is from this plate that the embryo grows. In the embryonic area the cells become grouped into three primitive layers known as the ectoderm, the mesoderm and the entoderm. In the course of subsequent growth the skin, certain mucous membranes and the central nervous system develop from the ectoderm; the blood, muscle, bones and certain organs from the mesoderm; and the lungs, alimentary mucosa, bladder, pancreas and parts of the liver from the entoderm.

The amniotic sac is filled with fluid and serves to protect the growing embryo which derives its nourishment from the yolk sac pending the development of a rudimentary placenta. The yolk sac is connected by a duct (vitelline duct) with the embryonic gut. With expansion the amniotic cavity gradually envelops the embryo at each end and along the flanks, and at the same time brings the yolk sac and the vitelline duct into contact with the body stalk to form the umbilical cord. Development of the cord is usually complete by the sixth week.

Development of the placenta

Buds of multiplying cells sprout out from the trophoblast where it comes into contact with the decidua. These buds or villi multiply in number and cover the entire ovum by the time it has been completely embedded in the implantation cavity. At the same time some of the villi become attached to the deep layer of the decidua (decidua basalis) and serve to anchor the ovum to the decidua. Other villi grow rapidly, penetrate the decidual-blood vessels, and as a result are continuously bathed by circulating maternal blood. This stage of development is reached about the third week of pregnancy (Fig. 4.3).

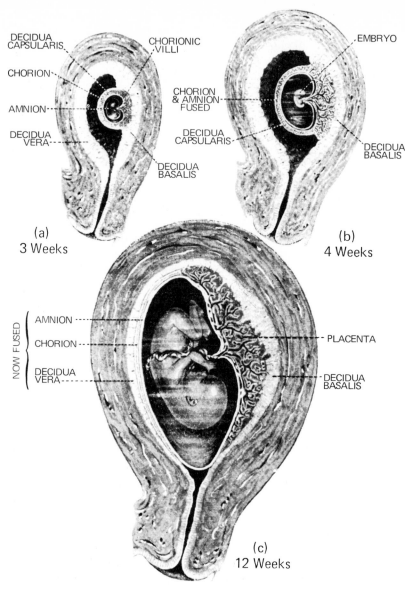

Fig. 4.3 Development of the placenta.

Umbilical cord

Thereafter the persisting chorionic villi multiply in number and increase in complexity. Each villus consists of a central core of fetal mesoderm and embryonic vessels in which fetal blood circulates and two cellular layers: an inner — Langhan's layer or cytotrophoblast — and an outer — the syncytium or syncytiotrophoblast. Fetal and maternal blood do not come into contact with one another, but Langhan's layer selects and absorbs substances necessary for the nourishment of the embryo from the maternal blood. Absorbed substances are conveyed to the embryo from the venous and waste products returned by the arterial vessels of the developing umbilical cord, which is continuous at one end with the chorion and attached to the embryo at the other.

Chorionic villi

In contrast with those in the uterine decidua the chorionic villi which cover the capsule of the trophoblast and which are nearest the uterine cavity degenerate and undergo atrophy. By the end of the third month the placenta acquires a discoidal shape consisting of some 15 to 20 clumps (cotyledons) of chorionic villi anchored to the decidua basalis and bathed in the maternal blood flowing through the spaces separating the chorion and decidua. Occasionally failure to disappear of a collection of chorionic villi in relation to the capsule of the trophoblast gives rise to an accessory placental lobe.

Twinning. In the great majority of instances of twin pregnancy resulting from fertilization of a single ovum (monozygote) there is one placenta, one chorion and two amniotic sacs. Exceptionally, however, two placentae may develop (Fig. 4.4). Where in a twin pregnancy fertilization of two ova has taken place (dizygote), there are two placentae which may, however, fuse and have the appearance of a single placenta. Fig. 4.4 illustrates that dizygotic twins may be born with separate placentae or with an apparently single placenta with two separate amniotic sacs (diamniotic) and two chorionic membranes (dichorionic). The monozyotic twins may be born with (a) separate placentae and membranes, (b) one placenta and dichorionic, diamniotic membranes, (c) one placenta with monochorionic membranes. Monozygotic twins originate from the splitting of one fertilized egg and are thus identical. The splitting can occur at different stages of development. Early splitting (2–3

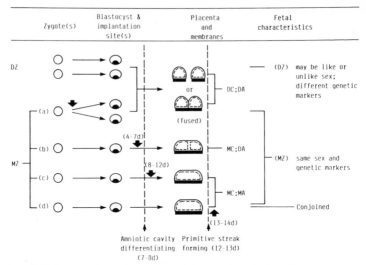

Fig. 4.4 Twins: zigosity and structure of the membranes. The chioronic membranes are shown with a full line and the amniotic membranes with interrupted lines. DZ — Dizygous; DC — Dichorionic; DA — Diamniotic; MZ — Monozygous; MC — Monochorionic; MA — Monoamniotic.
(With permission from C R Whitfield (ed) (1986) *Dewhurst's Textbook of Obstetrics and Gynaecology for Postgraduates*, 4th ed. London: Blackwell Scientific Publications.)

days) after conception will result in (a) or (b) twins (Fig. 4.4), intermediate splitting (4–7 days) situation (c), and late splitting (8–12 days) situation (d). When the splitting is delayed beyond 13 days the twins may be fused (conjoined or 'Siamese').

Decisions as to whether twins are identical or non-identical cannot therefore always be made by examination of the placentae and membranes. Twins of different sex must be dizygotic. In Europe, approximately 33% of monozygous twins are dichorial, 66% monochorial-diamniotic and 1% monochorionic-monoamniotic. It may require collection of blood from twins of the same sex in order to diagnose whether they are mono or dizygous. Tests would include blood grouping and DNA 'fingerprint' analyses.

Functions of the placenta

Knowledge concerning the functions of the placenta is incomplete but growing.

Fetal lung. The placenta acts as a fetal lung. In the placenta carbon dioxide is transferred from the fetal to the maternal circulation. Simultaneously the fetus obtains oxygen from the mother's haemoglobin.

Nutrition. The fetus derives its nourishment from the mother's blood. It is believed that Langhan's layer of the chorionic villi is capable of selective absorption of substances necessary for growth of the embryo and later of the fetus. Substances passing from the maternal blood into the fetal circulation include: amino acids, necessary for tissue development; glucose, needed for energy and growth; and calcium, phosphorus, iron and other minerals necessary for the formation of the skeleton, teeth and blood. Glucose is converted into fat by the fetus as required. In the early months of fetal growth, prior to normal liver function being established, glucose is stored as glycogen in the placenta where it is converted into glucose when required.

Excretion. Waste products of fetal metabolism such as urea and heat are transferred across the placenta to the mother's blood.

Protective barrier. The placenta acts as a protective barrier to the fetus by preventing the passage of certain but by no means all potentially harmful substances from the maternal to the fetal circulation. Very few infecting organisms can pass the placental barrier. Amongst the known exceptions are the virus of rubella, the virus of cytomegalic inclusion body disease, the virus of AIDS and the spirochaete of syphilis. The bacillus of tuberculosis and the protozoon of toxoplasmosis are also very rare exceptions.

The newly born baby frequently possesses a temporary passive immunity to infections such as diphtheria and measles. The immunity is acquired from the mother through transfer across the placenta of IgG antibodies to infections experienced by the mother. Transfer of fetal antigens in a reverse direction can take place. Rhesus-positive cells from a fetus may enter the circulation of the rhesus-negative mother and stimulate the formation of antibodies. Other substances which can penetrate the placental barrier include sedative, anaesthetic, antibiotic and antisyphilitic drugs.

Endocrine. The placenta functions as an endocrine gland secreting oestrogenic and other hormones. Maternal hormones can pass through the placenta to enter the blood of the fetus.

Disturbance of normal placental function can result in interference with healthy fetal development. Contributory factors include abnormal structure and size, degenerative changes and premature separation of the placenta.

THE FETUS

The first recognizable human characteristics appear about four weeks after conception. They consist of the rudimentary eyes and ears, and projecting buds representing the beginnings of limb formation. At this stage the embryo consists of a large head and a rather tapering body ending in a tail, weighs approximately 1 to 1.3 g and measures 9 to 12 mm in length. The head and tail almost meet because the embryo is markedly curved.

By the eighth week the hands and feet are recognizable; the external genitalia are developing, the tail has almost completely disappeared, and the head has assumed a normal human shape (Fig. 4.5). It has been customary to use the name embryo up until the end of the eighth week and thereafter to refer to the fetus but this distinction is arbitrary.

At 12 weeks the placenta is well developed, the umbilical cord shows normal spiral characteristics and the fingers and toes are distinguishable (Fig. 4.6). By this time the growing organism measures about 9 cm in length and weighs about 29 g. A uterus is present in the female. Centres of ossification are present in many bones. Lanugo first appears about the sixteenth week of gestation, and in a further four weeks vernix caseosa is present. Within some 24 weeks of conception hair appears on the head and the deposit of subcutaneous fat begins. During the subsequent 16 weeks of pregnancy the hair on the scalp increases in amount, the nails grow in length and the vernix caseosa becomes more plentiful. As the subcutaneous fat is laid down in increasing amount the face and forehead lose their creases, the skin acquires a smooth texture and pink colour, and the body as a whole becomes more rotund.

After a gestation period of 40 weeks the fetus measures approximately 51 cm in length and weighs about 3200 g, but wide variations occur. In general, male infants tend to be slightly heavier than female infants, and where the mother's age is under 30 years the weights of successive babies tend to increase.

Differentiation and organogenesis

During fetal development the various organ systems differentiate anatomically and progressively assume their individual function. This progress is extremely complicated but is of clinical importance under two groups of circumstances. If the fetus is delivered before its various organs are functioning sufficiently well to support independent life there is a grave risk that the infant will not survive

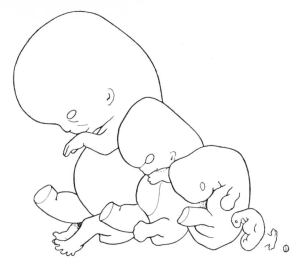

Fig. 4.5 The stages of growth from the end of the third week to the end of the eighth week in utero.

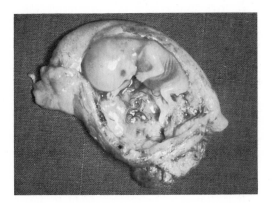

Fig. 4.6 Fetus of 12 weeks' gestation.

the separation from his mother's uterus. This subject is considered in further detail in Chapters 9, 10 and later chapters. If intrauterine development of one or more organ systems does not progress normally this may result in fetal death or the delivery of an infant with anatomical and functional abnormalities. This subject will be considered in greater detail in Chapter 11 which is concerned with congenital abnormalities. Where appropriate the disorder of fetal development which has caused the congenital abnormality will be described in the same section as the abnormality concerned. Further details of the anatomical development of the fetus will therefore not be discussed in this chapter but it is appropriate at this stage to consider those factors which influence prenatal growth and the means which are available for assessment of prenatal health.

Prenatal environment influences

One thousand years ago antenatal clinics were held in China to ensure tranquillity in mothers in order to promote mental health and tranquillity in their infants. The Chinese were more concerned with the mental than the physical progress of the fetus. We may be in danger of going to the opposite extreme. Recent investigations provide evidence in animals that environmental influences during pregnancy can affect the behaviour of that fetus in later development. In humans a relationship has been demonstrated between the activity of a fetus and his subsequent behaviour as an infant. The relative importance of intrauterine environment in shaping postnatal behaviour is, however, not clear and the need for appropriate management cannot therefore be assessed.

Assessment of the fetus

Menstrual age. Gestational age, that is age from conception, is generally calculated by reference to the date of the first day of the last menstrual period. Strictly this gives menstrual age and the relation to true gestational age depends on the interval between onset of menstruation and ovulation. Where this is known the mean interval between conception and delivery has been reported as 265 days. It is, however, more convenient to measure the duration of pregnancy as from the last menstrual period giving an average duration for a full-term pregnancy of 280 days. The first day of the last menstrual period is generally accepted as the date from which the gestational age is calculated to the nearest week. Although this method has the obvious merit of simplicity it has equally obvious fallacies. Mothers may not be sure of the date of their last period. Bleeding following the withdrawal of oral contraceptives may be mistaken for a true period. Early bleeding at the time of implantation of the ovum or due to a threatened abortion may similarly be accepted as menstruation. Other methods have been employed to measure the length of gestation.

Assessment by size. Bimanual assessment of the size of the uterus in the first trimester of pregnancy is a more reliable means of assessing fetal size and age than measurement of the height of the fundus above the symphysis pubis at later stages of pregnancy when factors other than fetal size affect the fundal height. Radiographs of fetal bones can give information about the appearance of centres of ossification and bone length from which fetal age is often calculated. It has been shown, however, that there is poor correlation between the bone age of twins although they are presumably of the same gestational age.

Ultrasound

The rapidly developing techniques of ultrasonography are proving particularly useful in the study of normal fetal growth and in the assessment of early fetal maturity. Measurement of the biparietal diameter of the fetal head can be made with a high degree of accuracy (Fig. 4.7). This measurement can be used to calculate fetal age and repeated examinations will give an indication of the rate of fetal growth. The accurate assessment of fetal age is of

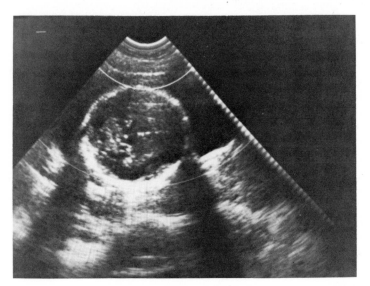

Fig. 4.7 Measurement of biparietal diameter by ultrasound. (Figs. 4.7, 4.8a and b and 4.9 have been kindly provided by Dr S R Wild.)

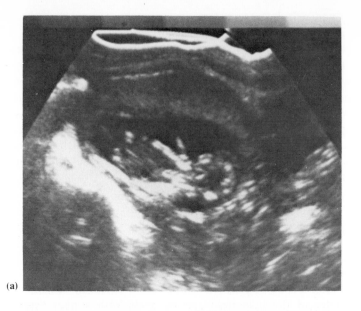

(a)

(b)

Fig. 4.8 Ultrasonogram of fetus; (a) 12-week pregnancy; (b) 22-week pregnancy.

importance to the interpretation of alphafetoprotein levels in serum or amniotic fluid in the detection of open neural tube defects as will be discussed in Chapter 11. Sufficient information has now been gathered about the pattern of growth of the fetus to establish the normal range (Fig. 4.8a and b) and it is now possible to detect abnormalities of early growth by serial ultrasonic measurement (Fig. 4.9). Measurement of crown–rump length in early pregnancy (12 weeks) can give a very accurate assessment of fetal maturity. In later pregnancy, measurements of trunk area in relation to skull area can give accurate assessment of fetal growth and development. Doppler ultrasound can be used to assess fetal and placental blood flow and can give an early indication of placental failure.

Real time scanning. The development of full grey tone scaling and of real time scanning which provides a moving picture as compared to the previous still frames have added greatly to the information which can be provided by ultrasonography. Improvements in the quality of the picture and the 'cine' effect of real time scanning are opening up new prospects of studying prenatal movement patterns and the factors which influence them. Increasing knowledge of such patterns leads to recognition of abnormal behaviour which can be recognized at 16 weeks or earlier before the mother can feel fetal movement. Such non-invasive methods of

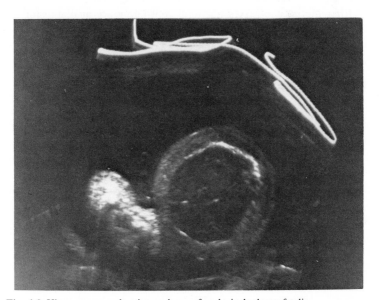

Fig. 4.9 Ultrasonogram showing oedema of scalp in hydrops fetalis.

examining the fetus are already leading to the provisional diagnosis of chromosomal and other developmental abnormality in the fetus before such a diagnosis can be established by other means. Ultrasonography is likely to become of increasing importance in our assessment of fetal health and well-being. Abnormalities of the fetus such as exompholos, hydrocephalus, hydronephrosis and congenital heart disease can be diagnosed very early in pregnancy. Some of these conditions may be treated before delivery.

Rate of growth

With an estimate of fetal age an assessment can be made as to whether uterine size conforms with that expected for that stage of pregnancy. If the rate of growth of the uterus is less than that expected it is probable that this is due to slow intrauterine growth of the fetus, which is said to be 'growth retarded'. This implies an increased risk to the fetus, and unless fetal growth improves the pregnancy may not end successfully. As there is a considerable variation in the rates of growth of normal fetuses it is most important to know whether the growth retarded fetus is a healthy but light fetus or whether growth is being retarded by some abnormal process. Excessive rates of uterine enlargement indicate possible abnormalities which require investigation.

Other methods of assessing fetal well-being are available for use where there is evidence of departure from the normal range of intrauterine growth.

Assessment of placental function

Urine oestriol. Placental function can be estimated by examination of the oestrogen content of maternal urine. Of the oestrogens present oestriol is the largest fraction, and as oestriol is produced by a combination of placental and fetal adrenal gland activity its output in the mother's urine is an indication of placentofetal function. Maternal urinary oestriol concentrations increase about the 32nd to 34th week of gestation. In about 90% of cases of retarded fetal growth oestriol excretion is decreased. Serial measurements are more useful than single. A falling value is a danger sign as is absence of the expected rise at 32 to 34 weeks gestation. Oestriol excretions below 5 mg in 24 hours indicate a high risk of early neonatal death.

Human placental lactogen (HPL). Human placental lactogen can be detected in maternal serum as early as the fifth week of gestation and rises steadily throughout pregnancy until the 38th week. Measurement which is carried out by a radioimmunoassay technique requires only 0.1 ml of serum.

In pregnancies complicated by diabetes mellitus or rhesus immunization both HPL measurement and urine eostriol estimations are more difficult to interpret.

Since the development of ultrasound techniques biochemical assessments of placental function have gradually become of less relevance.

Amniocentesis

Amniocentesis can be used to provide information about the fetus (Fig. 4.10).

Rhesus incompatability. Examination of amniotic fluid has been practised for many years in the antenatal diagnosis and management of rhesus incompatability in rhesus-negative mothers. By measuring the optical density (OD) of centrifuged amniotic fluid at a wavelength of 450 nm the concentration of bilirubin present can be calculated. This in turn gives an indication of the severity of the haemolytic process in the fetus. By reference to the curves originally prepared by Liley the obstetrician is given an indication

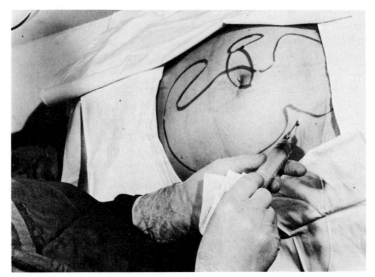

Fig. 4.10 Amniocentesis. (Photograph by courtesy of Dr J M Monaghan.)

as to when action is required. Repeat tests allow an assessment of the rate of deterioration and the risk of intrauterine death. Amniocentesis is not without risk, particularly of fetomaternal haemorrhage which may aggravate the maternal sensitization to the Rh or other blood group. It is therefore only carried out with ultrasound control and where the previous history of severely affected infants or the demonstration of rising antiglobulin titre in maternal serum indicates that the fetus is at risk. Dependent upon the amniotic findings and the maturity of the fetus either premature induction of labour or intrauterine transfusion may be indicated (Chapter 18).

Sexing. Amniotic fluid cells can be examined for sex chromatin after suitable staining. This is of value in families with a history of a disorder such as certain types of muscular dystrophy or of haemophilia which are inherited as sex-linked recessive conditions and males only are affected. If at an early stage of pregnancy it can be shown that the fetus is a male and therefore at risk the mother can be offered termination of pregnancy.

Chromosomes. Tissue culture of fetal cells found in amniotic fluid can be used to define the chromosome karyotype of the fetus. Where this is significantly abnormal as in the trisomies (Chapter 11) such as Down's syndrome therapeutic termination of pregnancy can be offered to the parents if appropriate. As such abnormalities are found more commonly in older mothers it is the practice in many centres to offer amniocentesis at an early stage of pregnancy to mothers over 40 years of age. Some would advocate its use routinely in mothers over 35 years of age.

Alphafetoprotein. Alphafetoprotein is raised in the amniotic fluid of pregnancies in which the fetus has anencephaly or an open spina bifida. As this rise can be recognized by the 13th week of gestation it is now possible to offer therapeutic termination to mothers with raised amniotic fluid alphafetoprotein. A further development of this test on maternal serum makes possible the screening of all mothers before the 16th week. In those with a positive or doubtful serum test amniocentesis and or ultrasound examination is carried out.

Lecithin:sphingomyelin ratio. Reference will be made in later chapters to the significance of phospholipid substances in the alveoli of the lungs which act as surface tension reducing agents. The principal substances involved are dipalmitoyl lecithin and phosphatidylglycerol. Studies of the lecithin content of amniotic fluid have shown a slow rise in concentration from the 26th to the 33rd week of gestation followed by a marked rise particularly after the 35th week. As the amniotic fluid concentration of another phospholipid, sphingomyelin, remains fairly static throughout pregnancy, the lecithin:sphingomyelin ratio is used as an index of fetal pulmonary maturity. When the ratio is less than 1.5 there is a high risk of pulmonary complications but little or no risk if the ratio exceeds 2. Measurement of amniotic fluid phosphatidylglycerol has been shown to be a more accurate predictor of fetal lung maturity.

Enzyme deficiencies. Examination of the enzyme activity of fetal cells cultured after amniocentesis can also be used to diagnose or to exclude the diagnosis of certain inherited disorders which are caused by deficiencies of particular enzymes. These include metabolic disorders such as the mucopolysaccharidoses, the cerebral lipidoses, glycogen storage disorders and some disorders of amino acid metabolism.

Risks involved. Amniocentesis following ultrasonography carries a 1% increase in the risk of aborting a pregnancy and this should be made clear to parents who wish to have this procedure carried out. The risk of those parents having an abnormal fetus must therefore exceed the risk of the procedure to justify amniocentesis being recommended. If ultrasound examination to locate the placenta and to establish the position of the fetus is not available the risk of puncturing the placenta and causing bleeding or of injuring the fetus directly are increased. Ultrasound appears to have no associated risk.

Indications for amniocentesis. As facilities for carrying out prenatal diagnosis will vary from one country to another and in different areas within a country the indications for requesting prenatal diagnosis will have to be governed to some extent by knowledge of the local situation. In general the present indications for amniocentesis should include a previous pregnancy resulting in an infant with Down's syndrome or a neural tube defect, a family history of detectable metabolic disorder or chromosomal abnormality and if the mother is a carrier of an X-linked disorder, a raised serum alphafetoprotein level, maternal age of over 38 years and evidence of rhesus blood group sensitization.

Fetal blood sampling. By inserting a fetoscope into the amniotic cavity through an incision in the mother's abdominal wall at the umbilicus, parts of the fetus can be inspected. This technique allows those with the appropriate experience to obtain fetal blood from the large vessels in the umbilical cord where it enters the placenta. Examination of fetal blood allows prenatal diagnosis of such conditions as thalassaemia major, haemophilia A and other major haematological problems. It also allows fetal blood to be obtained for blood grouping, sexing, chromosome karyotype analysis, assessment of enzyme activity and other biochemical measurements. Sampling of fetal umbilical venous blood by direct transplacental puncture with ultrasound guidance is a promising and potentially less hazardous new technique.

Chorionic villous biopsy

Recently developed techniques of chorionic villous sampling can provide samples of fetal chorion from about the eighth week of gestation. These samples can be used for chromosomal analysis, for estimation of enzymatic activity in some inherited metabolic disorders and for the identification of other inherited defects such as the thalassaemias using the techniques of DNA gene analysis. It is evident that earlier diagnosis is important but the relative risks of amniocentesis, fetal blood sampling and chorionic villous biopsy must be assessed.

Fetal monitoring

In the third trimester and particularly as pregnancy nears term the fetus becomes increasingly at risk from hypoxia and its complications. The risk is at its greatest during labour when continuous assessment is the only means by which the earliest signs of distress can be recognized reliably. Assessment at this stage is primarily aimed at ensuring that the fetus continues to be satisfactorily oxygenated and there are no factors which could interfere with the initiation of spontaneous respiration after birth. Fetal hypoxia results in alteration of several fetal functions and it is by monitoring these functions that an assessment of fetal health or fetal distress can be made.

Fetal heart rate. Auscultation of the fetal heart by listening over the mother's abdomen is the time-honoured method of measuring fetal health particularly during labour. Fetal bradycardia, particularly with a rate falling below 100 per minute is the principal method of diagnosing fetal distress in most parts of the world.

Cardiotocograph. In countries where electronic equipment and a dependable electricity supply is available this type of intermittent examination has largely been taken over by continuous monitoring of the fetal heart and simultaneous recording of uterine contractions (Fig. 4.11). Where the fetal heart does not recover to its base line within 30 seconds of the end of the contraction fetal distress is present.

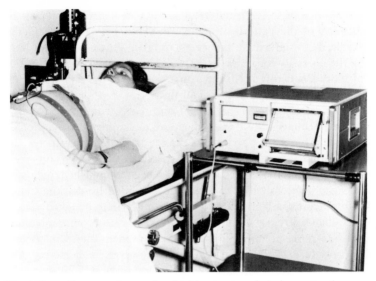

Fig. 4.11 Cardiotocograph recording fetal heart rate and uterine contractions.

Fetal electrocardiogram. When labour is sufficiently advanced a fetal electrocardiogram can be obtained with an electrode fixed to the presenting part of the fetus. Ultrasonic detectors employing the Doppler effect have also been used to record fetal heart rates.

Meconium staining. The other classical clinical sign of fetal distress is meconium staining of amniotic fluid in a vertex presentation. This sign can be used after rupture of the forewaters. Before the membranes rupture spontaneously or have been ruptured artificially meconium staining can be recognized by direct inspection with the amnioscope. In some centres, particularly on the continent of Europe, amnioscopy is carried out routinely in mothers who are ten days past their expected date of delivery.

Fetal blood $[H^+]$ (*pH*). Where there is a persistent bradycardia or tachycardia measurement of fetal blood hydrogen ion concentration, $[H^+]$ (pH) is indicated. Samples of capillary blood are taken after a small incision has been made in the fetal scalp. The fetal $[H^+]$ remains constant until just before delivery when there is a rise to between 45 and 55 nmol/l (fall of pH to between 7.35 and 7.25). A rise to 65 nmol/l or more (fall of pH to below 7.2) at this or an earlier stage of delivery indicates fetal acidosis due to accumulation of lactic acid. This occurs when the supply of oxygen to the fetus is inadequate and fetal $[H^+]$ (pH) can therefore be used as an indicator of hypoxia provided that there is no cause for maternal acidosis. Repeated fetal scalp blood sampling gives an indication of the pattern of change in [H⁺] (pH) and aids in the decision as to immediate management. It is claimed that not only may the necessity for immediate Caesarian section become clear but that more frequently it is shown that slowing of the fetal heart rate is not an indication of severe fetal distress.

Advantages of fetal monitoring. Controversy continues over the relative advantages and disadvantages of electronic fetal monitoring during late pregnancy and labour. Some mothers are disturbed by the equipment involved and the restriction imposed on their mobility although this restriction has been diminished by using telemetric devices. Other mothers are reassured by the knowledge that problems can be detected in time for action to be taken. There are conflicting reports from obstetricians of the benefits obtained from electronic monitoring and as to how many mothers require this procedure. The present tendency, however, is to increase the use of fetal monitoring and the benefits appear to outweigh the disadvantages.

Fetal respiration. The main objective of fetal monitoring is to prevent hypoxia which might interfere with cerebral function and the initiation of respiration after birth. Respiratory movement does, however, occur in the fetus before birth. This will be discussed further in Chapter 5.

Disorders affecting fetal growth

Hereditary factors may produce abnormalities of the fetus and newborn infant and these are considered in Chapter 11 under the heading of 'Congenital abnormalities'. Consideration is also given in Chapter 11 to those acquired factors such as infection and drugs transmitted across the placenta which if occurring at the time of organogenesis may produce physical abnormality with or without later fetal growth retardation. Disorders of fetal growth can occur which interfere with the normal development of the fetus without producing abnormality of individual organs. These disorders will be considered here as their recognition and management may contribute to the birth of a healthy newborn infant.

Maternal factors

British Births 1970 has provided information about many of the antenatal factors which are likely to result in impaired fetal growth. As shown in Figures 4.12 and 4.13 birth order and whether or not

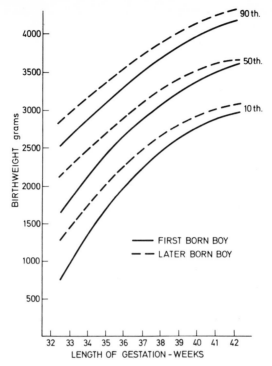

Fig. 4.12 The effect of primiparity on birth weight at all gestational ages (*British Births 1970*).

mother smoked during pregnancy have an effect on fetal growth resulting in lower birth weight.

Socioeconomic factors. Many of these factors can be included under the general heading of socioeconomic and it is important to realize that improvement in the standard of living and of the health education of a community is of prime importance in maintaining fetal health and reducing perinatal mortality. This is a function of national and local government and is slow in producing an effect.

High-risk pregnancies. Of more immediate significance is the recognition of high-risk pregnancies in which the fetus is in greatest danger (Chapter 3). Such recognition requires an alertness to at-risk situations by doctors and midwives and a realization by pregnant women of the need for regular antenatal care. In high-risk pregnancies the importance of attendance at a fully staffed and equipped centre is such that the patient must be persuaded of this and given every help to encourage her to attend.

The management of the fetus at risk is primarily in the hands

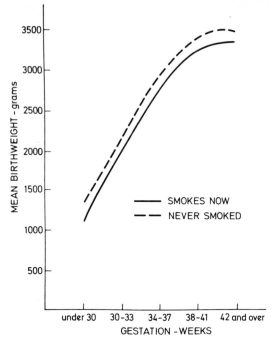

Fig. 4.13 The effect of smoking on birth weight at all gestational ages (*British Births 1970*).

of the obstetrician concerned but it is important that a close relationship be established between obstetric and paediatric teams so that each may be aware of the other's problems and the relative value of different possible means of management both antenatally and postnatally. Discussion about individual cases before and after delivery will help to evolve a common policy of action which should be kept under frequent review bearing in mind paediatric reports on the long-term follow-up of infants who have shown evidence of fetal growth disturbance or fetal distress. This subject is considered further in Chapter 21.

FURTHER READING

Clinics in Perinatology (1979) *Fetal Disease*, vol. 6. no. 2. Philadelphia: Saunders.
Davis, J. A. & Dobbing J. (eds) (1981) *Scientific Foundations of Paediatrics*. London: Heinemann.
Wald, N. J. (ed) (1984) *Antenatal and Neonatal Screening*. Oxford: Oxford University Press.
Widdowson, E. M. (1980) *Studies in Perinatal Physiology*. London: Pitman.

5

The newborn

ADAPTATION TO THE EXTERNAL ENVIRONMENT

The idyllic state of the fetus in utero with its complete dependence on the mother contrasts strongly with the degree of independence required of the newborn infant. Between these two stages of life the fetus is subject to a degree of physical trauma and deprivation which would cause us grave concern were it to occur under other circumstances. That the great majority of us have survived this shattering experience without harm is the best evidence available of the ability of the fetus to adapt successfully to the external environment.

Such adaptation is not without its problems and the ease with which the fetus achieves its conversion to an independent existence depends to a considerable extent on the intrauterine development of the fetus and the course of labour. The systems principally involved at birth are the respiratory, the cardiovascular and the nervous systems. Later, digestive, renal and hepatic, skin and musculoskeletal function become of more importance.

A study of adaptation to the external environment should begin with a consideration of fetal function in utero. Some aspects of this have already been mentioned in Chapter 4. Further attention will be paid here to those aspects of fetal development which are related to the establishment of respiration after birth.

Respiration

Fetal respiration

Study of the respiratory pattern of the human fetus in utero using ultrasound has revealed that fetal breathing movements occur and can be affected by extrinsic factors such as maternal smoking. Animal studies show that the normal pattern is related to the sleep state of the fetus as judged by fetal electroencephalography. The fetal lung is constantly producing a fluid which differs from amniotic fluid. Although some pulmonary fluid is expelled into the amniotic sac by fetal movement, most is swallowed by the normal fetus and amniotic fluid only enters the fetal lung under situations of stress when deep respiratory movements may be provoked because of severe fetal hypoxia. It has to be noted that there is a wide range of fetal blood-gas values in which such deeper respiratory movements are not triggered.

Fetal blood-gas exchange takes place in the placenta and is dependent on a good blood flow on both the maternal and fetal sides of the placenta. Even with satisfactory blood flows and normal maternal health, fetal blood oxygen concentrations are well below those in maternal blood. This is partly due to the large requirement of the placenta for oxygen and partly to the relative imbalance of fetal and maternal blood flow in differing parts of the placenta resulting in an uneven blood-gas exchange. There is, however, a sufficient safety margin achieved by variations in blood flow through the placenta without change in heart rate to compensate for small rapid changes in blood-gas values.

Fetal distress. Larger changes in fetal blood gases may be reflected in fetal tachycardia which is the first true sign of fetal distress and which may be sufficient to compensate for a temporary period of difficulty such as may occur during a uterine contraction. More prolonged or more severe difficulty with progressive hypoxaemia of the fetus is commonly manifest as bradycardia and results in acidaemia. This sign of fetal distress is an indication that the adaptive processes in the fetus have been stretched to their limit. Since the introduction of continuous recording of fetal heart rate and its relation to uterine contraction and the use of fetal scalp blood samples for measurement of $[H^+]$ (pH) more has been learned about the significance of change in fetal heart rate and its relation to intrauterine hypoxia. Techniques measuring beat to beat variation in fetal heart rate give a more sensitive indication of fetal difficulty.

Oxygen conservation. The cardiovascular system of the fetus is clearly closely involved in the regulation of fetal blood gases. Further adaptation to hypoxia may be achieved by selectively shutting down the circulation in parts of the body which are less important to fetal survival. Thus by vasoconstriction of the vessels supplying the skin, limbs, lungs and abdominal organs, blood flow and therefore oxygen uptake in these areas is reduced. This allows more of the oxygen present to be made available to the heart and brain. Some of the lactic acid produced in the underperfused areas, where anaerobic glycolysis is taking place, returns to the central circulation and produces a metabolic acidosis even in the absence of markedly lowered oxygen levels in scalp vein blood. This oxygen conserving adaptation mechanism is of significance in relation to the establishment of regular respiration after birth and will be discussed later.

Initiation of respiration

The first breath. Normal, mature vaginally delivered infants make their first respiratory movement within a few seconds of complete delivery. The time interval between the appearance of the nose and the first breath is usually between 20–30 seconds. Within 90 seconds of complete delivery the majority have commenced rhythmic respirations.

The strong initial inspiratory efforts and the subsequent rhythmic activities of the respiratory muscles are largely, if not entirely, dependent upon brain stem respiratory centres. In spite of a very large effort by many physiologists there is as yet no agreement as to the factors which initiate and maintain respiration. Table 5.1 summarizes the factors which can, under a variety of circumstances, initiate or influence the patterns of neonatal respirations, but none of these individual factors is absolutely essential. For example, some infants commence breathing normally when their blood-gas status is normal, whilst others do not make any respiratory movement until they have become moderately asphyxiated. There are a number of factors which influence the ability of the respiratory centres to respond to each or any of these stimuli: for example, maternal anaesthetic and analgesic drugs, low environmental temperature, high environmental temperature, gestational age, ante- and intrapartum asphyxia, intracranial or brain stem haemorrhage, vascular thrombosis and cerebral oedema with increased intracranial pressure.

Once breathing is established the pattern of respiration is primarily determined in the medulla. Pulmonary ventilation is regulated by the chemical state of the arterial blood, particularly by the Pco_2 and $[H^+]$ perfusing chemoreceptors in the medulla. Breathing may also be stimulated by decrease in Po_2 acting on the chemoreceptors in the carotid bodies. This hypoxic drive may assume great importance if the medullary centres are insensitive.

Table 5.1 Stimuli which may contribute to the initiation and maintenance of respiration in the newborn assuming intact nerve pathways between receptors and functional respiratory centres and from these centres through the spinal cord and lower motor neurones to the respiratory muscles.

Thermal	Loss of heat at about 600 cal per minute; cold stimulus
Pain	Skin, muscle and tendon receptors
Pressure	Gravity — decreased pressure from that in utero
	Increased intrathoracic pressures during delivery
	Increased intracranial pressures during delivery
	Changes in intratracheal and intrathoracic pressure
Tactile	? Trigeminal area particularly important
Receptors in lungs and pleura	Hering-Breuer reflexes
	Head's reflex
Receptors in muscle, tendon and joints of limbs, spine and chest wall	Stimulated by alterations in posture during and after delivery
Auditory	
Visual	
Olfactory	
Cord clamping:	
Increased arterial pressure	Carotid baroreceptors
	Stretch receptors aorta and carotid
Decreased Pao_2	Aortic and carotid body chemoreceptors
Increased $Paco_2$	Direct effect on respiratory centre
Increased $[H^+]$	

Lungs and heart

Pulmonary fluid. During the passage down the birth canal some of the fluid contained in the fetal lungs is expelled by pressure on the chest. Following onset of respiration the remainder of the fluid is absorbed by the lymphatic system of the lungs.

Chest expansion. The muscular movement of the first breath increases the capacity of the chest and allows air to flow into the pulmonary alveoli as they begin to fill with air.

Pulmonary bloodflow. Changes take place in the blood vessels in response to an increase in the oxygen content of the blood perfusing them. Pulmonary arterioles dilate with reduction in pulmonary vascular resistance and increase in pulmonary blood flow. These changes do not take place instantaneously but the healthy newborn will expand his pulmonary circulation to a degree which allows an adequate exchange of oxygen and carbon dioxide within a few minutes of birth. The ductus arteriosus constricts in response to increasing oxygen concentrations as do the umbilical arteries. These effects are mediated by prostaglandins in the arterial walls. Further adaptation continues over the next few days and includes closure of the foramen ovale. The infant's blood volume will be augmented by transfusion of up to 90 ml of blood from the fetal side of the placenta unless this is prevented by early clamping of the cord or holding the infant above the level of the placenta before the cord is clamped. With cessation of the placental circulation the infant's systemic blood pressure rises.

Surfactant. The muscular movement required to take the first few breaths is very much in excess of that required for later regular respiration. Newborn infants are capable of producing negative intrathoracic pressure of the order of 40 to 70 cm of water but most infants achieve primary expansion of their lungs with negative pressures of the order of 15 to 25 cm of water. The surface tension produced by the film of fluid lining the alveoli would naturally cause the alveoli to collapse completely when air is allowed to escape in expiration were it not for the presence of surfactant, a substance which reduces surface tension. Surfactant is a phospholipid produced in the fetal lung as part of the pulmonary fluid (Chapter 9). Because of its presence alveoli do not collapse completely once expanded and the lung maintains a residual capacity of the order of 15 to 30 ml per kg of body weight. After the high negative pressures required to initiate respiration, lower pressures of about 4 cm of water are sufficient to maintain respiration.

Respiratory centre. In the healthy newborn infant at delivery the sensory stimuli and blood-gas alterations are sufficient to arouse in the brain motor impulses which produce the initial muscle movements in the diaphragm and intercostal muscles required to create the intermittent negative intrathoracic pressures which allow air to enter and leave the alveoli. The centre of this reaction is the brain stem and medulla and any factor which depresses central nervous function will interfere with the onset of respiration. Although a falling oxygen tension and a rise in carbon dioxide tension at first stimulate the respiratory centre, persistence of these trends leads to depression of function. An infant who has been chronically hypoxic during labour may be delivered with a respiratory centre which is already non-responsive, and further falls in oxygen have no stimulating effect. Similarly, if the infant's nervous system has been depressed by sedative drugs given to the mother or by injury during delivery, it will fail to react to the stimuli reaching it after birth.

The airway. Other difficulties in establishing normal respiration may occur if the infant's airway is not clear of fluid when the first breath is taken. Aspiration of amniotic fluid, mucus, blood or meconium may occur and these may prevent air reaching some or even all of the alveoli. Abnormality of the motor nerves, the muscles of respiration and the thoracic cage may also cause problems. Several of these factors may be combined, particularly in low birth weight babies in whom there may be the added problem of deficiency of surfactant.

Anaerobic metabolism. The newborn infant fortunately has the ability to withstand postnatal hypoxia for longer periods than would be tolerated by an older infant or child. This period is reduced in those infants who have been hypoxic before delivery. Anaerobic metabolism releases lactic acid, and infants who have to rely on anaerobic metabolism will develop a metabolic acidosis. When glucose is normally metabolized in aerobic metabolism a large quantity of energy is released, together with water and carbon dioxide. In anaerobic glycolysis, glucose is only partially metabolized to lactic acid and releases only a very small fraction of its potential energy. The brain is the organ which is most likely to suffer damage during periods of hypoxia. In order to preserve an infant's future chance of normal development adequate tissue oxygenation and perfusion must be established before brain damage occurs. Knowledge of the condition of the fetus prior to delivery is essential to those who are to care for the infant at birth.

Resuscitation

Preparation. Whereas the majority of infants achieve respiration spontaneously after birth, midwives and doctors who attend deliveries must be trained and equipped to resuscitate the infant who does not start to breathe or who after a few gasps stops breathing. It is convenient to have a resuscitation trolley, which should be kept in an easily accessible place which is well heated, free from draughts and well lit. In many labour wards a special bay with an overhead radiant heat source is set aside for this purpose. At any delivery one person must accept responsibility for assessing and resuscitating the infant with or without the help of others. Who the person is matters less than that he or she should be experienced, know what they are going to do, how to do it and the risks involved. They should be present before delivery, aware of the progress of labour and the state of the fetus. The equipment available including means for keeping the infant warm should be checked.

Clearing the airway. It is essential to record the time lapse from delivery of the infant to onset of spontaneous respiration. For this purpose it is useful to have a large clock indicating seconds and minutes. The face and nose are wiped clean as soon as the head is delivered, and when the trunk has been delivered the infant is received on to a warm towel and the head is kept lower than the body and turned to one side to allow the pharyngeal fluids to escape. This can be helped by gentle aspiration of the pharynx. Overzealous suction or excessive movement of the tubing in the infant's mouth may cause local injury to mucous membrane and create new problems including inhibition of respiration rather than aiding resuscitation. If suction is provided mechanically the negative pressure should not exceed 100 mmHg ($\equiv$ 136 cm H_2O). The stimulus of aspiration together with the stimulus provided by changes in temperature and blood gases are generally sufficient to initiate respiration.

Oxygen. If the initial movements are poor and if the heart rate is slowing, oxygen or oxygen enriched air should be given to the infant through a suitably sized face-mask or through a catheter passed into a nostril.

Apgar score

These simple resuscitative procedures should have been completed within 1 minute of birth and the opportunity should then be taken to assess the infant's state more completely. The assessment score originally introduced by Apgar has proved its value and is commonly employed (Table 5.2). By adding the scores of 0, 1 or 2 for each individual assessment a total score ranging from 0 to 10 is made. This score together with the time from birth at which it was made should be recorded for comparison with subsequent scored assessments should these become necessary. Either one or two minutes after delivery is suitable for the initial assessment.

Repeat assessment. Infants with Apgar scores in excess of 7 at 1 minute are breathing satisfactorily and no assistance is required. Where the score is in the range of 4 to 7 further action is dictated

Table 5.2 Apgar score sheet

Name .... Date				Time from birth minutes		
	0	1	2	1	5	
HEART RATE	Absent	Below 100	Above 100			
RESPIRATORY EFFORT	Absent	Slow. Irregular	Good crying			
MUSCLE TONE	Limp	Some flexion of extremities	Active. Good tone			
RESPONSE TO CATHETER	No response	Grimace	Cough or sneeze			
COLOUR	Blue. Pale	Body pink. Extremities Blue	Completely pink.			
			Total			

by the infant's general condition and particularly his heart rate. If the rate is over 100 per min and not falling the simple measures discussed above should be repeated. The Apgar score should be repeated and if the score is falling the procedures described in the next paragraph should be instituted. Many infants with Apgar scores of 4 to 7 at 1 minute will show improvement over the next 3 or 4 minutes, and if the score is 7 or more by 5 minutes no further action is required.

Artificial ventilation

An infant with an initial Apgar score of less than 4 or a score that is falling towards this number is very unlikely to improve without further resuscitative measures. Laryngoscopy should be carried out immediately and the posterior pharynx aspirated. If this does not produce an immediate response with onset of normal respiration an endotracheal tube should be passed and intermittent positive pressure ventilation (IPPV) using oxygen at a pressure limited to 30 cm water applied. This procedure is described in greater detail in Chapter 20. When the heart rate is above 100 per minute, the infant pink, and spontaneous respiration established, the endotracheal tube can be withdrawn.

External cardiac massage. If the heart stops beating or if the rate is falling below 40 per minute external cardiac massage must be applied in addition to artificial respiration. Grasp the infant with both hands placed so that the finger tips are over the thoracic spines and both thumbs over the manubrium just below the sternal angle. Give four to five firm presses with both thumbs at about one press/second followed by an inflation of the lungs. Repeat until the heart rate is recovered.

Alkali. Respiratory acidosis is corrected by adequate ventilation. If there is evidence of metabolic acidosis antenatally from scalp vein sampling and if the infant does not achieve spontaneous respiration within one or two minutes of IPPV, 5 ml of 8.4% sodium bicarbonate solution diluted in 5 ml 10% dextrose solution can be given slowly through a needle inserted in the umbilical vein. Failure to establish respiration following this indicates severe cerebral depression or a major cardiorespiratory disorder. If the infant can be maintained in a satisfactory state of IPPV this must be continued using a suitable ventilator. Insertion of an umbilical arterial catheter will allow arterial blood-gas sampling to monitor progress and to administer additional therapy if necessary (Chapter 19). Other investigations such as X-ray of chest may be required to exclude the possibility of diaphragmatic hernia and/or pneumothorax and to assess pulmonary aeration and cardiac size (Chapter 11).

Heat loss

After birth the normal infant if placed on his mother's abdomen will derive heat from her.

The risk of an infant losing heat in any involved resuscitative procedure is high and a very careful watch should be kept on skin and rectal or oesophageal temperature. Keeping the room temperature at or above 25 °C helps but it is not sufficient to prevent hypothermia. The infant should be dried and wrapped in a warm towel paying particular attention to covering the large surface area of the head. Wrapping baby's trunk in foil may further reduce heat loss. Extra local heat is generally required and can be given by an overhead infrared heater, an electrically heated pad or warm water-bottles depending on the available facilities. Care must be taken to prevent skin burns. It takes surprisingly little local heat to damage the skin of the asphyxiated infant. The fact that there is often severe peripheral vasoconstriction means that local heat application whether radiant or direct is not disseminated by the normal vascular mechanisms. Heat loss may occur during the transfer from labour ward to a nursery. The infant should be well wrapped or transferred in a heated, portable incubator.

Domiciliary delivery

Ideally mothers booked for domiciliary delivery should include only those in whom there is confident expectation of normal delivery without need for resuscitation. Abnormalities occurring during pregnancy or the first stage of labour are in general an indication for arranging hospital delivery rather than for planning major resuscitative procedures in the home. Midwives and doctors attending domiciliary deliveries must be equipped and trained to deal with unexpected problems of resuscitation. This can and should include the ability to pass an endotracheal tube, and those concerned with domiciliary midwifery must maintain their expertise in this technique. Intermittent positive pressure ventilation (IPPV) can be supplied from a hand pump or by blowing with the cheeks rather than the lungs. If an endotracheal tube has not been passed, IPPV can be given using a suitable round infant face mask and bag such as the Laerdal (Fig. 5.1).

Emergency situations. Situations can and do arise when delivery occurs in places in which there are no facilities for resuscitation. Bearing in mind the general principles of the methods already discussed all but the most severely hypoxic infants can be resuscitated. Drainage of fluids from the mouth is encouraged by placing the infant in a 30° head down position and holding open the lower angle of the mouth with a finger. If spontaneous respiration does not occur, mouth to nose respiration should be started (Chapter 20).

Drugs. The use of respiratory and cardiac stimulants is unnecessary and potentially fatal and is no longer accepted as part of normal resuscitation procedure. Where mothers have been given pethidine or morphine within 6 hours before delivery the respiratory depressant action of these drugs can be counteracted by the use of naloxone (Narcan Neonatal). The dose, 0.01 mg/kg, can be given into the umbilical vein, which is then 'milked' towards the infant or can be given by intramuscular injection and repeated after 15–30 minutes if no response is observed.

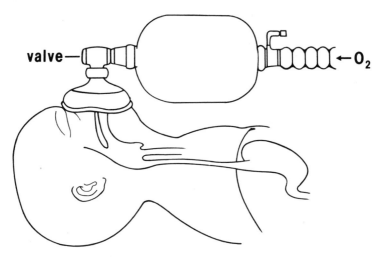

valve

← O$_2$

Fig. 5.1 Bag and mask ventilation.

Some infants begin to breathe but shortly afterwards become apnoeic. Many such infants have metabolic acidosis and respiration is re-established when the biochemical abnormality is corrected.

Prognosis

The prognosis of infants who require resuscitation at birth depends primarily on the underlying condition which has caused delay in onset of respiration. If this should be brain injury or chronic prenatal hypoxia the prognosis is not as satisfactory as in those infants where there has been short-term hypoxia or depression of a normal brain by drugs. It is therefore dangerous to generalize about prognosis but from what has been said it follows that a short episode of perinatal hypoxia is seldom a cause of neurological damage whereas neurological damage may well be a cause of delayed onset of respiration. This subject is discussed more fully in Chapter 12.

Temperature Control

Reference has already been made on many occasions to the liability of the newborn infant to lose heat. This applies particularly to those parts of the world where the air temperature is normally below 30 °C. In climates where the temperature rises above 30 °C much higher temperatures may occur indoors; under such circumstances newborn infants may become overheated and their body temperature rises. Recognition of the difficulty which infants have in maintaining a stable temperature is essential to understanding the management of the newborn and particularly of the preterm infant.

Heat loss

Heat is lost from the skin by radiation, convection, evaporation and conduction. Evaporation of fluid from the skin is most marked where there is movement of air across the wet infant. Exposure of the infant increases all these channels of heat loss. The greater proportional surface area of the small infant and the relative absence of the insulating layer of fat in the preterm infant all contribute to heat loss. As skin temperature falls a gradient is established and heat will then be lost from the deeper tissues and the infant's central or core temperature will fall. The infant is capable of producing extra heat in response to an initial small fall in temperature but the capacity for heat production is quickly overtaken by the even greater liability to heat loss. A marked fall in core temperature is associated with a fall in metabolic activity, reduction of heat production and a further fall in body temperature. Thus a vicious circle is set up. Eventually a point of no return is reached and the infant will die.

Heat production

The infant produces heat by metabolic activity in the muscles and elsewhere. The newborn, however, is not able to shiver and increase heat production by this method when chilling occurs. Lying close to his mother allows a baby to obtain heat from her, helps to maintain body temperature and reduces the need for heat production.

Brown fat. An alternative source of heat is available in the form of catabolism of brown fat which has a high mitochondrial content and is capable of rapid conversion to energy. Brown fat is present in the newborn between the shoulder blades, behind the sternum, in the neck and around the kidneys and suprarenal glands. The chief function of these collections of fat is to supply local heat and a source of fuel which the infant can utilize quickly when extra heat is required. Release of heat from brown fat in response to cooling is mediated through the sympathetic nervous system and noradrenaline.

Use of energy. It is important to remember that continuing heat production is dependent on a regular source of energy. This is normally the diet. If any infant's temperature falls an increasing proportion of the energy contained in the diet will have to be used for heat production and the infant will not have sufficient energy left for normal growth. Failure to gain weight may therefore be due to heat loss followed by the need for increased heat production.

Environment and body temperature. Because of the ease with which newborn infants and particularly a low birth-weight newborn infant will lose heat if exposed to an environment at a lower temperature than its body temperature it is important to recognize situations in which heat loss is occurring. This can most readily be measured by comparing the skin or surface temperature of the infant with its deep or core body temperature. Skin temperature may be measured by a standard mercury thermometer or more conveniently by a thermocouple with continuous recording of the temperature on a dial which may either record the movement of a pointer over the scale or may print out the temperature in numerals.

An accurate assessment of deep body or core temperature is more difficult to achieve but it is generally acceptable to use a high rectal temperature or an oesophageal temperature to indicate core temperature. Comparison of the skin and core temperature will indicate whether the infant is losing or gaining heat. The object is to maintain a core temperature of 37 °C and not to allow the skin temperature to divert from this by more than 0.5 °C. If the skin temperature falls below 36.5 °C heat loss will begin to occur and the further the skin temperature falls below the rectal temperature the greater will be the call on the energy supplies of the infant to supply heat to maintain the core temperature. This is demonstrated in Figure 5.2.

The core temperature can be maintained over a range called the thermoregulatory range. This lies between points C and B which are measurements of environmental temperature and will differ for each infant depending upon his ability to provide extra energy. Point C is the temperature below which the infant is unable to provide sufficient energy to maintain his core temperature; should the skin temperature fall below this the core temperature will also fall.

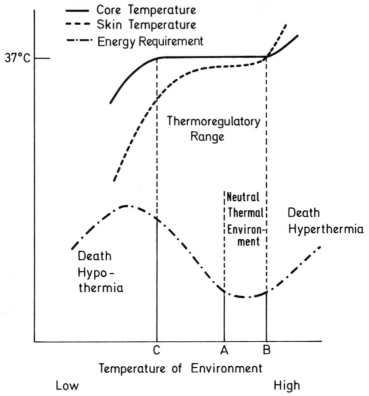

Fig. 5.2 The effect of environmental temperature on energy requirement and body temperatures.

Neutral thermal environment

Points A and B represent the range of environmental temperature over which the infant has to use the minimum amount of energy to maintain his core temperature. This is called the neutral thermal environment. It will be noted that point B is the upper end of the neutral thermal environment and also the upper end of the thermoregulatory range. Environment temperatures above this point lead to a rise in skin and core temperature which would eventually result in death of the infant from hyperpyrexia. The actual temperatures corresponding to points A and B for any infant depend on a variety of factors including the amount of clothing, the degree of air movement over the baby, moisture on the baby's surface, the conductivity of the materials on which baby is being nursed, the presence or absence of heat reflectors and the temperature of the air to which baby is being exposed. No absolute levels for neutral thermal environment can therefore be given which will cover every situation.

Incubators

The principal object of nursing a baby in an incubator is to allow close observation and ready access to the infant in an environment which can be controlled to correspond to the neutral thermal environment. For the very smallest infants this may require environmental temperatures of 36 °C or more and care has to be taken to ensure that this temperature is maintained. If the incubator is in a room at a temperature of 25 °C considerable fluctuations in temperature within the incubator will take place when the incubator is opened for nursing or other procedures. Clothing the infant, keeping him close to his mother or covering him with a heat reflecting shield will lower the neutral thermal environment but may reduce access and prevent full observation. In each individual situation a suitable compromise has to be reached. The nursing aspects of this important subject are considered further in Chapters 6, 9 and 10.

Digestion

The newborn infant cannot thrive unless supplied with energy, essential amino acids, vitamins and certain trace elements. Whereas these were all supplied transplacentally in utero the newborn has to root, fix, suckle, swallow and digest his mother's milk before absorption and utilization can proceed. There is considerable evidence that many of the components of human breast milk are more readily absorbed than the equivalent components of other milks.

Maturation of enzymes. The enzyme systems required for this digestion have not been required in utero and are not all fully prepared in the baby at birth. The term infant can digest and absorb 90% of the fat in human milk even although there are very low production rates for pancreatic lipase and amylase and for bile salts. It is now known that there are alternative sources of effective lipase and amylase capable of digesting fats and starches.

Lingual lipase is synthesized and secreted by the serous glands of the tongue from before 25 weeks gestation and acts in the acidic environment of the stomach. Infants fed intragastrically rather than intrajejunally are better able to digest and absorb fat probably as a result of lingual lipase activities. In the newborn, including the preterm newborn, gastric digestion by this means has been estimated to contribute 60 to 70% of the hydrolysis of ingested fats. There are also at least three enzymes in human milk: a lipoprotein lipase, a bile-salt-stimulated esterase, and a nonactivated lipase. These lipases ensure that human milk fat is well tolerated and digested, unlike most fats supplied in artificial formulae. Heat treatment of human milk can diminish human milk lipase activity. Milk fat globules are resistant to the action of pancreatic lipase and of milk bile salt stimulated lipase, but are readily hydrolysed by lingual lipase, which penetrates into the core of the fat particles and hydrolyses triglyceride. Human milk bile-salt-stimulated lipase (BSSL) is present in 'preterm' human milk whereas lipoprotein lipase appears after delivery. The combined action of intragastric lipolysis by lingual and gastric lipases and intestinal hydrolysis of fat by the bile-salt-stimulated lipase of human milk can effectively substitute for low pancreatic lipase activity and low concentrations of bile salts.

Starches and glucose polymers are hydrolysed by salivary amylase, small intestinal brush-border glucoamylase and mammary amylase. Salivary amylase is active in the gastric fluid of preterm infants. Human breast milk contains amylase which has also been shown to be stable in the gastric and duodenal content of the newborn infant. The physiological role of these amylases is at present uncertain, but it is known that feeding glucose polymers to preterm infants can prove an effective way of increasing energy intakes.

There are no protein digestive enzymes in human milk and upper gastrointestinal tract. It is interesting to speculate that in the immediate newborn period this may be necessary to allow the passage to the jejunum and ileum of undamaged immunoglobulins and growth promoting factors.

Control of diet. Human breast milk is least likely to produce disturbances such as diarrhoea and perianal excoriation which occur more commonly with cow's milk preparations. The modifications of cow's milk discussed in Chapter 8 have reduced digestive disturbances considerably.

Elimination

The elimination of waste products involves the skin, the bowel, the liver, the kidneys and the lungs. In the absence of hypoxia, hypoglycaemia and hypothermia even the smallest newborn is capable of evacuating normal meconium, stool and urine provided that there is no mechanical obstruction. The role of the skin in thermoregulation and water loss has already been described, as has elimination of CO_2 from the lungs. The physiological changes occurring in the liver and kidney are of vital importance to the infant.

Hepatic function

Apart from its importance as a biochemical factor in which new proteins and other substances necessary for tissue growth are prepared, the liver has a major part to play in the elimination of toxic products of body metabolism. Several products may share the same detoxification process and may therefore compete with one another for priority if the process is overloaded.

Conjugation. Several substances including some drugs can be excreted by the liver only after they have been joined to another substance such as glucuronic acid, a reaction called conjugation. Bilirubin is a typical toxic end product which can be rendered nontoxic by conjugation with glucuronic acid to form bilirubin diglucuronide. Conjugation of bilirubin which is soluble only in fat solvents produces the water-soluble bilirubin diglucuronide which is not harmful to tissues and which can be excreted in the bile. The conjugation is catalysed by the enzyme glucuronyl transferase. For the first few days of life this enzyme may not be present in adequate amounts; the liver is then incapable of dealing with all the bilirubin presented to it and jaundice becomes evident (Chapter 15).

Synthesis. The ability of the liver to produce proteins may be stretched beyond its limits, particularly in the presence of infection or other cause of increased tissue breakdown or protein loss in the newborn period. Should the serum protein level fall sufficiently oedema will occur. The production of some proteins such as prothrombin is dependent upon an adequate dietary supply of precursor, in this case vitamin K. Absence or deficiency of the proteins involved in the coagulation of blood can lead to excessive bleeding. Hypoxia, hypoglycaemia or infection will all reduce liver function and accentuate any or all of the problems mentioned.

Albumin. Substances such as bilirubin have to be attached to albumin to allow their transport in plasma. Albumin binding sites are limited and other substances compete for the available sites. A rise in $[H^+]$ (fall in pH) renders bilirubin less tightly bound to albumin and more liable to pass into tissues such as the brain where it can cause cell death. The ability of the liver to provide albumin is therefore of importance in the prehepatic stage of bilirubin metabolism.

Renal function

The lower rate of glomerular filtration found in the newborn is mainly due to high vascular resistance which reduces renal blood flow. A progressive decrease in intrarenal vascular resistance during the first few weeks of life allows greater blood flow and increased filtration.

Solute load. At birth the renal cortex is relatively underdeveloped and the juxtamedullary nephrons have a higher blood flow than the cortical nephrons. The reduction in glomerular filtration rate prevents overloading of the proximal tubules whose function is immature at birth. As a result of these differing aspects of renal function the newborn's kidney is poorly suited to excrete a saline load but is better able to conserve sodium and water although the capacity to concentrate the urine is limited. Difficulty in excretion of ammonium compounds and titratable acid impairs the capacity to correct metabolic acidosis which occurs readily in the newborn particularly in preterm infants.

Maturation. The capacity of the kidney to mature after birth does not appear to be influenced by preterm delivery and is related to the load presented to it. Ninety-five per cent of healthy infants will pass urine within 24 hours of delivery. Urine output is of the order of 20 to 35 ml per day in the first two or three days of life while fluid intake remains low and rises to 100 to 200 ml per day by the end of the first week.

Lack of reserve. In spite of the limitations of renal function discussed above the kidneys of the newborn are almost always able to maintain a satisfactory state of health and growth. It is under conditions of dietary overload, infection or other stresses that the lack of reserve renal function becomes of major significance.

Erythropoiesis

The high number of red blood cells, 5.5×10^9 per litre (5.5×10^6

per mm³) and the high concentration of haemoglobin (Hb), 17 g per dl (17 g per 100 ml) necesarry for adequate oxygenation of the fetus are not required after birth with the establishment of a more efficient mechanism of breathing using the lungs.

Physiological anaemia. After a temporary rise in the first day or two of life due to shift of plasma water to the extravascular compartment there is a steady fall in both the red cell count and the haemoglobin. This is due to a sharp reduction in erythropiesis during the first nine days of life followed by a slow gradual recovery which is not complete until the third month of life. The associated fall in haemoglobin to 11 g per dl (11 g per 100 ml) is described as physiological anaemia of the newborn. In preterm infants the fall is more marked and the haemoglobin may be only 7 g per dl (7 g per 100 ml) by the eighth or ninth week. Although sharing a common cause this is often called anaemia of prematurity. Such anaemias are not preventable by giving iron supplements from birth but added iron may be used after the first month of life.

White blood cells. The white blood cells also undergo considerable change during the first few days of life and these changes make interpretation of white cell counts difficult at this age. In general neutrophils rise from about 8×10^9 per litre (8000 per mm³) at birth to around 13×10^9 per litre (13 000 per mm³) at 20 hours and then fall to about 4×10^9 per litre (4000 per mm³) by 72 hours and remain at this level. Lymphocytes fall from about 6×10^9 per litre (6000 per mm³) at birth to 3×10^9 per litre (3000 per mm³) at 72 hours and then rise slowly to 6×10^9 per litre (6000 per mm³) by ten days.

FURTHER READING

Cockburn, F. & Drillien, D. M. (1974) *Neonatal Medicine.* Oxford: Blackwell.
Forfar, J. O. (Ed.) (1976) Aspects of neonatal metabolism. In: *Clinics in Endocrinology and Metabolism.* London: Saunders.
Hey, E. (1975) Thermal neutrality. *British Medical Bulletin,* **31**, 69.
Klaus, M. & Fanaroff, A. A. (1979) *The Physical Environment in Care of the High Risk Neonate,* 2nd edn. Philadelphia: Saunders.
Roberton, N. R. C. (Ed.) (1986) *Textbook of Neonatology.* Edinburgh: Churchill Livingstone.

6

Nursing care of the healthy newborn

The newborn baby is responsive to his environment and to the love, care and emotional responses of his parents. Midwives have an important role as they must impart their skills and experience to parents as well as supporting them in the care of their baby. The ward should have a friendly, relaxed atmosphere and procedures should be adapted to the individual needs of each mother and baby. Midwives need to be flexible in their approach. Conflicting advice should be avoided as this is confusing and distressing to parents. Rigid routines should be avoided. The care that the mother and her baby receive makes an important contribution to the parents' emotional attachment and gradual development of the parent-child relationship. Mothers of very small or sick infants feel isolated and anxious and this may affect their whole attitude and relationship with their child in the future. The special problems relating to the nursing of low birth weight infants are discussed in Chapter 10.

The mothering instinct

The mother-baby relationship must be considered before dealing with the physical needs of the newly born infant. The mothering instinct is dominant during the months of pregnancy and immediately following delivery. All thought is centred around the baby's safety and physical requirements. Nearly all mothers have an intuitive knowledge about babies but they may 'mother' their babies in their own individual way. Separation of the mother and child at birth especially in hospital should be avoided as far as possible. The newly delivered mother must be given time to fondle and handle her baby shortly after birth in the delivery room.

The baby should be put to the breast as soon as possible after delivery in such a way that there is skin to skin contact. The first feed is extremely important and helps to initiate lactation but also promotes the vital relationship between mother and baby. The newborn baby is usually alert and responsive in the first hour after birth and will show when it is ready to suckle by 'rooting'. This early success encourages the mother.

The rooming-in system of nursing the mother and baby side by side is practised and assists in the prevention of cross-infection. Mother and baby are not separated and the mother can watch over her baby, pick him up, nurse him and feed him when he demands it. It is, however, essential to ensure that the new mother has sufficient rest during the day and sleep at night.

Nursery staffing

Neonatal nursing demands a very high standard of nursing care. Those involved must have keen powers of observation, alertness and a readiness to make quick decisions. The neonatal nurse must have a high sense of responsibility and a devotion to her task. Not all nurses are suited for this type of work particularly as the attributes already mentioned must be coupled with gentleness and extreme patience. The use of monitors, ventilators and other electronic equipment calls for a type of expertise which was not formerly expected of nurses. It is now well recognized that working in a neonatal intensive care unit can be very stressful to nursing and medical staff. Training in midwifery or in general children's nursing or a combination of these is not sufficient in itself to qualify a nurse for work in special care nurseries or neonatal intensive therapy units, and further special training is required.

In order to achieve a national standard, courses in neonatal nursing must now be approved by the National Boards in Scotland, England and Wales. There are many such courses available throughout the country.

Midwives. Student midwives receive theoretical and practical education in the care of the newborn which is part of the curriculum in the midwifery training course. Midwives are therefore particularly well suited for further training in nursing in special-care baby units. Trained midwives in maternity departments often work in nurseries as part of their further postcertificate education. In order to maintain a continuing high standard of care it is essential that the senior nursing staff in a nursery should be appointed to posts in the nurseries and not be part of a circulating pool of trained staff. In each nursery there should be sufficient trained permanent staff to ensure that at least one senior member is on duty at all times of the day and night.

Nursery nurses. The recommendations of the expert group on special care for babies with regard to staffing ratios have already been considered in Chapter 2. Difficulties may arise in achieving the high nurse:patient ratios advised if reliance is placed on employing only trained midwives to fill these places. The skills of nursery nurses after in-service training are suitable for some of the duties in special care baby units.

Registered nurses, particularly those with a children's nursing certificate, can fill most of the posts in a special care nursery.

Staff-patient ratio

For administrative purposes within the NHS normal babies are not counted as occupying beds whereas babies who are classified as 'sick' do count as occupying beds. An allocation of beds for 'sick babies' is made in each maternity unit and such beds or cots generally form a special care nursery. Because of this difference in administrative attitude staff:patient ratios have to be considered in relation to special care nurseries separately from the care of well babies. In many hospitals the same nursing staff may be looking after both groups of babies and wide differences in staff:patient ratios therefore appear to occur. The report of the expert group on special care for babies comments that nurse staffing ratios should be flexible ranging between 1 and 1.5 nurses per cot in special care nurseries, rising to 4 nurses per cot in intensive care nurseries. The expert group also made recommendations about the ratio of experienced nurses to those still training in special care for babies. It must be borne in mind that the above staffing ratios may have to be adjusted to meet changing conditions of service.

Liaison

The role of the family doctor and health visitor is of prime importance and with the integration of the health services since 1974 some progress has been achieved in removing barriers between hospital and community. The liaison health visitor plays a key role in establishing the link between a hospital and the community. She is often attached to a local group practice and has a wide knowledge of her patients and their home problems. She may visit the mothers and babies herself in the wards and obtain additional information from the nursing and medical staff. Any special problems are discussed and the health visitor imparts this information to her colleagues if this particular patient is outside her own area. The family doctor also gains a great deal from this liaison through the group practice attachment. The report of the Committee on Child Health Services (Court Committee) recommends that a 'child health visitor' should have contact with the expectant mother in pregnancy and in the first days of the baby's life to give continuity of care from birth.

Nursing staff

As part of their training student midwives will spend some time working in a special care nursery but the majority of their training and experience will concern the well baby and his mother. Contact with mother may have been made first in the antenatal clinic and it is a pleasure for both the expectant mother and the midwife to know each other before mother is admitted to the labour ward.

Nursing care of the mother and baby in the puerperium is radically different from the role of the nurse in the general field. The vast majority of newly delivered mothers are not ill and within a few days are ambulant and independent. There is minimal patient dependency and sometimes the new student midwife may find this a situation which is difficult to accept and which requires a different attitude on her part. The new mother requires a great deal of support and advice in coping with her baby and adjusting her emotional feelings. She requires very deep human understanding, sympathy and professional skill. The value of an experienced sister midwife at this time is tremendous, working closely with the hospital and family doctor.

Delivery room

The design and construction of delivery rooms should take into account the special requirements of the newborn infant. In particular the air temperature may fluctuate and air currents occur. Movement of air over the wet skin of a newborn infant causes evaporation and loss of heat even when the air itself is warm. A cold draught is even more likely to cool the baby. Placing a newborn infant under the warm-air intake of an air-conditioned room may cause as much heat loss from evaporation as heat gain from the warmth of the air. Delivery rooms must be kept warm and the temperature should never fall below 25 °C and preferably should be nearer 30 °C. Mothers and staff may feel uncomfortable in the higher range of temperature quoted, and if a temperature above

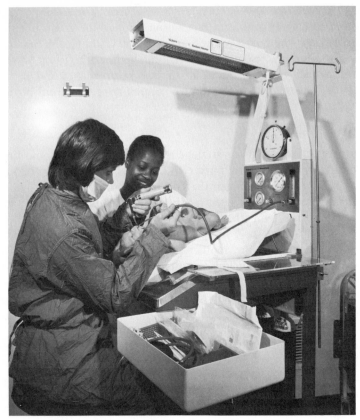

Fig. 6.1 Infant resuscitation unit. The mask should cover the operator's nose. (Photograph by courtesy of Vickers Medical.)

25 °C is not tolerable it is essential that the area where the baby will be resuscitated has an extra source of heat such as an infrared heater. The heater can be a fixture or on a mobile trolley so that its position can be changed (Fig. 6.1).

Preparation for delivery. Before delivery takes place the cot and blankets into which baby is to be placed should be warmed and extra heat supplied if necessary. The resuscitation equipment is checked. This should include the following:

A clock showing minutes and seconds
Mucus extractors
Source of suction
Suction catheters
Cotton-wool balls (sterile)
Face-mask and bag

Oxygen supply
Endotracheal tubes
Infant laryngoscope
Various cannulae syringes and needles
Ampoules of 8.4% sodium bicarbonate and 10% dextrose
Neonatal Naloxone
Umbilical venous and arterial catheters of various sizes.
Stethoscope

Delivery. Assuming that labour and the first stages of birth have progressed normally, when the baby's head is delivered the midwife should quickly feel for the umbilical cord which may be round his neck. It may be possible to slip the loop of cord over the baby's head or down over the anterior shoulder as it is being delivered. The cord should be clamped and cut before delivery only if it is very tight or looped more than once around the neck in which case it could strangulate the baby during birth. The baby's oxygen supply is completely cut off when the cord is prematurely cut and subsequent delay in delivery of the shoulders could result in anoxia and stillbirth. The midwife swabs each eye using separate large, dry sterile cotton-wool balls to remove any contaminated secretions from the birth canal. There are different schools of thought regarding this procedure and some do not approve of wiping the eyelids at birth. Others advocate the use of prophylactic eye drops such as silver nitrate 1% or sulphacetamide drops 10% (Albucid) immediately following birth to prevent gonococcal ophthalmia. While waiting for rotation of the shoulders external mucus may be wiped from the nose and mouth with a sterile gauze swab.

Suction. When the baby is completely born he is held with the head tilted down for a few moments to allow drainage of fluid and mucus from the trachea and pharynx. This mucus should be aspirated from the baby's mouth by the midwife. The healthy baby cries at once and no further treatment is required. If the mouth still contains secretions further suction of mucus should be carried out. Should the airway be completely obstructed anoxia will result. Mucus extraction must therefore receive priority over other procedures at this time. A simple mouth-operated mucus extractor with a trap can be used and there are several disposable varieties on the market which are very effective (Fig. 6.2). Fears of transmission of AIDS virus (HIV) have caused some units to discontinue use of mouth-operated suction. Various types of mechanical suction apparatus are also available. The mucus extractor must be directed over the dorsum of the tongue into the pharynx for not

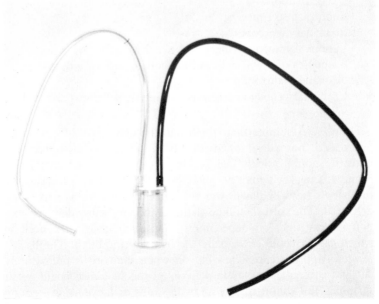

Fig. 6.2 Disposable mucus extractor

more than 5 cm. Gentleness must be exercised to avoid trauma to the delicate lining of the nasopharynx. Excessive suctioning of the pharynx can stimulate the vagus nerve and produce secondary apnoea in an otherwise healthy baby.

Assessment at birth. Once baby has been delivered an immediate assessment of his general condition should be carried out paying particular attention to the interval between delivery and the onset of regular respiration. A clock should be started as soon as the infant has been delivered. The method of assessment originally devised by Apgar and named after her is widely used and has proved its value (Chapter 5).

Resuscitation. At every delivery, before the infant is born, one member of the team should be given responsibility for the resuscitation of the infant. If the person responsible is a midwife who has not been trained in the passage of an endotracheal tube she should know how to give air or oxygen by a bag and mask and understand the indications for calling for further help. These indications would be, an infant with an Apgar score of 3 or less at any stage, an infant in whom the Apgar score was falling in spite of oxygen administered by face mask and an infant where the Apgar score had not reached 7 by five minutes. Should delivery occur as an emergency in a place where no resuscitative equipment is available mouth to nose respiration should be used if artificial resuscitation is required (Chapter 20).

The cord. The time at which the cord is cut varies according to the wishes of the parents and the practice of the obstetrician concerned. Delay in cutting the cord until pulsation has ceased allows the infant to receive a transfusion of placental blood provided that the infant is not held above the level of the placenta. The cord is clamped with Spencer Wells artery forceps 5 cm from the umbilicus. A second clamp is applied 6 cm from the umbilicus and the cord divided between the two forceps. The baby is placed on the mother's abdomen so that she can touch and see her baby. Drying the baby with a warm towel is essential to prevent evaporative heat loss. The mother should be given her naked baby to cuddle immediately. This is a very exciting and emotional time for both parents. A mother will try to establish eye to eye contact and will gradually touch and stroke her baby. This early contact helps to promote bonding. The baby should then be wrapped in a warm towel and placed in the cot near the parents. The cord is finally occluded by one of three methods.

Sterile disposable plastic cord clamps are applied about 1 cm from the umbilical skin and closed by pressure with the fingers. The cord is then cut approximately 1 cm beyond the clamp to prevent it slipping off. The clamp may be removed after 24 to 48 hours (Fig. 6.3).

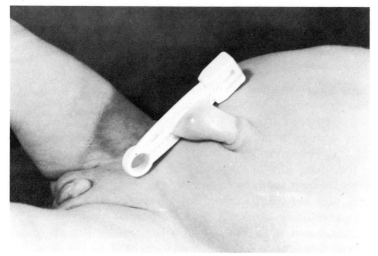

Fig. 6.3 Disposable cord clamp.

Rubber bands which are placed around the cord by the use of forceps and tape. It is useful to have a sterile pack containing the following ready for use: rubber bands size 28, fine tape about 15 cm long, straight Spencer Wells forceps. The pack containing the above equipment is opened. The middle of the tape is clipped at the point of the forceps and one half laid along the length of the forceps. The rubber band is then looped round the tape and forceps four times just below the point of the forceps. The tape is then released from the end of the forceps and the ends approximated. The tape is now in position through the folds of rubber band. The forceps with the rubber band in situ are applied about 4 cm from the umbilicus. The forceps already on the cord are removed. Steady traction is applied to the tape and the rubber band is drawn over the cord stump to within 1 cm of the umbilical skin (Fig. 6.4). The excess cord is cut between the rubber bands and the forceps and the tape removed. As with the clamp, the rubber band may be removed after 48 hours if the cord has shrivelled satisfactorily.

Ligation. The cord is clamped and cut 5 cm from the umbilicus. Ligatures made of nylon material which is very strong and suitable are available. The first sterile ligature is placed 2.5 cm from the umbilicus and the second ligature between the umbilicus and the first ligature. The excess cord is cut between the first ligature and the forceps and as a precaution against haemorrhage the forceps may be reapplied to the end of the cord.

Rubber bands and umbilical clamps provide continued pressure as the Wharton's jelly shrinks and thus reduce the possibility of haemorrhage. They are thus potentially safer than ligatures.

Examination of the baby

A preliminary examination of the baby should be carried out in the delivery room to establish the infant's sex and to look for any congenital abnormality which requires immediate treatment. The more detailed examination of the baby which takes place during the first 24 hours of life is described in Chapter 7.

Should the genitalia appear in any way abnormal no statement about the baby's sex should be given to the mother by the midwife until baby has been examined by an experienced doctor. Medical advice should be sought for any abnormalities found.

Identification of the baby. It is most important that an entirely dependable system of identifying each baby be operated in a maternity unit and that this be applied as soon as possible after

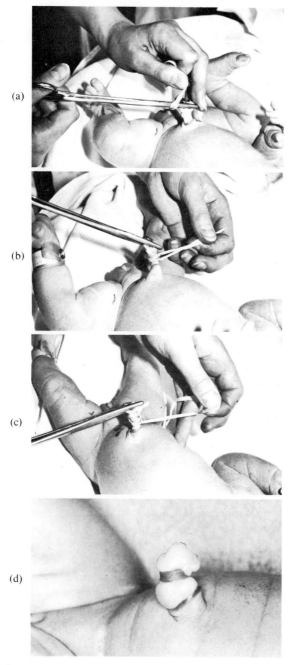

(a)

(b)

(c)

(d)

Fig. 6.4 Stages in the application of a rubber band to the cord.

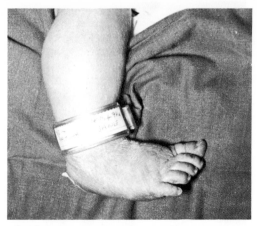

Fig. 6.5 Name band.

birth in the presence of the baby's parents. It must be completed before the infant leaves the delivery room. One of the most commonly used methods is to write the infant's surname and date and time of birth on a small pink or blue card according to sex. The card is then inserted into a transparent bracelet which is clipped round the infant's wrist or ankle (Fig. 6.5). As the special press stud closing such bracelets cannot be opened the bracelet can be removed only by cutting it off.

Other methods of identification such as taking finger or footprints are popular in some parts of the world.

Apart from those who have been anaesthetized for operative deliveries most mothers are well enough to be shown their baby and check the identification label and sex prior to being transferred to the ward from the delivery room. The father can also participate. This is a most reassuring and satisfying experience for both parents. On discharge from hospital the label is removed by the Nursery Sister, checked by the mother and given to her for safe keeping.

Records. It is essential that accurate records are made throughout labour, so that the complete record of antenatal care, labour and the immediate postdelivery phase can be passed on to staff of the neonatal nursery when the baby is transferred. In addition to details of identification the following are of special note:

    Antenatal assessment
    Type of delivery
    Drugs given to mother in labour

Condition of baby at birth, Apgar score, resuscitative measures and drugs given.

Care after resuscitation. Once respiration is satisfactorily established, the preliminary brief examination has been completed and the identification bracelet applied, mother, if well, should be given an opportunity to hold her infant. As will be mentioned in Chapter 7 parents may wish to watch their baby being examined and wish to examine him. Mother will certainly wish to cuddle her baby and should be encouraged to put him to the breast should she wish to do so. During this period of mothering a midwife should be present to make sure that the infant is not allowed to become cold and to remove him should mother fall asleep.

If the delivery room is not as warm as the recommended temperature of 25 °C it will be necessary to use an additional source of heat. Baby is placed in a cot which has been prepared previously and kept warm. The cot is labelled and the record on the cot label checked with the record on baby's bracelet in the presence of another nurse. When the baby's temperature is stable mother and baby are transferred to the ward. The newborn baby should be observed closely with particular reference to possible aspiration of mucus. The umbilical cord must be carefully checked for bleeding at least hourly during the first 6 hours and preferably until the end of 12 hours. The baby is allowed to rest following delivery for approximately 2 to 3 hours prior to further examination, weighing and initial cleansing. Skin temperature is taken in the groin or axilla with a low-reading thermometer to ensure that the baby is maintaining his body heat. A skin temperature of less than 36 °C is an indication for careful assessment of the infant by a paediatrician and for additional warmth.

Weight, length and head circumference. The baby's weight must be very carefully recorded and checked by a second midwife as great anxiety and distress can be caused by an error. Length must be measured accurately preferably using a neonatometer. The maximum circumference of the head in the occipitofrontal plane should be measured using a disposable tape measure. In order to avoid error associated with moulding during delivery the measurement should be repeated on the third day (Chapter 7).

Initial cleansing. After birth the baby is frequently covered with vernix caseosa, blood, meconium and other secretions. It is customary to clean the newborn baby but such cleansing requires exposure and handling during which heat loss will readily occur unless suitable precautions are taken. The infant skin with its covering of vernix and fatty acids is an excellent barrier to micro-biological attack and there is disadvantage in removing these materials from the skin surface. The initial cleansing should not be carried out until the baby has settled after delivery and has a normal and stable temperature. The room used must be at 30 °C and free from draughts. Cleansing can be carried out in the cot and does not involve immersion of the baby in water as in subsequent bathing. Sterile cotton wool swabs are used to wipe off excess vernix. If necessary the swabs can be moistened in water. In the initial and subsequent cleansing special attention should be paid to the skin creases.

After cleansing, the cord should be treated with a swab mois-tened in 70% isopropyl alcohol and Sterzac (hexachlorophane) powder applied. The buttocks may be coated with an emollient cream to make subsequent removal of meconium easier. The temperature should be checked.

Clothing. The nurseries and wards should be maintained at a temperature of at least 20 °C and therefore clothing for baby can be kept to a minimum. Clothes should be simple and boilable. The baby at all times must be able to move freely without constriction of tight wrappings. There is now a complete range of disposable baby clothes but they are not yet entirely satisfactory and are expensive to use. Disposable napkins are probably the only dispos-able items which are widely used and proving to be satisfactory. Vests with envelope shoulders allow greater ease in dressing the baby. Gowns should be short and fasten with tape down the back. Terry towelling napkins if in plentiful supply are excellent but they must be properly laundered. Mittens and bootees must also be made of boilable material and have carefully finished inside seams. When the inside seam is left unstitched there is a danger of loose threads being wound round the fingers and toes. Cases of gangrene have been reported following constriction of fingers by loose threads. Although there is a complete range of disposable bed linen these items are expensive and it is doubtful if they will ever be as efficient as conventional linen. Blankets made from cotton cellular material can be boiled and laundered easily. Pillows are not used in neonatal nurseries.

Cots. A variety of cots is now available. The more expensive have a metal supporting frame on castors with cupboard space for all baby's toilet requirements and shelves for use during nursing procedures. On top of these a transparent plastic bassinet can be placed flat or at preset angles of tilt. Such cots are designed to

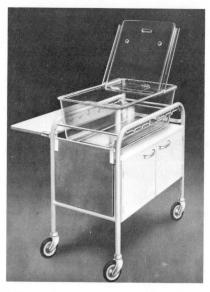

Fig. 6.6 Cot suitable for special care nurseries. (Photograph by courtesy of Hoskins and Sewell Ltd.)

contain all the baby's linen and bathing requirements. A typical example is shown in Figure 6.6. Simpler cots may have a tubular metal frame supporting a perspex or canvas bassinet. Some such cots have a small storage box at one end. The main advantages of these cots are their relative cheapness and the smaller space which they occupy. When not in use the frame of some can be folded up. They are therefore easy to transport. Each type of cot will require a mattress which should be covered in a waterproof washable material. The cot and mattress should be thoroughly cleansed between use by different babies.

Rooming-in is widely used so that the baby can be with his mother during the day. Some hospitals encourage mothers to keep their babies in bed beside them. The baby requires frequent feeding on demand which can prove tiring for the new mother. The process of adjustment can produce extreme exhaustion and emotional stress in the mother and this may require the infant to be nursed in an adjacent room for short periods.

Midwives' observations

In the care of any infant after delivery the midwife has a major responsibility in making and recording observations about his health and progress. She must be quick to recognize early signs of deviation from normal and make sure that these are recorded and reported. The medical staff rely to a very great extent on nursing observations about the behaviour of infants in their clinical assessment of the need for investigation and treatment. While it is essential the midwives should understand the comparatively wide range of normal behaviour they must seek help if they are in doubt about an infant. Senior midwives and doctors will not be critical of a student midwife who reports what she believes to be abnormal but which is in fact a normal variant. It is better to be safe than sorry.

Daily observations

General well-being. A healthy thriving newborn infant is active, has good muscle tone, cries lustily, feeds well, feels warm and has no central cyanosis. Departure from this state indicates some abnormality.

Temperature. Temperatures are recorded at least once daily. Low-reading thermometers with a scale down to 25 °C must be used. If the axillary temperature falls below 36 °C the baby should be moved to a warmer room and a full medical examination carried out with the possibility of infection in mind. Temperatures should be recorded half-hourly or preferably continuously using a thermocouple and servo-controlled heater. If these are unavailable, rectal temperatures should be obtained with care until the rectal temperature returns to 37 °C.

Weight may be recorded daily or at birth, third day, fifth day and daily thereafter. There is normally a reduction in body weight during the first few days of up to 10% of the birth weight. It should begin to increase by about the fourth day. Great care must be taken not to allow the mother to become obsessed by the baby's weight.

Stools. Meconium which has been present in the bowel from the 16th week of pregnancy and which is dark green in colour is generally passed within 24 hours of birth and for the first two or three days. When feeding is commenced the stool alters to a greenish brown colour, the changing stool. After the third or fourth day the stools of the breast-fed baby are yellow in colour, soft in consistency and about three or four per day are passed. The artificially fed baby has more formed grey-coloured stools with a slightly offensive odour. Green stools can occur in a healthy baby and are merely a sign of a rapid transit through the bowel.

Other observations. Urine is normally passed during the first 24 hours of life if the bladder has not already emptied during delivery. A record should be made of the time of passing of the first urine and the frequency of subsequent passage. Any abnormality of colour should be reported. The midwife must also record the onset of pallor, jaundice, cyanosis or purpura. Small mouthfuls of regurgitated milk should not be recorded as vomits but anything greater should be recorded and reported with particular note of the approximate volume, colour and consistency of the vomit and its relation to feeding. Difficulty in respiration particularly when feeding may indicate nasal obstruction particularly if accompanied by subcostal indrawing. Noisy respiration, if associated with frothy mucus, is an early sign of possible oesophageal atresia which requires immediate investigation.

If doubts about a baby's condition or behaviour arise the opinion of a more experienced nurse or doctor should be sought.

Feeding

It is interesting to note that in spite of all the advances in preparing formulae for artificial feeds breast milk remains unsurpassed. Oliver Wendell Holmes said that a pair of good lactating breasts were of far more value than the two cerebral hemispheres of a learned professor's brain. It is the duty of all midwives to promote breast feeding but it is a very personal matter between the mother and her baby. Good antenatal preparation is essential (Chapter 8).

The early feeds should be carefully observed by an experienced midwife so that the correct help and supervision is given. The mother should be relaxed and in a comfortable position. The correct fixing of the baby at the breast is extremely important and assists in establishing successful breast feeding. The sucking time at the breast should never be controlled or restricted in the early days of feeding. The more frequent the feeds the quicker lactation is established.

Care of the breasts. Some mothers find a supporting brassiere helpful. The only skin preparation required is daily washing, avoiding the use of soap on the nipples. Soap removes the natural secretions from the nipples and therefore predisposes to soreness. A lanolin based cream may be of benefit to some mothers and should be applied to the nipples after feeding. If the baby is being fed by bottle a record must be kept of the type of feed, frequency of feeding and the amount taken. The mother should be relaxed and in a comfortable position and should enjoy close contact with her baby. Records must be kept of vomiting and regurgitation of feeds.

Daily care

The baby needs a careful daily examination until the 10th day. Eyes must be carefully examined for signs of infection and if clean they are left alone. The face should be washed with a swab moistened in water. Nose and ears should also be inspected.

The mouth may be examined daily for signs of thrush infection. The skin flexures must be carefully dried and inspected daily as moisture left in these areas can cause excoriation and subsequent infection.

The umbilical cord should be examined. It should dry and separate about the sixth or seventh day. The umbilical area must be carefully cleansed with a swab moistened in 70% isopropyl alcohol, hexachlorophane 3% powder applied and any inflammation, discharge or odour reported immediately.

The buttocks must be carefully washed with water and gently dried each time the baby is changed. If they become excoriated a barrier cream may be applied.

FURTHER READING

Docherty, R. C (Ed.) (1979) *The Book of the Child: pregnancy to 4 years.* Edinburgh: Scottish Health Education Unit.
Macfarlane, A. (1977) *Psychology of Childbirth.* London: Fontana.
Myles, M. F. (1985) *A Textbook for Midwives*, 10th edn. Edinburgh: Churchill Livingstone.
Nash, B. (Ed.) (1978) *The Complete Book of Baby Care.* London: Octopus Books.
Sweet, B. R. (1982) *Maye's Midwifery*, 10th edn. London: Baillière Tindall.

7

Examination of the healthy newborn

Once her baby has been delivered and respiration has been established mother's chief concern will be, 'Is my baby all right?' This generally has double significance implying concern not only for her baby's immediate survival but also her anxiety about possible abnormalities which might affect his future well-being.

Preliminary examination

Midwives and doctors must share mother's natural concern and prepare to answer her questions after a rapid examination of the infant to exclude major abnormalities and to establish the sex. This preliminary examination may be carried out in full view of the mother. Mothers gain great pleasure in handling their infants after delivery and may wish to examine them themselves. This should be encouraged provided that heat loss is prevented. A midwife or doctor should be close by to answer mother's questions about her baby particularly with reference to anything that is puzzling or worrying her.

Significant congenital abnormalities are discussed in Chapter 11.

In this chapter we shall describe the features of a healthy newborn infant and discuss some minor departures from normal which can be considered as variants of normal and which are not generally included under the title of congenital abnormalities.

FIRST DAY EXAMINATION

The rapid examination of the newborn infant carried out in the delivery room is insufficient for a full assessment of baby's state of health, and a more detailed examination should be carried out by a competent physician within the first 24 hours of life. In maternity hospitals this examination is commonly carried out by a paediatric house physician. Much help can be given to the doctor by the midwives or nurses caring for the infant, who should report any abnormalities of appearance or behaviour noted by them. Similarly any anxieties about her infant expressed by the mother should be made known to the doctor examining the infant. Before the examination is started the doctor concerned should also read the history of the mother's pregnancy and delivery and learn about any significant family history.

Place of examination

Warmth, freedom from draughts, space, good lighting and easy access are essential so that the infant can be fully exposed without risk of heat loss thus allowing a complete physical inspection. It is generally easier to examine an infant on a firm flat surface rather than in the depths of a cot. The surface should be covered with paper or other disposable material to prevent cross-infection from one infant to another.

Records

A detailed examination is of limited value unless an accurate record is kept of the findings. This record may be made on a standard form suitable for transfer of the information contained to an information retrieval system. Much of the value of the routine physical examination of infants in the past has been lost because adequate records have not been kept or the information has been recorded in a manner such that subsequent collation of data was difficult. Experience with a standardized neonatal record in several centres in Scotland has led to a common record sheet (SMR 11) being used by units for a total of 56 000 births per annum (Fig. 7.1). This information together with that collected with regard to mother's pregnancy (SMR 2) is coded and stored in computer form which allows for rapid retrieval of information with regard to individual units and for comparison with other units. Ultimately it is hoped that this neonatal record will form the basis for an ongoing record of that individual's health.

Object of examination

The first day examination is intended to provide an assessment of the infant's state of development and well-being and to detect any evidence of departures from normal in form or function which might require treatment immediately or at a later stage. It also provides a base line against which an assessment of progress can be made and with which comparisons can be made at subsequent examinations including the examination which will be made at the time of the infant's discharge from the maternity hospital.

Repeat examinations

The physical examination will be essentially the same at the 24 hour and the discharge examination but certain features may be more appropriate at one of these examinations and these will be mentioned separately. One or both of these examinations may be conducted in mother's presence. Particularly in respect of the examination at the time of discharge mothers are happy to see that their infant has been thoroughly assessed. Should any finding indicate the advisability of further examination the reason for this should be discussed with mother. Her co-operation is more likely to be achieved if she appreciates why a further examination is being requested. At the same time it must be appreciated that undue anxiety can be caused by a request for a repeat examination for a trivial cause. It is essential that mothers can be given a chance to express their anxieties and that their questions be accepted and answered seriously although they may seem unreasonable to those with greater knowledge of the newborn.

Identification

At the outset of any examination of a newborn infant the examiner should check the identity and sex of the infant and verify that the record of the examination is labelled with the correct name, sex and reference number.

General inspection

The inspection of the infant must include an overall appraisal of the infant's prenatal growth and nutrition with an assessment of the degree of maturity reached. Following this a more systematic examination of the regions of the body and of the various systems should be carried out. Assessments of maturity of development of low birth-weight infants is dealt with in Chapter 9.

PLEASE PRESS FIRMLY WITH A FINE TIPPED BALL-POINT PEN

SMR11

NEONATAL RECORD (Revised 1982)

Hospital of Birth (Name or Code No.).

....

Case Reference No.

Maternal Reference No.

Surname

Infant Forenames..

Telephone No. ....

Home Address..

....Post Code

Religion...............Occupation of Mother..................

Father's Age........Occupation of Father.....................

Family Doctor..

Address...

.............................Telephone No ....

MATERNAL RECORD

Age.........Parity (Previous) Nos.   ....
                                     L.B.   S.B.   Abor.

Marital Status   1. Married   8. Other
                    2. Single   9. N/K

Health in Pregnancy   Normal   Abnormal

Specify...

....

....

Drugs in Pregnancy....................Gestation............

....

....

Previous Obstetric History.................................

Date	Place	Gest.	Delivery	Sex	B.W.	Outcome

SEROLOGY

	Blood Group		Antibody		WR/Kahn
	ABO	Rh	Type	Titre	
Mother					

Rh Genotypes
Amniocentesis
Infant Blood Group

1. O Rh—ve   5. B Rh—ve   9. N/K
2. O Rh+ve   6. B Rh+ve
3. A Rh—ve   7. ABRh—ve
4. A Rh+ve   8. ABRh+ve   45

Coombs Test   1. Positive   2. Negative   9. N/K   46

Family History

Past History of Mother

Obstetrician .... Ward...............

Paediatrician or G.P. ....

LABOUR RECORD

Onset   1. Spontaneous   2. Induced   3. None   9. N/K

Duration   1st Stage...................2nd Stage.................

Foetal Distress 1. Yes. Mont'd   3. No. Mont'd   5. Doubtful
                2. Yes. Not Mont'd 4. No. Not Mont'd 9. N/K

Drugs Given   1. Analgesic   2. Anaesthetic   8. Other   9. N/K

Specify................................Time...................

Drugs given in labour.......................................

Mode of Delivery

      0. Vertex   3. Forceps Low   6. Caesarean
      1. Manipulation   4. Forceps Other 8. Other
      2. Breech   5. Ventouse   9. N/K

Comments...

Complication of Delivery

Placenta Weight......................
      Condition   1. Normal   2. Abnormal   3. Doubtful   9. N/K

BIRTH RECORD

                                          1. Hospital
Specify Place   2. Home
                                          8. Other
                                          9. N/K

E.D.D. ....Sure   Not Sure   N/K

Gestation (by dates)............. ....

Membrane Rupture/Delivery Interval........................

Time   Hrs.   Date of Birth

Apgar Score   1 min./5 min.
                     (for 9 and 10 enter 9)

Time to First Breath (mins.)

Time to Establish Respiration (mins.)

Resuscitation

1. Nil (with clear airway, funnel O_2) 5. Intubation, IPPV (with drugs)
2. Mask, IPPV (no drugs)   6. Drugs only
3. Mask, IPPV (with drugs)   Specify:
4. Intubation, IPPV (no drugs)   8. Other   9. N/K

Birth Weight (g)

Number of births this
pregnancy and Birth Order   NUMBER: BIRTH ORDER

Sex   1. Male   2. Female   9. N/K

O.F.C. .... cm.

Length (Crown–Heel)   cm.

      (Crown–Rump)   cm.

No. of Umbilical Vessels

Gestational Age by Assessment of baby by scoring method
(Completed Weeks)

Guthrie Test   1 Yes   2. No   9. N/K

B.C.G.   1 Yes   2. No   9. N/K

Transfers within hospital (2 only)

0. None   8. Other   1st
1. Post Natal Cot   9. N/K
2. SCBU   2nd

Number of days in SCBU

Local Option

Fig. 7.1 Combined case sheet and computer record (SMR 11) for use with newborn infants.

Normal	Abn.	Doubtful	N/K
1	2	3	9

C.V.S. Femoral pulses
Murmur (Absent 1)
Heart sounds
Chest Auscultation
Abdomen
Spleen
Kidneys
Liver
Genitalia
Anus
Spine
Arms
Hands
Legs
Feet
Hips
Posture & Movement
Muscle tone
Grasp
Moro
Cry (not heard 8)
Head
Facies
Eyes
Ears
Nose
Mouth
Palate
Neck
Skin
Umbilicus

Date   Signature

Exam. _____ _____ First

_____ _____ Final

Jaundice   1. Absent   2. Mild (5—11.9; 86—204)
(bilirubin mg%; µmol/l)   or not measured

3. Moderate   4. Severe   9. N/K
(12.0—19.9; 205—340) (20.0+; 342+)   1

Absent	Present	N/K
1	2	9	Any age

Infection   2
Significant Hypotonia   3
Cyanosis (Central)   4
Oedema   5
Convulsions   6
Recurrent Apnoea   7
Assisted Ventilation after 30 mins.   8
Feeding Difficulty   9
Vomiting   10
Diarrhoea   11

TRANSFER BETWEEN HOSPITALS (Neonatal Only)
TRANSFER 1
Receiving
Hospital Code No.   12

Case Reference No.   17

Paediatrician
or G.P.   27

Date of Admission......................   33

Admitted to 1. Post Natal Cot   2. SCBU   8. Other   39

Number of days in SCBU   40

TRANSFER 2
Receiving
Hospital Code No.   42

Case Reference No.   47

Paediatrician
or G.P.   57

Date of Admission......................   63

Admitted to 1. Post Natal Cot   2. SCBU   8. Other   69

Number of days in SCBU   70

Age (Days)........................   Weight at Discharge   75

Date of Discharge   79

DIAGNOSIS

− V 3   85

....   91

....   97

....   103

....   109

....   115

                                                                121

....   127

....   133

....   139

DISCHARGE RECORD
Feed   1. Breast   4. Not Applicable
        2. Bottle   8. Other   72
        3. Breast and Comp. 9. N/K
Condition 1. Normal   4. Dead   8. Other   73
        2. Doubtful   5. Dead P.M. 9. N/K
        3. Cong. Abn. 6. Cong. Abn.
Discharge (Final)   & Other
1. Home with Mother   5. Residential or
2. Home after Mother   Foster care
3. To care of relative   6. Dead
4. To other ward or hospital 8. Other   74
   (Medical or Surgical) 9. N/K
FOLLOW UP   1. None   2. This Hospital   3. Elsewhere   4. Multiple

Coding completed............   Letter written.............

Operations 1. ....
(2 only)   2. ....

                                            145

                                            149

                                            153

Local Option   154

                                            164

Defining the normal

In this chapter while discussing the routine examination of the normal healthy newborn infant we shall also describe some of the minor variations of normal which do not justify the term abnormality. To describe a 'normal' healthy newborn infant would be to describe a whole range of sizes, shapes, weights and colours depending on racial, familial and individual factors.

Length and weight. As far as length and weight are concerned measurements of large numbers of infants of different gestational ages provide material for statistical analysis, and for each gestational age the distribution curves of weights can be plotted. If it is then accepted that the smallest 10% and the largest 10% are excluded, the intervening 80% are said to be of appropriate weight for dates. This can also be expressed by saying that those infants lying between the 10th and 90th percentiles of weight for that gestational age are of appropriate weight for dates. Charts showing the range of weight, length and head circumference at each week of gestational age are readily available (Fig. 7.2). The percentile distributions for weight, crown–heel length and head circumference for male and female term infants are given in Table 7.1. By international agreement an infant weighing 2500 g or less at birth is said to be low birth-weight (Chapter 9).

Gestational age. A term delivery is one which takes place between the 37th and 42nd weeks of gestation. Preterm and post-term infants are those who fall outside this range.

Measurement

Examination of the infant includes the measurements required to assess that infant against the standard in use. Changes in the nutritional status of a population of mothers and in feeding practices can bring about changes in the patterns of infant growth. Because of this, growth standards may require to be periodically revised. Alternatively it is recommended by some authorities that an internationally recognized set of data should be agreed and accepted as a universal standard.

Measurements of the infant must be accurate and reproducible. As far as possible the techniques used should correspond with the techniques used to measure the infants who formed the population used to establish the standards. As weight is the easiest to obtain it is unfortunately often the only measurement made. Crown–heel length or crown–rump length together with head circumference are equally important but are more difficult to measure.

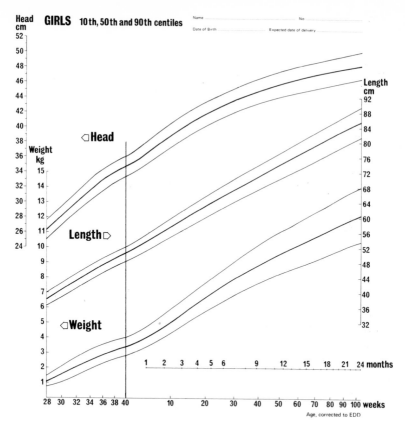

Fig. 7.2 Chart prepared by Drs D Gairdner and J Pearson showing 10th, 50th and 90th centiles for head circumference, length and weight from 28 weeks gestation to 100 weeks after birth. (By courtesy of the authors and the editor of *Archives of Disease in Childhood*.)

Table 7.1 Distribution by percentiles of weight, length and head circumference of term infants. (Based on figures from the Harvard School of Public Health.)

50th	Males			Percentiles Females		
	10th	50th	90th	10th	50th	90th
Weight (g)	2860	3400	4130	2810	3360	3900
Length (cm)	48.1	50.6	53.3	47.8	50.2	51.9
Head circumference (cm)	33.5	35.3	37.0	33.4	34.7	36.0

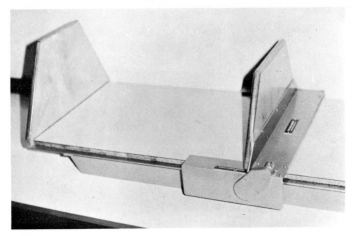

Fig. 7.3 Measuring table.

Length should be measured with the infant supine and the knees lightly pressed down to obtain maximum leg extension. The head, trunk and limbs must be in line. By using a measuring table (Fig. 7.3) with boards at the head and feet the crown–heel length can be measured as the distance between the boards. Similarly crown–rump length can be easily measured. Measuring boards are, however, bulky and cannot be introduced into cots. A neonatometer is a more suitable method of measuring length in the newborn (Fig. 7.4). Where such aids are not available measure-

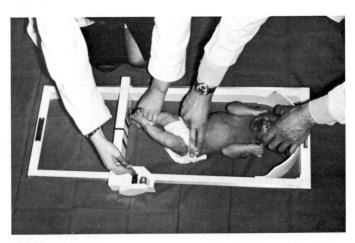

Fig. 7.4 Neonatometer.

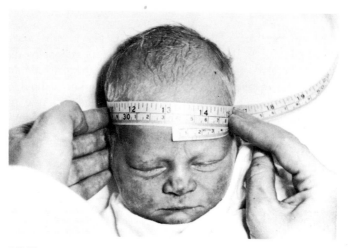

Fig. 7.5 Measurement of occipitofrontal circumference.

ments can be made against a firm ruler of suitable length or with a tape measure.

Head circumference is generally measured with a tape measure (Fig. 7.5). Moulding of the head during delivery will affect the head circumference and it is more appropriate for this measurement to be taken on the third day. The maximum circumference of the head in the occipito-frontal plane should be measured. With any tape or instrument used precautions must be taken to prevent the possibility of transfer of organisms from one infant to another.

Recognition of discrepancy. It is useful to have the basic measurements discussed above available at the time of the first detailed examination. This does not preclude their being taken separately as the disturbance caused may upset the infant and make physical examination more difficult. Whenever they are taken it is essential that the midwife or doctor making the measurements should be trained in the use of equipment involved and be capable of recognizing discrepant results so that these can be checked before they are recorded. Overall assessment of the infant under examination will include both a visual estimation of size and reference to the measurements taken. Should these appear to be discrepant the identity of the infant and the name on the documents must be compared to make sure that they coincide.

More detailed inspection should follow to compare the relative size of the head, trunk and limbs and to check for any evidence of asymmetry.

Posture

Posture and movement should be observed. The healthy newborn infant when lying in the supine position will generally show partial flexion of the arms and legs (Fig. 7.6) and the head is commonly turned a little to one side. Even without a napkin to hold them apart the hips are partially abducted. If turned into the prone position the flexion of the limbs becomes more marked so that the buttocks are raised and the knees take much of the weight of the lower body. The head is turned to one side (Fig. 7.7).

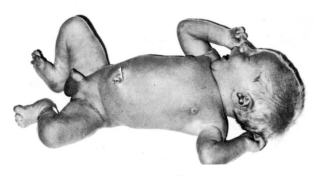

Fig. 7.6 Posture of term infant in supine position.

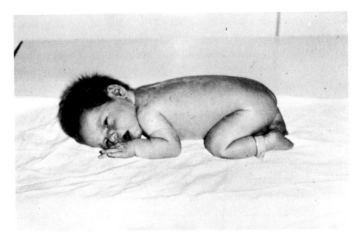

Fig. 7.7 Posture of term infant in prone position.

Movement is most evident in the face and limbs. Asymmetry, unusual movements or lack of movement should be noted. The response to stimuli will be considered later under Neurological Examination, but at this stage any evidence of irritability or undue apathy should be looked for.

Skin

Inspection of the whole infant should continue with observation of skin colour with particular reference to pallor, cyanosis, haemorrhage, jaundice, rashes or birthmarks.

Vernix caseosa. At birth the skin is covered with vernix caseosa (Fig. 7.8). This is a greasy substance which is secreted by the fetal sebaceous glands and which disappears in the course of a few days if not removed by bathing.

Lanugo. Fine, scarcely perceptible hair known as lanugo (Fig. 7.9) can frequently be detected, being most obvious in dark-haired babies (Fig. 7.10).

Peeling. Some degree of exfoliation of the skin may take place a few days after birth. Peeling is usually most marked on the hands and feet. The skin of light-for-dates infants is often dry and scaly.

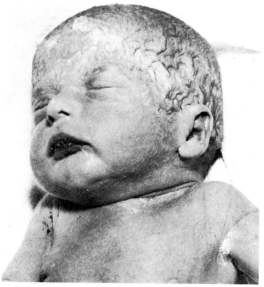

Fig. 7.8 Vernix caseosa.

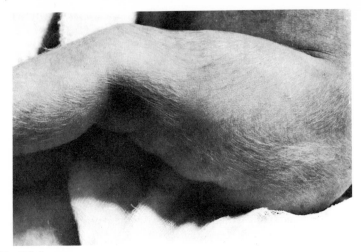

Fig. 7.9 Lanugo.

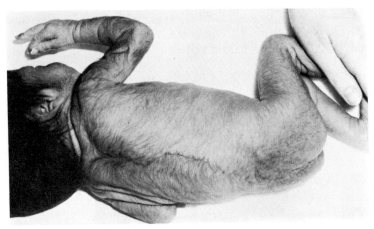

Fig. 7.10 The plentiful dark hair often present at birth in babies of Eastern races.

Hair. Much of the hair of the scalp present at birth may fall out during the first few weeks of life. The exact colour of the hair in the early weeks of life rarely persists into later childhood.

Colour. Skin colour changes quite rapidly with changes in blood flow through the skin capillaries, vasoconstriction causing pallor, vasodilatation redness and slowing of the circulation peripheral cyanosis. The changes are not always uniform.

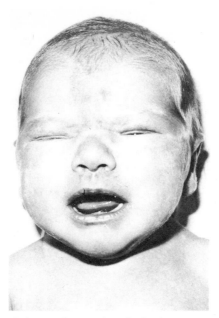

Fig. 7.11 Stork mark (naevus flammeus) on forehead.

Harlequin. A striking clinical picture occasionally results with one half of the body, e.g. the right side red and the left white. This is called the 'harlequin sign' and is not of significance.

Cyanosis. A blotchy discoloration of the skin is generally an indication of poor peripheral circulation and the cause should be looked for. If cyanosis is present its distribution should be noted and in particular whether it is uniformly distributed or present only in the periphery. The distribution and character of haemorrhage, e.g. petechiae or ecchymoses, should be recorded for comparison with the findings at later examinations. Skin abrasions or incisions must be noted.

Stork marks. Many babies show 'stork marks', or naevi flammei (Fig. 7.11), which are temporary areas of redness over the root of the nose, the upper eyelids or the nape of the neck. They disappear gradually but may reappear when the baby is hot, as after a hot bath, or following crying.

Milia. Small white opalescent spots on the nose and surrounding structures are called milia (Fig. 7.12). They are blocked sebaceous glands which clear spontaneously. No treatment is required and it is important to distinguish milia from skin pustules.

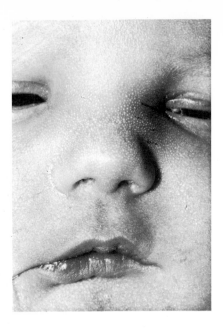

Fig. 7.12 Milia.

Birthmarks. Small birthmarks which are mainly haemangiomas often disappear within a few years without treatment although they may increase in size before regressing. This applies particularly to cavernous haemangiomas.

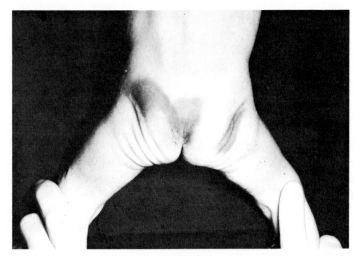

Fig. 7.13 Blue patches

Blue patches are areas of a deep bluish pigmentation over the buttocks and back seen in dark-skinned races (Fig. 7.13).

Rashes

The skin of the newborn is readily irritated by a wide range of physical and chemical agents. As a result rashes are common but are frequently transient and it is not always easy to identify the specific cause. Transient erythema often occurs over pressure points particularly where there has been any friction.

Urticaria neonatorum (sometimes inappropriately called erythema toxicum) is a common rash seen in the first week of life (Fig. 7.14). It resembles papular urticaria and consists of blotchy red areas with a raised central papule which is pale and which can be felt by the

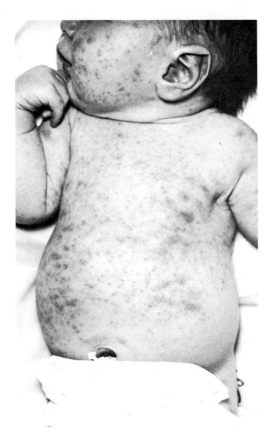

Fig. 7.14 Urticaria neonatorum

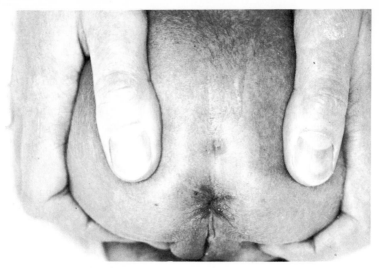

Fig. 7.15 Sacrococcygeal dimple.

finger. This condition is not infective and requires no treatment. It must not be confused with staphylococcal skin pustules.

Buttocks. The buttocks may be a site of erythema which generally occurs because of close contact with a moist stool on the napkin. In severe cases ulceration of skin may occur. Such lesions are less frequently seen in breast-fed infants and may occur on change to cow's milk feeding. The erythema and ulceration is most marked over the prominence of the buttocks and is absent in the immediate perianal area as opposed to monilial skin infection which spreads outwards from the anus. Treatment of simple erythema is by avoidance of contact with stool by nursing baby prone with the buttocks exposed to the air.

Sacrococcygeal dimple. Another common finding in this area is a sacrococcygeal dimple which is a small sinus, the bottom of which can be seen by everting the skin (Fig. 7.15). No treatment other than local hygiene is required. This simple condition has to be distinguished from the deeper forms of pilonidal sinus lying further up the sacrum. As these may communicate with the theca careful examination is called for.

DETAILED EXAMINATION

Following the general inspection of the whole infant a more

detailed examination is undertaken. It is generally more convenient to start at the head and work systematically down the body.

The head

Head size and shape are assessed by both inspection and palpation. It was earlier noted that measurement of occipitofrontal circumference is more meaningful if deferred until the third day by which time much of the moulding often present at birth will have subsided.

Caput. Bruising and oedema of the scalp over the presenting part of the skull will remain evident for two or three days after birth. The skin should be inspected for any laceration which could be a potential source of entry of infection.

Moulding. The shape of the head may have been considerably distorted by moulding during delivery. Moulding can occur because of the pliability of the sutures and the relative softness of the cranial bones particularly in preterm infants. The resultant shape depends on the degree of flexion of the head during delivery. In a vertex presentation the head is lengthened in the mentovertical axis (Fig. 7.16) whereas in a breech presentation the frontooccipital

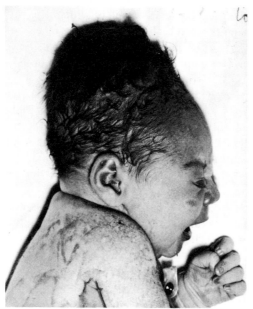

Fig. 7.16 Head moulding in vertex delivery.

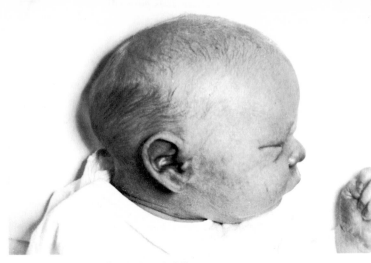

Fig. 7.17 Head moulding in breech delivery.

axis is lengthened (Fig. 7.17). Overriding of the edges of the cranial bones may occur at the suture lines to make such moulding possible. Such changes in shape naturally call for a change in shape of the underlying blood vessels some of which may rupture. In the absence of signs of cerebral dysfunction or of rising intracranial pressure even marked degrees of moulding are, however, not of consequence. The shape of the skull returns to normal within a few days.

Fontanelles are wider areas of fibrous tissue occurring where two or more sutures join. The anterior and posterior fontanelles lie at either end of the saggital suture. The coronal sutures join the anterior fontanelle and the posterior fontanelle is joined by the lambdoidal sutures.

Plagiocephaly. Asymmetrical development of the skull produces the condition called plagiocephaly (Fig. 7.18). This commonly corrects itself to some extent but investigation is required if the condition appears to be progressive as unilateral craniosynostosis may be present. Temporary or permanent unilateral neurological abnormalities (hemi syndromes) may be an associated feature.

Craniotabes. Small areas of the parietal bones near the suture lines may be unusually soft and can be felt to click in and out on pressure. When localized this condition is harmless and is called craniotabes.

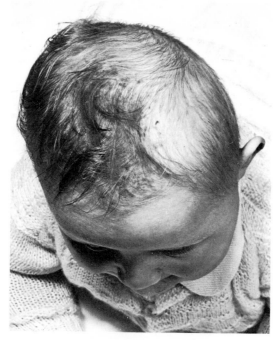

Fig. 7.18 Plagiocephaly.

Cephalhaematoma, which is a collection of altered blood below the periosteum of one of the cranial vault bones, is rarely present in the first day of life (Chapter 13).

Ears

Before examining the facial features it is advisable to inspect the ears both for the general pattern of their development and for their position.

Accessory auricles. Small accessory auricles (Fig. 7.19) may be found on the line between the angle of the mouth and the ear. They commonly lie immediately anterior to the ear. If they have a sufficiently narrow peduncle they can be treated by ligation of the base so that the arterial blood supply is occluded.

Face

The variations in facial features with different racial and familial

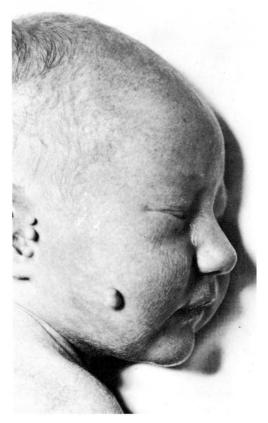

Fig. 7.19 Accessory auricles.

backgrounds make it advisable to see the parents and siblings before deciding whether an infant's facies is abnormal. Some characteristics of abnormal facies are considered in Chapter 11.

The facial expression can be a useful guide to an infant's general state of health and should therefore be observed. Experience soon teaches the examiner to differentiate between the normal pattern, that of the overreactive irritable infant and that of the seriously ill infant.

Eyes

The eyes are difficult to examine but with patience can be seen in most infants. Future eye colour cannot be stated at birth as all infants have a greyish-blue iris. Eye movements are not fully co-ordinated and therefore momentary squinting is likely to occur. Tears are rarely seen and a discharge from the eyes generally indicates some degree of conjunctival irritation or blockage of the nasolacrimal duct. Small subconjunctival haemorrhages disappear without treatment. Vision at birth is present but limited. Ophthalmoscopic examination in the newborn is difficult and requires an expert skilled not only in the technique but also in the interpretation of findings. Cataracts are difficult to identify at birth unless well formed.

Epicanthus, a fold of skin over the inner canthus of the palpebral fissure, is common in young infants and generally disappears as the infant grows older. The length of the palpebral fissure varies but is abnormal if it does not allow the eyelids to part sufficiently for the dilated pupil to be uncovered completely.

Hypertelorism. The distance between the inner edge of each eyeball is normally the equivalent of the diameter of the eyeball. This can also be stated as the distance between the centre of each pupil being twice the diameter of the eyeball. Wider separation is called hypertelorism.

Nose

Determination of the patency of both nasal airways should be part of the routine examination of the newborn. This can be done by ensuring that the mouth is closed and then occluding each side of the nostril in turn. Slight indrawing of the chest wall may result as the nasal passages are narrow but gross distress and indrawing indicate a blocked airway.

Mouth

Examination of the mouth begins with an assessment of mandibular development with particular reference to underdevelopment or gross asymmetry.

'Sucking blisters' (Fig. 7.20) on the lips can be accepted as normal and occur particularly in babies fed at the breast.

Tongue. The size and position of the tongue are of considerable significance as glossoptosis (Chapter 11) is a potential cause of airway obstruction. The frenulum is attached near the tip of the tongue and rarely interferes with normal tongue movement at this stage of life. As described in Chapter 8 movement of the tongue

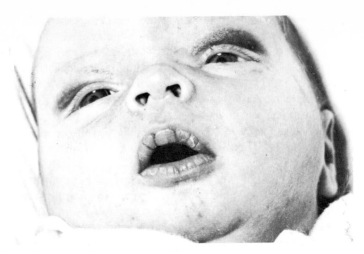

Fig. 7.20 Sucking blisters.

pressing the nipple or teat against the roof of the mouth is essential in feeding and the ability to do this should be checked.

Palate. At the same time the hard and soft palate should be inspected. Small greyish white areas on either side of the midline posteriorly on the hard palate are called *Epstein's pearls* and are a normal finding. The soft palate should be capable of closing off the nasopharynx.

Teeth. Occasionally one or more teeth, generally low incisors, are present at birth (Fig. 7.21). They are often loose and either fall out or are readily removed if they are causing damage to mother's nipples.

Neck

The neck of the newborn is short and therefore difficult to examine. The range of movement is greater than in adult life and infants' heads can be turned to look directly over either shoulder. Soft tissue swellings or abnormal range of movement should be noted.

The chest

Following examination of the head and neck attention most naturally passes to the chest, beginning with a general assessment of shape, size, symmetry and movement.

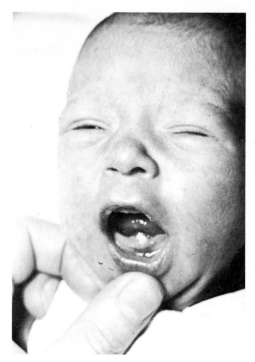

Fig. 7.21 Tooth at birth

Nipples. The position of the nipples, their form and contour and the presence of accessory nipples should be checked.

Breast. Breast engorgement may occur in both male and female infants. It reaches a maximum between the third and fifth days and regresses spontaneously although the breasts may remain enlarged for several weeks. Secretion of colostrum occasionally occurs. Provided that infection is avoided the condition is harmless and requires no treatment.

The ribs are held more nearly horizontal in the newborn increasing the antero-posterior diameter of the chest and limiting movement of the thoracic cage. As the diaphragm therefore becomes a more important factor in respiratory movement inspection of the chest must take this into account. Some indrawing of the lower ribs which are softer than in later childhood is likely to occur on inspiration. The descent of the diaphragm displaces the abdominal contents and pushes the abdominal wall forward.

Respiratory movement can most easily be seen and counted in the upper central abdomen below the xiphisternum. The rate varies considerably with activity but is of the order of 40 cycles per minute at rest. Rates above 60 per minute should be considered abnormal.

Percussion is of value only if carried out with a very light tap. With light percussion the area of cardiac dullness can be recognized. Absence of this dullness is of significance indicating emphysema or displacement of the heart.

Auscultation of the breath sounds is helpful in giving information about the volume of air entry in each part of the lung.

The cardiovascular system

Cyanosis indicates hypoxaemia and if there is no respiratory or haematological problem to account for this, this is likely to be due to shunting of venous blood from the pulmonary to the systemic circulation (right to left shunting).

Pulses. The radial and femoral pulses should be palpated and compared for both volume and timing. An abnormally high pulse pressure may be an indication of patency of the ductus arteriosus. Absence of femoral pulses or brachiofemoral delay indicate further investigations to exclude aortic coarctation.

Blood pressure is an important measurement which is frequently not measured because of lack of appropriate equipment or skills (see Chapter 19).

Apex beat should be located by palpation. If not felt within the nipple line on the left side it should be felt for more widely on both sides of chest.

Heart sounds. The site of maximum intensity of the heart sounds aids localization of the position of the heart.

Murmurs do not of themselves indicate cardiac abnormality unless they persist or are accompanied by other evidence of abnormality. No murmur may be heard in an infant with a major cardiac defect.

The abdomen

Before turning baby over to examine the back of his thorax it is generally convenient to continue with the examination of the abdomen. Inspection is most important to observe the degree of prominence of the abdomen, comparing particularly the upper and lower segments.

Distension. Upper abdominal distension is common after feeds. Absence of lower abdominal distension, marked peristalsis or gross distension without peristalsis are abnormal and indicate the need for immediate investigation (Chapter 11).

The cord

Inspection of the cord including the number of vessels which it contains should have been made at the initial examination in the labour ward but should be repeated. At the same time the efficiency of the clamp, elastic band or ligature is checked. Shrinkage of the cord with drying occurs rapidly after birth as the umbilical arteries close depriving the tissue of a blood supply. Separation of the cord generally takes place between the fifth and tenth days. Exposure of the cord and local application of antiseptics prevents delay in separation. A discharge from the cord stump after separation warrants further investigation to exclude infection and persistence of a urachus.

Granuloma. A collection of granulomatous tissue at the site of separation has to be distinguished from an umbilical polyp which is persistence of part of the mesenteric duct which requires surgical removal. A cord granuloma can be treated by local application of a copper sulphate crystal or silver nitrate stick.

Hernia. Umbilical hernia may be present at birth but more commonly develops within the first month particularly in low birth weight infants. Spontaneous remission is common by one year of age.

Palpation. Palpation of the abdomen in the newborn requires patience and a delicate touch. By waiting for the abdominal wall to relax and wrapping the fingers around the abdominal contour more is gained than by irritating the baby with prodding finger tips. Examination is generally simplest during a feed but care must be taken not to cause vomiting.

The liver is normally palpable in the epigastrium and the edge can be felt around to the right costal margin in the midaxillary line on inspiration. The left lobe of the liver is sometimes mistaken for the spleen.

The spleen. The spleen when enlarged presents more laterally than in older children and its tip points to the left rather than the right loin. Ability to palpate the tip of the spleen on deep inspiration is not always an indication of abnormality but should be considered along with other findings.

Kidneys. During the first day or two before the bowel is fully distended both kidneys may be readily palpable and experience is required to decide whether they are enlarged. After the third day only the lower pole of the kidneys is palpable unless they are enlarged or the abdomen is unusually soft.

The bladder is an abdominal organ in infancy and is easily palpable or outlined by percussion when full. It should not be palpable after the baby has passed urine.

Femoral pulse. Examination of the groins should include palpation of the femoral arteries and comparison of the timing of the pulse stroke with that felt in the brachial artery.

Masses. The site, size, contour, consistency and mobility of any mass must be noted.

Genitalia

The external genitalia will already have been examined at birth when the sex was decided. Further more detailed inspection and palpation is now necessary. Identification of the urethral opening is important in both sexes. In term males both gonads should be palpable and capable of being brought into the scrotum.

Hydrocele of the tunica vaginalis is common generally with small collections of fluid. These disappear within a few days. Larger collections of fluid particularly around the cord should lead to examination for inguinal hernia (Chapter 11).

Penis. There is considerable variation in the size of the penis and scrotum and in the anterior attachment of the skin web between penis and scrotum. The foreskin is adherent and should not be retracted. Urine should pass in a free stream without ballooning of the prepuce.

Labia. The female genitalia show considerable differences from the form found later in childhood, the clitoris and labia minora being more prominent. A thick white vaginal discharge may be evident shortly after birth. Small skin tags are not significant and generally disappear spontaneously. Vaginal bleeding as a result of oestrogen withdrawal is not abnormal unless the blood loss is excessive.

The limbs

Following examination of the anterior part of the trunk, the limbs should be examined paying attention to the relative lengths of upper and lower segments and comparing the two sides.

Digits. The fingers and toes must be counted and separated to examine for webbing. Digits should be felt for the number of phalanges and the nails should be inspected.

Palms. Examination of the palm of the hand gives information about the shape and form of the creases but prints are necessary before the ridge pattern can be seen accurately.

Hip joints

Assessment of the range of movement at each joint should conclude with examination for the stability of the hip joints. With the infant lying supine the pelvis is stabilized by the left hand while the right hand holds the left femur between the thumb and fore or middle finger with the end of the finger lying over the greater trochanter (Fig. 7.22). With the femur held vertically pressure is applied downward and outward and then the femur is abducted and pressed inward. If the joint is unstable the head of the femur will be felt to ride forward and inward as it re-enters the acetabulum. This movement may be accompanied by a low-pitched clunk. High-pitched clicks without the sensation of the head of the femur leaving or re-entering the acetabulum are not significant. With the leg held in abduction the greater trochanter is pushed gently forward by the fore or middle finger of the right hand. The femur is then adducted and if a clunk occurs dislocation is present. After

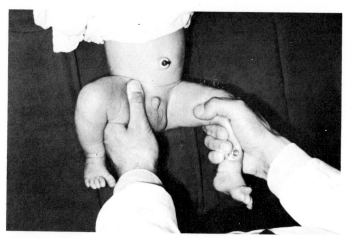

Fig. 7.22 Examination for congenital dislocation of the hip.

the left hip has been examined the position of the hands should be reversed and the right hip examined.

Unstable hips. The presence of instability of the hip joint on the first day of life does not necessarily indicate liability to subsequent dislocation of the joint. Many unstable joints, particularly following breech delivery, become stable within a few days. It is prudent to reexamine the hips after 24 to 48 hours and if in doubt request an orthopaedic opinion.

Dislocated hips. At the original examination a hip may be found to be lying in the dislocated position without pressure being applied. Such a situation is always abnormal. In true dislocation abduction at the affected hip joint is limited and difficulty in abducting either hip to 80° should always raise suspicion of congenital dislocation. The management of the dislocatable and the dislocated hip is discussed in Chapter 11.

The back

The infant should now be turned into the prone position and careful inspection and palpation be made of the back including the buttocks and natal cleft. By running a finger down the spines of the vertebral bodies abnormalities of the vertebral column can often be detected more readily than by visual inspection. Examination of the thorax is completed by auscultation of the lungs from behind.

Posture

Having completed the anatomical examination attention is paid to those aspects of the infant's posture and movements which can be used as an assessment of his behaviour and motor function. A detailed description of the techniques required for the full neurological assessment of the newborn will be found in more specialized publications. Every routine examination should, however, include a less detailed neurological examination of the following type.

Muscle tone

After observation of the infant's posture in the supine and prone position, noting particularly the degree of activity, the pattern of movement and any obvious asymmetry, muscle tone is assessed by passive manipulation of the limbs. Greater resistance is normally found to extension as opposed to flexion. In the mature baby when the arms are extended and then released they return to their flexed position. Similar movements take place when the leg is extended in the supine position.

Other specific responses are elicited when the appropriate stimulus is applied. The response may be suppressed if the infant is drowsy or has been disturbed and is crying. Skill and patience are required in carrying out these tests and in interpreting the results.

Reflexes

The grasp reflex in both hands and feet is elicited by pressing a finger lightly against the palm or sole (Fig. 7.23). The tightness of the grasp is often sufficient to allow immediate progress to testing for the traction response but it is generally safer to do this by holding the infant's wrist and pulling him slowly to the sitting position. The infant flexes his elbows as if trying to assist the movement and there may be an attempt to hold the head in line with the trunk as it is raised.

The crossed extension response is elicited by extending one leg and tickling the sole. A positive response is a movement of extension possibly with adduction of the other leg.

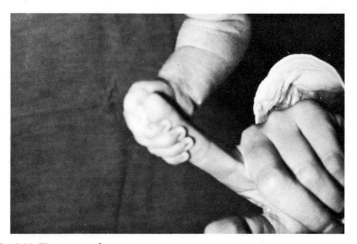

Fig. 7.23 The grasp reflex.

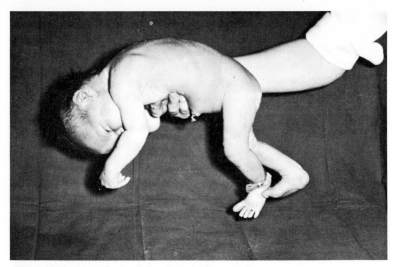

Fig. 7.24 Position of term infant in ventral suspension.

Stepping movement. When held erect with the feet on a firm surface a full-term infant attempts to straighten the trunk and make stepping movements with his legs.

Ventral suspension. Before laying the baby down the position adopted when held in ventral suspension should be examined (Fig. 7.24). The spine and limbs are normally flexed but there may be momentary extension of the neck.

Moro reflex. As the infant is returned to his cot in the supine position the Moro response can be elicited by a sudden movement such as allowing the head to fall back unsupported for a short distance. The normal reaction is a sudden extension and abduction of the limbs followed by a slower adduction and flexion to the resting position.

The rooting response is tested by touching the infant's cheek, the normal reaction of an alert hungry baby being to turn eagerly to the side stimulated in the hope of finding a nipple.

Asymmetrical tonic neck reflex. Passive rotation of the head to one side is used to test the tonic neck reflex in which the limbs on the side to which the head is turned extend while the limbs on the opposite side are flexed. This reflex is not always easy to elicit but may be observed to occur spontaneously when the infant turns the head to one side.

Eye movements. If eye movements are visible when the head is rotated a movement of the eyes in the opposite direction may be seen. This is sometimes called the doll's eye phenomenon.

Glabellar reflex. Percussion over the root of the nose produces a screwing up of the eyes, the glabellar reflex.

The responsiveness of an individual infant to the tests indicated depends on a large number of factors including the degree of alertness, of hunger, of contentment or frustration. Interpretation of results must bear such factors in mind and the significance of absence of the expected response be tested by repeat stimulation under more favourable circumstances.

Other observations

Further important information about an infant can be gained by noting his ability to maintain a constant temperature, by assessing the speed with which he returns to a normal resting state after being disturbed and by watching his vigour while feeding. At the same time reports on urine output, number and nature of stools, vomiting and undue crying should be available.

Second examination

Some of these features will be of more value at the second examination when charts of progress will be available. If the second examination takes place on the sixth day or later other special examinations such as collection of capillary blood for the Guthrie test for phenylketonuria and other metabolic and endocrine disorders will be appropriate.

FURTHER READING

Cockburn, F. & Drillien, D. M. (1974) *Neonatal Medicine.* Oxford: Blackwell.
Gandy, G. M. (1986) Examination of the neonate including gestational age assessment. In: *Testbook of Neonatology,* ed. Roberton, N. R. C. Edinburgh: Churchill Livingstone.
Gordon, N. (1976) *Paediatric Neurology for the Clinician.* London: Heinemann.
O'Doherty, N. (1979) *Atlas of the Newborn.* Lancaster: Roche Products Ltd and MTP.
Standing Medical Advisory Committee and Standing Nursing and Midwifery Advisory Committee Report (1986) Screening for the detection of congenital dislocation of the hip. London: DHSS.
Walker, C. H. M. (1977) Neonatal records and the computer. *Archives of Disease in Childhood,* **52,** 452.

8

Feeding

In order to maintain a rate of growth approaching that achieved by the fetus before birth the newborn infant must be adequately fed. Any method of feeding which provides the basis for normal growth and health and which keeps the infant and mother happy is acceptable.

Changing fashion

The current return to popularity of breast feeding particularly among educated mothers in developed countries can only be welcomed as a beneficial effect of change in fashion. It has to be balanced however, by the adverse effect of fashion and advertising on mothers in the cities of developing countries where bottle feeding is looked upon as a change towards practice in more developed countries. Health professionals have much to learn in the skills of health education, particularly where these relate to feeding habits. We need to pay more attention to the study of factors which affect mother's choice of feeding and learn how to influence these more successfully. It is also essential that we have a sound basis of fact for any methods which we advocate and that we should be prepared to modify or alter our views should circumstances prove that they are no longer applicable.

Priorities

In the world situation, although infant mortality remains high and malnutrition is a major problem in many countries, our chief problem is a population explosion. Even under adverse conditions infant nutrition does not present an insuperable problem. The human race existed for thousands of years without an understanding of nutritional requirements. We must not allow the wealth of scientific information now available about dietary requirements to obscure the relatively simple needs of an infant for food.

Measuring success

Most mothers find infant feeding, whether by breast or bottle, uncomplicated, enjoyable and successful. If she sees that her baby is thriving and contented mother too will be happy and will not be interested in theoretical calculations as to what her baby 'should' be having.

Knowledge of the anatomical, physiological, biochemical and psychosocial aspects of the feeding of infants is not essential to a mother feeding her infant but is necessary for those to whom she may turn for advice and reassurance.

Changing requirements

Infant feeding is a progressive affair involving different requirements and different foods as the infant grows and develops. As this book is concerned with the care of the newly born infant attention will be focused on the establishment of feeding and its continuation during the first month of life.

As we are dealing with the early days of feeding when problems of delivery may be as important as the content of the food delivered we feel that it is appropriate to begin with a consideration of the sucking, swallowing and digestive mechanisms of a newborn infant. These mechanisms are similar for both breast- and bottle-fed infants but there are differences.

Rooting

The rooting reflex is initiated by contact of the infant's cheek with mother's nipple. This reflex mediated by the trigeminal nerve ensures that the infant's head turns towards the stimulus and that the mouth opens to accept the nipple. When the infant is hungry this reflex is enhanced so that stimuli applied anywhere on the face supplied by the trigeminal nerve will result in the infant's mouth being directed towards the stimulus. It is important that the infant is not confused by stimulating one cheek with the nipple while pushing or stroking the other cheek.

Sucking

The healthy newborn infant is capable of performing the complicated manoeuvre of taking milk from his mother's nipple from the time of birth. The infant draws the nipple well into his mouth so

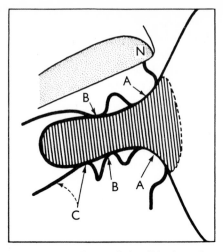

Fig. 8.1 Fixing on the breast: A, lips applied well back on the areola; B, Gum margins pressing over the sinuses; C, Rolling movement of the tongue squeezing the nipple against the hard palate; N, Anterior nares clear of breast allowing air entry.

that the areola of the nipple lies at the level of his gums (Fig. 8.1). This is termed fixing on the breast. By closing the gums and by a rolling movement of the tongue milk is then squeezed from the milk ducts which are compressed against the infant's palate. Milk enters the pharynx and passes by co-ordinated muscular action into the oesophagus and stomach. The gums and tongue are relaxed while the milk ducts refill and a further cycle commences.

During each cycle the mouth is sealed anteriorly by the closure of the lips and the nasopharynx is closed off by the soft palate. Between sucks the mouth is closed posteriorly by apposition of the tongue and soft palate and the infant can breathe.

Feeding difficulty

Nasal obstruction. If the nose is completely or partly obstructed nasal breathing may be impossible or difficult and the infant has to stop feeding in order to breathe through his mouth. Nasal airway obstruction is a common cause of feeding difficulty.

Muscular incoordination. Normal sucking and swallowing requires a coordination of several movements. This coordination is mediated through brain-stem reflexes which are not fully developed in immature infants and which may be inhibited by sedative drugs and intrapartum hypoxia.

Cleft palate. Infants with structural abnormalities such as cleft lip or cleft palate have difficulty in sealing the lips round the nipple or in producing the stripping movement required to remove milk. Special feeding arrangements may be required. It is always worth a carefully supervised trial of breast feeding in the mature infant with cleft palate.

Immaturity. In immature infants the milk may have to be delivered by a fine tube passed through the nose into the stomach or jejunum. Extremely small or very ill infants may not even tolerate such tube feeding and their needs have to be supplied intravenously. This subject will be considered further in Chapter 9.

Swallowing

The fetus swallows small volumes of liquor amnii from about the fifth month. The stomach is relatively small at birth but capable of considerable expansion in the first week or two after birth. As soon as the infant cries after birth air enters the stomach and passes on through the small intestine reaching the colon by three hours. At each sucking movement air as well as milk is swallowed, the smaller the volume of milk the greater is the volume of air likely to be swallowed and vice versa. Particularly during crying considerable quantities of air may be swallowed. Most of the swallowed air is eructated but some may pass through the intestines to be discharged at the anus as flatus.

The stomach

The gastric contents are normally passed on to the intestine via the pylorus but gastric emptying may take place in the reverse direction in the form of vomiting which is readily induced in young infants. Considerable digestive activity takes place in the stomach during the first few weeks of life. Whereas the whey portion of milk leaves the stomach within an hour or so casein curds may remain there for several hours. Most modified cow milk formulae now have a whey: casein protein ratio similar to that of human milk (60:40), whereas unmodified cow milk has a ratio of 20:80.

The role of milk, salivary, lingual and gastric enzymes is described in Chapter 5.

Digestion

The small intestine is the principal site of digestion and absorption. In the newborn infant the processes involved are virtually identical with those occurring in the adult but some differences relating chiefly to the maturity of the enzyme systems involved have implications as far as feeding at this age is concerned. Lactase, the enzyme which splits milk sugar (lactose) into its components glucose and galactose, is not present in optimal quantity until term. Preterm infants may therefore have difficulty in dealing with large quantities of lactose. Less of the fat splitting pancreatic enzyme lipase is present initially in preterm infants but by one week the amount present is at least as great as that found in term infants. Pancreatic trypsin which breaks up protein into its constituent peptides and amino acids is produced by the fetal pancreas and secreted into the small intestine from about 14 weeks. It is interesting to speculate that the lack of protein digestive enzymes in human milk and upper gastrointestinal tract in the newborn may be necessary to allow the passage of undamaged immunoglobulins and growth factors.

Stools

Mothers are frequently concerned about the appearance or smell of their infant's stool.

Meconium

Meconium, which is passed during the first one to three days after birth, is a dark green sticky paste consisting of swallowed amniotic fluid, desquamated cells and digestive juices. It is odourless.

Changing stool

As food residues reach the lower bowel a mixture of meconium and stool called a 'changing', or 'transitional', stool is passed. By the third or fourth day the infant is passing stools composed of dietary residue, digestive juices and desquamated cells.

Milk stools

In the breast-fed baby the stool is yellow and has a 'yeasty' smell.

The stool of the baby fed on modified cow's milk formulae is often paler at first becoming a greyish-green colour and has a more definite faecal smell. Defecation is involuntary and may occur several times a day. In the breast-fed baby the frequency of normal defaecation is between seven times per day and once every seven days.

NUTRITIONAL REQUIREMENTS

The nutritional requirements of an infant have to be considered under various headings including the total amounts of fluid, energy protein, fat, carbohydrate, minerals and vitamins necessary for normal health and growth. In addition the frequency of feeding and the content of each individual feed is of importance. By using a feed which contains the necessary constituents in the correct proportions, and by taking an appropriate volume, the infant is supplied with all the necessary nutritional requirements. If in addition the food is palatable and satisfying to the infant, presented at a suitable temperature and available at short notice the ideal situation is achieved.

Such, in essence, is the situation when an infant feeds from his mother's breast. In the case of the breast-fed infant volume of feed is the only assessment of adequacy of feed whereas in a bottle-fed infant it is also necessary to know the composition of the feed in order to check its nutritional efficiency. Human breast milk composition is used as the standard for comparison with the compositions of modified cow's milk and other formulae.

Human milk

Advantages of breast feeding

The infant fed at its own mother's breast benefits not only from the nutritional properties of the milk but also from the immunological protection against infection which mothers provide specifically for their babies. In addition the close contact between mother and infant aids the bonding between them and provides both with a very satisfying emotional experience. The hormonal changes induced in the mother by regular suckling at the breasts inhibit ovulation and thus constitute a form of contraception and contribute to better spacing of pregnancies.

Each of these advantages will be considered in more detail.

Nutritional value of human milk

Variability. Human breast milk varies in its constitution as the time from delivery increases. The mother who is delivered preterm produces milk of a different constitution from that produced by a mother who is delivered at term. Milk produced early in the day differs from that produced later in the day and the fore milk produced at the beginning of a feed differs from the hind milk produced at the end of a feed. This variability of human milk appears to be acceptable to infants and may confer advantages of which we are not yet fully aware. Certainly no substitute preparation can provide an equivalent degree of variability. For a fuller discussion on this interesting subject reference should be made to the books quoted at the end of this chapter.

Adequacy of human milk. Many countries have a set of Recommended Dietary Allowances (RDA). For young infants these are generally based on the nutritional content of adequate volumes of breast milk with an added safety margin. Because of this artificial addition of an additional percentage of each factor breast milk is then made to appear suboptimal against such artificial standards — an entirely incongruous situation. There is ample evidence to support the acceptance of breast milk as a complete source of nutrition during the first four to six months of life of a term baby. For preterm babies there is evidence to suggest that milk from his own mother is adapted to suit the particular requirements of her infant and can provide adequate nutrition. It is only for the very low birth weight infant that special preterm formulae containing a greater total energy content than human milk is necessary. These special formulae also contain a greater total protein and whey, sodium, calcium, phosphorus, copper and zinc content than mature human milk and are usually fed in conjunction with fresh maternal expressed breast milk (EBM). The constitution of colostrum and breast milk will be considered in more detail later in this chapter.

Immunological advantages

Studies of the role of breast milk in protecting infants against infection particularly of the gastrointestinal tract have shown that several factors are involved.

Immunoglobulin. Secretory immunoglobulin A (IgA) is the most important immunoglobulin in colostrum and breast milk. It is resistant to protein digestion and prevents the passage of intestinal organisms and antigens across the mucosal surfaces of the gastrointestinal tract. Destruction of bacteria by IgA only occurs in the presence of lysozymes and complement which are present in human milk.

Lactoferrin. The iron binding protein lactoferrin if not saturated with iron has an inhibitory effect on the growth of *E. coli* in the bowel.

Cellular activity. Colostrum contains about 2000 cells per millilitre. Most of these are macrophages. Some have the ability to synthesize lysozyme, lactoferrin and complement. Some lymphocytes are capable of synthesizing IgA specific to infections to which the mother has been exposed.

Bifido bacillus. This is the principal organism found in the alimentary tract of breast-fed infants and this appears to reduce the risk of colonization by other more potentially harmful bacteria. The bifido bacillus is a normal commensal organism of the lactiferous sinuses of the breast and is very sensitive to antibiotics. It may be absent when a mother has been given antibiotics prenatally and unavailable to colonize the infant's gut. This advantage is also lost when supplements of cow's milk based feeds are introduced.

Growth factors. Recently the presence in colostrum and milk of a variety of stimulators and regulators of growth has been recognized. These substances are low molecular weight proteins which stimulate cells to grow and divide and also stimulate protein synthesis. In human colostrum and milk epidermal growth factor (EGF), insulin-like growth factor (IGF) and a number of other factors capable of stimulating growth in a wide range of different body organs have been identified. The relative importance of these factors in normal human infant development is not yet known.

Allergy. Feeding confined to breast milk of human origin prevents the exposure of the infant to foreign food antigens. It may reduce and probably delays the subsequent incidence of allergic disorders such as eczema and asthma. Sudden infant death syndrome has many causes but there is evidence to suggest that it occurs less frequently in infants who are entirely breast fed.

Bonding

The emotional bond between mother and infant is at its firmest during the process of feeding. Many mothers and nurses feel that although bottle feeding allows close contact between mother and infant there is an even closer and more intimate contact when the mother nurses her infant at her breast. The satisfaction of successful breast feeding brings psychological advantages to mothers and appears to do so also to their infants. Satisfactory bonding in the early stages of infancy is a firm basis on which to build future mother-child relationships.

Colostrum

During the first two or three days after birth the maternal breast secretes colostrum, which increases progressively in volume and alters in composition until by the third or fourth day milk is being produced together with colostrum which declines in volume thereafter. Colostrum is a translucent fluid with a high protein content but less sugar and fat than milk. The large globulin fraction includes immunoglobulins, some of which may be absorbed by the infant. IgA is one of the most important globulins and can act in a protective manner in the bowel against viruses and bacteria.

Constitution of breast milk

As milk flow increases the protein content falls slowly until it reaches a stable level of about 2% at the end of the first week of life and thereafter there is a slow fall to levels of about 1% at one year. At the same time there is a rise in the content of lactose. Fat content is variable both within an individual feed and at different times of the day. Any figures given for the content of human milk have therefore to be averages and these are shown in Table 8.1. The energy content is of the order of 280 kJ/dl (67 kcal per 100 ml).

With the basic information given above and a knowledge of the volume of breast milk taken by healthy infants who are growing

Table 8.1   Average constitution of human and cow's milk

Constituent	Human milk (per dl)	Cow's milk (per dl)
Protein	1.40 g	3.40 g
Casein	0.55 g	2.70 g
Lactalbumin	0.85 g	0.70 g
Lactose	7.00 g	4.60 g
Fat	4.00 g	4.00 g
Minerals	0.20 g	0.70 g
Water	88.0 g	88.0 g
Energy	290 kJ	280 kJ

normally an indication of an infant's nutritional intake can be made.

Volume

By the end of the first week of life an average daily intake would be 150 ml per kg of body weight but this may rise to 190 ml per kg by the end of the first month. Thereafter there is a fall to 150 ml per kg by the fourth month. Intake is highest at the period of maximum growth.

Average intake

Taking an average fluid volume of 150 ml per kg per day and using breast milk as a guide the figures shown in Table 8.2 give the average intake for a healthy infant growing normally and can be accepted as the nutritional requirements of such an infant. Not all infants require the same dietary intake for health and growth and it is important to realize that there is a range of normality, some infants requiring more, some less than the average. The infant's progress remains the best short-term measure of the adequacy of his diet.

Table 8.2   Average daily intake of an infant feed on 150 ml/kg of human milk

	Daily intake (g/kg body weight)
Protein	2.00
Carbohydrate	11.00
Fat	5.25
Energy	420 kJ (100 kcal)

Information with regard to vitamin requirements has to take into account maximum as well as minimum levels. Minerals cannot be considered in isolation from one another or from other constituents of the diet. Recommended daily intakes of selected vitamins and minerals are shown in Table 8.3. Absorption of iron and vitamin D from human milk may be more efficient than from cow's milk and it is probable that the supplements of iron and vitamin D previously advocated for breast-fed infants are not necessary given that the mother's diet is adequate and that she is not grossly malnourished.

Table 8.3   Average daily requirement in infancy

Vitamin A	1500 iu
Vitamin C	15 mg
Vitamin D	400 iu
Calcium	600 mg
Iron	6 mg

Long-term effects

The long-term effects of variations in diet in infancy cannot be assessed rapidly and may only become evident as the infant passes through childhood into adult life. Such long-term effects may be due to changes in the mineral or vitamin content of the diet and in some instances to the precise nature of the protein, fat and carbohydrate. Changes may be noted in bone structure, in dental enamel, in the tendency to obesity or hypertension. Infant feeding may have some relation to subsequent character and behaviour. As such problems may be related to factors other than diet in infancy it is not always easy to give recommendations as to optimal requirements.

PHYSIOLOGY OF LACTATION

The breast

The change in contour of the breast at puberty is due to deposition of fat. At the same time there is development of the areola and nipple with some increase in the duct system. Further development of the duct system occurs in early pregnancy and the alveolar system, which consists of secretory cells, differentiates in the middle trimester. Colostrum is present in the breast from the 16th week of pregnancy. No milk is usually produced until after delivery.

The lactating breast

The lactating breast (Fig. 8.2) has 18 to 20 segments each consisting of large numbers of secretory alveoli. These are drained by small ducts which join others to form a large duct in each segment. This large duct eventually leads to a separate opening in the nipple. The walls of the duct contain smooth muscle which can propel milk towards the nipple. Proximal to the nipple the lacti-

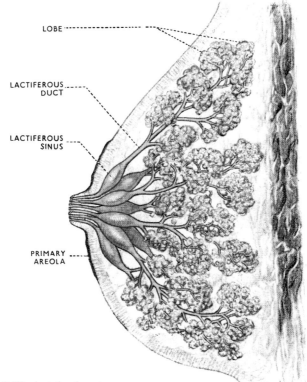

LOBE

LACTIFEROUS
DUCT

LACTIFEROUS
SINUS

PRIMARY
AREOLA

Fig. 8.2 The lactating breast.

ferous sinus, a distensible segment of the main duct, acts as a small temporary reservoir for milk. When the infant fixes at the breast and draws the nipple well into his mouth the sinuses lie under the areola between the infant's gums. Pressure by the gums helps to eject milk.

Control of lactation

The growth and development of the breast and the production of milk are controlled by hormones the most important of which are oestrogens and prolactin. After delivery the maternal plasma concentration of oestrogens falls and this fall together with the higher plasma concentrations of prolactin produced during labour are probably the factors responsible for the initiation of lactation. Once the breast has begun to secrete milk suckling appears to be the strongest stimulant to further milk production. In the early postpartum period lactation used to be inhibited by oestrogens administered to the mother. This practice is no longer acceptable because of the risk of venous thrombosis.

Draught reflex. Milk secretion takes place in the alveoli continuously but muscle sphincters at the nipple prevent leakage between feeds. A variety of stimuli, principally placing the infant to the breast, produces a reflex propulsion of milk from the alveoli and relaxation of the nipple sphincters. This is called the draught reflex (milk flow or milk ejection reflex) and is often recognized by the mother as a prickly sensation in the breast. Once the draught reflex has been initiated milk may continue to flow from both breasts even when the infant is not sucking. Ideally the draught reflex is initiated shortly after the infant fixes on the breast and fortunately most mothers and infants achieve this without difficulty. If the mother is not relaxed at the beginning of a feed the draught reflex may be delayed and the infant is likely to become frustrated.

Relaxation. The successful establishment of breast feeding depends to a considerable extent on the mother's ability to relax before and during a feed. She can be greatly helped in this by the attitude of those around her and by being in a pleasant, comfortable situation. If antenatal instruction has prepared her well and if her attendants are confident and sympathetic a mother is much more likely to be relaxed and to feed her baby at her breast without problems. The example of other mothers calmly and happily feeding their infants has a strong influence and it is often noted that the incidence of breast feeding in a lying-in ward rises as newcomers try to imitate the example of other mothers and infants who are clearly enjoying breast feeding. Emotional factors have a big part to play in determining the success of feeding baby at the breast.

Contraception

Ovulation is delayed to a variable degree in different mothers by full breast feeding and this provides a method of contraception. In more primitive societies, where infants are likely to be nursed throughout the day and night at the breast, the intervals between feeds are never long and there is a link between the shorter interval between feeds and the likelihood of suppression of ovulation.

Combined oral contraceptives containing oestrogen and progestogen are contraindicated during lactation. The combined oral contraceptive can reduce the volume and alter the quality of milk and a larger dose of hormone is transferred to the breast-fed infant than would be the case with the progestogen-only pill. This transfer of artificial steroids to the infant should be avoided. By contrast the progestogen-only pill appears a suitable choice for lactating women. Progestogens when administered alone appear to reduce neither the volume of milk nor the duration of lactation and some reports suggest that both may even be increased. Studies have shown that the progestogens norethisterone and levonorgestrel are transferred in minute amounts to the milk and are most unlikely to present any hazard. The contraceptive combination of lactation plus the progestogen-only pill is nearly 100% effective. It is possible to start the progestogen-only pill in the immediate postpartum period, usually seven days after delivery. This therapy does not affect lactation or increase the risk of venous thrombosis.

Instruction

Mothers do not know, without an example to follow, how to get their babies to fix at their breasts. Instruction is required. Even those mothers who have attended regularly at antenatal classes on breast feeding find it reassuring to have a sympathetic nurse to help them at the first few feeds. This is a situation requiring calm and patience and time must be allowed so that this can be achieved. The appointment of a midwife with personal experience in breast feeding with the sole task of educating mothers and assisting them when breast feeding has much to commend it.

In a quiet, settled atmosphere mother must be shown how to arrange herself and her baby so that both can lie or sit at ease. Mother should hold her baby in the crook of her arm supporting baby's back and buttocks (Fig. 8.3). Baby's head is directed towards the nipple which should be allowed to touch baby's cheek. The rooting reflex is then stimulated and baby will hunt for the nipple. Mother may help by holding the breast between the fore and middle finger thus protruding the nipple and areola (Fig. 8.4) so that they pass well into baby's mouth. It is important to ensure that baby's nasal airway is not obstructed and that he can breathe freely.

Establishing breast feeding

Placing baby at mother's breast immediately after delivery is an

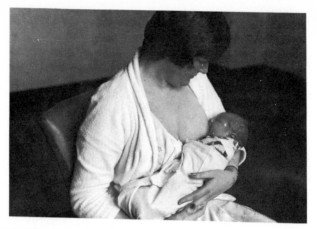

Fig. 8.3 Comfortable position for breast feeding.

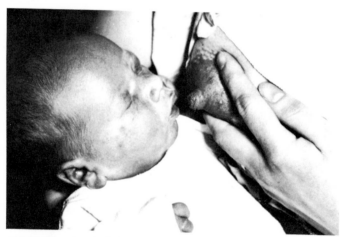

Fig. 8.4 Guiding the nipple into baby's mouth.

excellent way of beginning mother-child bonding. Oxytocin is released from the mother's posterior pituitary gland in response to the cry of her infant and to a direct reflex stimulation from the infant sucking her nipple. This release of oxytocin hastens the contraction of the uterus and expulsion of the placenta. If not put to the breast at this early stage the first feed should be offered within 2 to 3 hours after delivery at a convenient time with short periods at each breast. There appears to be more advantage than disadvantage in continuing feeds of short duration but at frequent intervals until the milk comes in as this helps to establish a good draught reflex with free passage of colostrum and later of milk. If during the first few days of life the infant is not satisfied by breast feeds the infant should be offered the breast more frequently. Later in the first week of life complementary feeds if necessary should preferably be of expressed breast milk. Every effort should be made to avoid introducing a cow's milk based feed. Unless there is a very poor supply of milk from mother's breasts the decision as to whether or not to continue with breast feeding is often best deferred until mother has returned home as some mothers find that their milk supply increases when they return to more familiar surroundings.

Engorgement

The onset of lactation on the third or fourth day after delivery is accompanied in some mothers, particularly primiparae, by a variable degree of engorgement of the breast. Accumulation of milk causes parts of the breast to become tense and tender and there may be oedema of the overlying skin.

Manual expression. The milk may not flow when the infant feeds but may be removed by manual expression of the breast (Fig. 8.5). Hot bathing of the breast may make this easier. Mothers who have been taught the technique of manual expression in antenatal classes

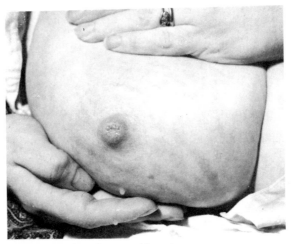

Fig. 8.5 Manual expression of engorged breast.

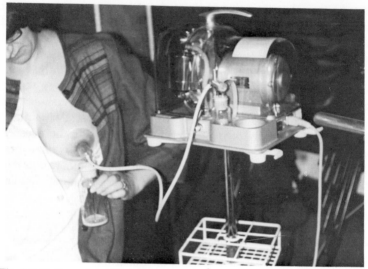

Fig. 8.6 Mother using a Humolactor.

and who practise it as soon as they feel tension rising in the breast have little difficulty in overcoming engorgement and subsequently maintain a free flow of milk. Others find a hand pump or mechanical aids such as the Humolactor helpful (Fig. 8.6).

If the breast is allowed to become severely engorged milk production may be permanently suppressed in the segments affected. The pain of severe engorgement and the poor subsequent lactation put some mothers off further attempts at breast feeding. It is essential, therefore, that this subject be discussed antenatally and that mothers are taught how to cope with the problem before it becomes severe.

Milk flow

The flow of milk during a feed is not constant, being largest in the first minute during which up to 50 ml may be taken. Following this rapid flow there are further phases of flow at gradually lengthening intervals. During the intervals the infant may stop sucking temporarily and then induce a further flow by a rapid movement of his jaw and settle again to the slower regular sucking action. The bottle-fed infant develops a completely different pattern of suckling.

It is probable that the breast is not completely emptied at each feed. Prolonged overfilling appears to reduce the volume of milk secreted. Frequent emptying of the breasts increases milk production.

Demand and supply

The more frequently baby is allowed to suckle the greater the stimulation to further milk production. This was well demonstrated many years ago when Budin studied the milk output of a wet nurse who was feeding from two to five children simultaneously on different dates (Fig. 8.7). As the demand increased so did her milk supply. It would be difficult to obtain comparable up-to-date figures, but the ability of mothers to breast feed twins successfully is a useful reminder of the way in which breast milk supply reacts to an increase in demand (Fig. 8.8). Where breast feeding does not appear to be satisfying the infant more frequent feeds of short duration are more likely to be successful than longer times at the breast at longer intervals.

Alternating the breasts

If a mother feeds her baby on the right breast first she may be able to satisfy his needs and should put him to the left breast at the next feed. If the infant is not satisfied at the first breast he should then be placed at the other breast but it is unlikely that he will get as much milk from the second as from the first breast. This is because the draught reflex initiated by his sucking at the first breast occurs in both breasts but generally the nipple sphincters relax only in the

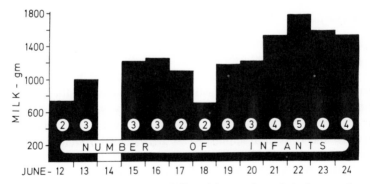

Fig. 8.7 Milk output by wet nurse (delivered four weeks earlier) given varying number of infants to suckle (Budin 1907).

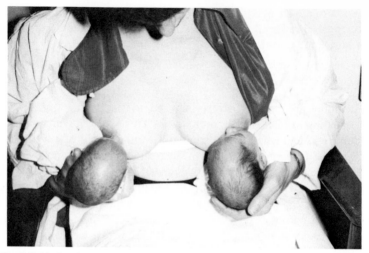

Fig. 8.8 Mother breast feeding twins.

breast at which he is feeding probably because of the warmth of his mouth. By the time he is placed at the second breast the draught reflex may be more difficult to initiate and less milk be expelled. The second breast will probably have a considerable volume of milk left at the end of the feed and should be used first at the next feed.

If the supply of milk appears to be diminishing it is important that the infant be put to both breasts at each feed. On the other hand if supply is too plentiful only one breast should be used at each feed.

Demand feeding

The importance of the draught reflex has been stressed because of its place in the establishment of breast feeding. As with other involuntary reflexes there is ample evidence that it can become conditioned to a variety of stimuli experienced by the mother. Among these, in addition to the stimulus of the infant being placed at the breast, are hearing her infant cry, knowing that it is the usual feed time and warmth applied to the nipple area. Should the reflex be initiated and suckling not start within a few minutes the infant may have difficulty in inducing the reflex again if put to the breast within the next hour. Until a satisfactory regimen is established baby should be put to the breast when he appears hungry or if mother senses the draught reflex. This may result at first in frequent feeds at irregular intervals and is a strong indication for leaving infants beside their mothers so that feeding can take place on demand. Mothers must be reassured that the frequency of feeds diminishes after the first few days and that they should have no difficulty in establishing a routine which suits both infant and mother when she returns home.

Continuation of lactation

The length of time during which lactation continued in women who in the past offered their services as wet nurses shows that milk secretion will continue for many years provided that the stimulus of an infant feeding from the breast continues. There is evidence that if in a period more than one infant was being fed milk production increased while the demand increased but decreased again if the wet nurse again fed only one infant.

The full advantage of breast feeding is only obtained if the baby continues with breast feeding for from four to six months. Breast feeding for even the first two weeks only however confers considerable advantage to the infant.

If an infant is given other foods or fluids he will take less from the breast and with decreasing demand the supply of milk diminishes and eventually ceases. For the comfort of the mother breast feeding should not be stopped suddenly.

In situations where it is necessary to inhibit lactation, such as after a neonatal death, restriction of fluid intake and occasionally an oral diuretic and analgesia with paracetamol will be necessary. Oestrogen therapy should not be used to inhibit lactation.

Expressed breast milk

For infants who are not able because of immaturity or other reason to take milk directly from their own mother's breasts it is still possible for them to have the nutritional and immunological advantages of breast milk if they are fed on their mother's expressed breast milk (EBM). As some of the potential advantages of breast milk are destroyed by heat it is preferable that the milk should be collected as cleanly as possible into sterile containers and fed to the infant with minimum delay to avoid the risk of contamination and to prevent the need for sterilization by heat. Milk can be collected from mothers by use of the Humolactor or by the collection of milk which drips from the breast not being suckled. Direct feeding using mother's EBM is generally only practicable if mother is living in the maternity unit or can visit it at least once a day. For mothers who have returned to homes at a distance milk can be collected at home and if it cannot be delivered to the maternity hospital within 24 hours it should be stored in a deep freeze if available or in the coldest section of a refrigerator until it can be dispatched to the maternity hospital. If the milk is to be fed to her own baby only it can then be thawed and used without further treatment. Mothers may be able to contribute more milk than their own baby requires to a human milk bank.

Milk banks. Many maternity hospitals now organize milk banks to which mothers are encouraged to supply surplus milk which can be used for any infant requiring more human milk than his own mother can supply. It must be remembered that this milk which will come from mothers at varying stages of lactation will vary considerably in its constitution. Pooled human milk is therefore not necessarily the ideal milk for any particular infant and its limitations must be accepted.

Pasteurization. When milk from several mothers over a period of time is pooled the risk of bacterial contamination is increased and some form of heat treatment to reduce the bacterial content becomes necessary. As mentioned above heat is capable of destroying some immune factors in milk and boiling is therefore to be avoided. Pasteurizing the milk by maintaining the milk at 63 °C for exactly 30 minutes is reported to achieve a satisfactory reduction in bacterial count and to destroy human immunodeficiency virus without significant destruction of immune properties. The Oxford Human Milk Pasteuriser (Fig. 8.9) provides a suitable means of pasteurizing human milk. The detailed organization of human milk banks requires very careful planning and the preparation of detailed instructions for both mothers and the nursing staff involved.

Choice of feed

Before birth

It follows from what has been stated so far that the management of breast feeding starts with preparatory instruction to the mother when she attends the antenatal clinic. Opportunity can be taken to discuss the paediatrician's view on breast feeding when he meets mothers in the antenatal classes as suggested in Chapter 3. Even

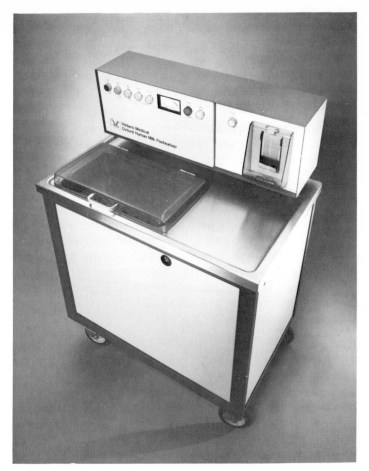

Fig. 8.9 Oxford Human Milk Pasteuriser. (Photograph by courtesy of Vickers Medical.)

more useful may be talks and demonstrations to girls at school. As the father's attitude can be very important in encouraging or dissuading his wife to breast feed the boys should also be included.

Physical effects

Encouragement to breast feed can be overdone and harm may result from an overzealous exposition of its advantages. Breast-fed babies are less prone to infections, particularly of the gastrointestinal tract, and are less likely to develop tetany associated with raised levels of phosphate and lowered levels of calcium in the blood. On the other hand breast-fed infants are more liable to deficiency of vitamin K resulting in haemorrhagic disease and, in some instances, are more likely to become jaundiced.

Emotional effects

Breast- and bottle-fed babies will both thrive if receiving a satisfactory intake. Mother and baby are in close contact with each other in either method. The mother who breast feeds her baby successfully has, however, a greater sense of achievement and this may help to establish a more satisfactory emotional relationship with her infant. Equally it must be recognized that the mother who is forced to breast feed may develop an antipathy not only to breast feeding but even to her infant. The establishment of satisfactory feeding and a happy relationship between mother and infant is more important than theoretical considerations of the relative advantage of one feed over another. Breast feeding is not the ideal solution in every situation. It is unfortunate, however, that it is not always given a trial.

Contraindications to breast feeding

In addition to the situation in which mother chooses not to put her baby to the breast there are a small number of circumstances in which mothers should be advised against breast feeding. These in general are conditions in which mother's health would be harmed to a greater extent than the infant's health would benefit from breast feeding.

Maternal illness. When breast feeding is well established a mother has an additional load on her metabolic activity of up to 4200 kJ (1000 kcal) a day. Mothers with chronic respiratory, renal, or cardiac disease may find this extra effort difficult to achieve. In addition mothers with potentially infective disease may be a source of risk to their infants and consideration has to be given as to whether it is safe for mother to handle the child until the infection has been brought under control. Several drugs taken by the mother may be excreted in her milk but the small concentrations transferred in the milk only rarely have any clinical effect on her infant. For instance it has been demonstrated that mothers on well-controlled treatment with Warfarin can safely breast feed their infants. Table 8.4 gives an indication of the drugs which can be

Table 8.4 Drugs and breast feeding

	Anti-inflammatory	Antibacterial agents	Cardiovascular	Endocrine drugs	Nervous system drugs	Other drugs
Not advised	Indomethacin Phenylbutazone High-dose salicylates	Chloramphenicol Isoniazid Nalidixic acid Tetracyclines	Phenindione Reserpine	Carbimazole Iodides Oestrogens	Lithium Meprobamate	Anthraquinone Antineoplastics Atropine Ergotamine Senna
Doubtful	Low-dose salicylates	Aminoglycosides Co-trimoxazole Ethambutol Sulphonamides Nitrofurantoin	Beta-blockers Nicoumalone Thiazide diuretics Warfarin	Oral hypoglycaemics Progestogens Thyroxine High-dose corticosteroids	Carbamazepine Phenytoin Primidone Sodium valproate High doses of: barbiturates benzodiazepines phenothiazines	Propantheline
Advised	Codeine Dextropropoxyphene Flufenamic acid Ketoprofen Paracetamol Pethidine	Cephalosporins Clindamycin Erythromycin Lincomycin Metronidazole Penicillins Rifampicin	Clonidine Digoxin Heparin Methyldopa	Insulins Low-dose corticosteroids	Barbiturates Benzodiazepines Chloral Dichloralphenazone MAOI Phenothiazines Tricyclics	Antacids Antihistamines Bisacodyl Bulk laxatives Recommended doses of iron and vitamins

Adapted from Gray, O.P. & Cockburn, F. (eds) (1984) *Children — A Handbook for Doctors*. London: Pitman.

transferred in breast milk and whether there is an absolute or relative contraindication to breast feeding.

Low birth-weight and congenital abnormalities occurring in the infant may make feeding from the breast difficult. If the problem is temporary mother can be encouraged to empty her breasts by manual expression or Humolactor and her milk can be given to her infant by bottle or tube until her infant is able to fix at the breast.

Faulty advice. The reasons given by many mothers for wishing to give up breast feeding after a short trial are often based on faulty advice given by those with no real interest in supporting mother's attempt to feed her baby herself. Very often the antenatal preparation has been inadequate and mother has not been helped enough to gain confidence in her ability to breast feed.

Health education

Much of the failure to convince mothers of the advantages of breast feeding is a reflection on the inadequacy of current health education at all ages. Too little is known about the most effective way of persuading mothers to alter their attitude and therefore their behaviour with respect to the way in which they feed their children during infancy and early childhood. There is, however, increasing evidence that the type of food which they choose may have a long-term effect on the child's health and growth and probably influences the type of diet which the child will take as an adult. Thus excessive intake of sugar, salt and saturated fatty acids in infancy may be the initial stage leading to obesity, hypertension and atheroma in adult life. Much more research is required into these possibilities before they can be totally accepted. Meanwhile, there would appear to be no harm and probably benefit in increasing the amount of nutritional advice given to mothers and beginning with encouragement to breast feed their babies.

ALTERNATIVE FEEDS

Alternative methods of feeding when breast feeding is not chosen are readily available and, as they are widely advertised, better known by the mother. Two factors have to be considered, the type of milk and the method of delivery. These will be considered separately beginning with the milk. The milk of other mammals is not identical to human milk and whichever milk is chosen some modification is likely to be required to render it suitable for human infants.

COW'S MILK

Because cow's milk is readily available in one form or another in most parts of the world it is the commonest milk to be used. The average composition of cow's milk when compared with human milk is shown in Table 8.1. The energy content of the two milks is the same. Total fat content varies in both but on average is similar. There is, however, a difference in the protein, carbohydrate and fat components. Human milk has less total protein but more lactalbumin (whey protein). Casein is present in higher concentration in cow's milk and this makes the total protein content of cow's milk greater. Milk sugar (lactose) is the carbohydrate in both milks and is present in human milk in a higher concentration. There is a higher proportion of long-chain unsaturated fatty acids in human milk than in cow's milk with lower concentrations of linoleic and linolenic acid in cow's milk. Cow's milk contains the same minerals as human milk but in greater quantities.

Modification

Unmodified cow's milk or reconstitution of unmodified dried milk powders or evaporated milks are not suitable for babies under six months of age and are particularly unsuitable in the neonatal period.

Modification of cow's milk to make it more suitable for infants has been practised for many years but it is only recently that the modifications have produced milks which are similar in chemical constitution to human milk (Table 8.5). Absolute equality cannot be achieved and there is a risk that the more that milks are modified the greater the chance that essential nutritional factors may be lost.

Modern milk preparations can be loosely grouped into those which are partially modified and those which are fully modified. In the former the protein is altered only by the heat process involved in evaporation or drying the milk; some of the fat may be removed and the energy content restored by addition of lactose or maltidextrins. Examples of such feeds are Cow & Gate Baby Milk Plus and Ostermilk Complete Formula.

The preparation of fully modified milk involves more complicated processes in which much of the casein is removed and replaced by whey milk protein which contains a higher content of lactalbumin. Part of the milk fat is replaced by vegetable fat. The

Table 8.5 Nutritional comparison of infant formulae available in the UK.

COMPOSITION PER 100ml		MATURE HUMAN MILK		DEMINERALISED WHEY-BASED FORMULAS				MODIFIED MILK FORMULAS					COW'S MILK[d]
		DHSS[a]	MAC[b] et al	OSTERFEED BABY MILK[c] (FHP)	PREMIUM[c] (CG)	SMA GOLD CAP[c] (W)	APTAMIL[c] (M)	OSTERMILK COMPLETE FORMULA[c] (FHP)	OSTERMILK TWO[c] (FHP)	PLUS[c] (CG)	SMA WHITE CAP[c] (W)	MILUMIL[c] (M)	
MACRONUTRIENTS													
Protein ◊	g	1.34	1.45	1.45	1.5	1.5	1.5	1.7	1.8	1.9	1.5	1.9	3.4
Casein	%	—	32	39[a]	40	40[a]	40	77[a]	77[a]	77[a]	82[a]	80	77[a]
Whey	%	—	68	61[a]	60	60[a]	60	23[a]	23[a]	23[a]	18[a]	20	23[a]
Fat	g	4.2	3.8	3.82 (veg oils + milk fat)	3.6 (veg oils + milk fat)	3.6 (veg oils + beef oleo)	3.6 (veg oils + milk fat)	2.6 (veg oils + milk fat)	2.4 (veg oils + milk fat)	3.4 (veg oils + milk fat)	3.6 (veg oils + beef oleo)	3.1 (veg oils + milk fat)	3.9
Saturated	%	50.1	52	39.5	41.1	46.7	52	39.5	48.8	41.1	46.7	53.7	63.2[a]
Unsaturated	%	48.5	48	60.5	56.2	53.1	48	60.5	51.2	56.2	53.1	46.3	36.6[a]
Carbohydrate ‡													
Lactose	g	7.0	7.0	7.0	7.3	7.2	7.2	2.8	5.3	7.3	7.2	6.0	4.6
Maltodextrin	g	—	—	—	—	—	—	5.8	3.0	—	—	1.3	—
Amylose	g	—	—	—	—	—	—	—	—	—	—	1.1	—
Total	g	7.0	7.0	7.0	7.3	7.2	7.2	8.6	8.3	7.3	7.2	8.4	4.6
ENERGY	kcal	70	68	68	66	65	67	65	62	66	65	69	67
	kJ	293	285	284	275	274	281	273	260	275	274	288	280
MINERALS													
Calcium	mg	35	33	35	54	44	59	61	65	85	56	71	124
Chloride	mg	43	43	45	40	40	38	56	58	60	47	44	98
Magnesium	mg	2.8	4	5.2	5	5.3	6	6	6.4	7	4.1	6	12
Phosphorus	mg	15	15	29	27	33	35	49	53	55	44	55	98
Potassium	mg	60	55	57	65	56	85	70	79	100	74	85	155
Sodium	mg	15	15	19	18	15	18	25	26	25	20	24	52

	Units												
TRACE ELEMENTS													
Copper	μg	39	40	43	40	50	46	39	38	40	50	27	20
Iodine	μg	7	7	4.5	7	6.9	4	10	11	7	3.4	2.1	ND
Iron	μg	76	150	650	500	670	700	650	650	500	670	400	50
Manganese	μg	ND	0.7	3.4	7	16	4.2	3.3	3.1	7	16	13	ND
Zinc	μg	295	530	350	400	500	400	330	310	400	500	400	360
POTENTIAL RENAL SOLUTE LOAD §	mOsm/l	88	91	93.5	96	92.1	101	112	120	130	100.8	121	225
VITAMINS													
A retinol	μg	60	53	100	80	79	61	97	95	80	79	57	40
B₁ thiamin	μg	16	16	42	40	80	40	39	38	40	80	32	40
B₂ riboflavin	μg	31	42.6	55	100	110	50	53	51	100	110	50	200
B₃ pantothenic acid	μg	260	196	230	300	210	400	220	220	300	210	240	360
B₆ pyridoxine	μg	6	11	35	40	50	30	33	32	40	50	42	40
B₁₂ cyanocobalamin	μg	0.01	trace	0.14	0.2	0.11	0.15	0.13	0.13	0.2	0.11	0.2	0.3
Biotin	μg	0.76	0.4	1.0	1.5	1.5	1.1	0.97	0.95	1.5	1.5	1.1	2.1
Folic acid	μg	5.2	0.18	3.4	10	5.3	10	3.2	3.1	10	5.3	5	5
Niacin	μg	230	172	690	400	1000	400	650	640	400	1000	240	80
C ascorbic acid	mg	3.8	4.3	6.9	8	5.8	6.0	6.4	6.2	8	5.8	7.5	1.5
D cholecalciferol	μg	0.01	0.01	1.0	1.1	1.05	1.0	1.0	1.0	1.1	1.05	1.0	0.02
E d-α-tocopherol	mg*	0.35	0.56	0.48	0.81**	0.64***	0.7	0.46	0.45	0.81**	0.64***	0.8	0.09
K phytomenadione	μg	ND	1.7	2.7	5.0	5.8	4.0	2.6	1.5	5.0	5.8	4.0	ND

§ Method of Ziegler and Fomon, 1971: Calculated values.
◇ Total Nitrogen x 6.38.
‡ Figures as declared by manufacturers. Values for Farley's products are quoted as disaccharide.
• 1mg Vitamin E (d-α-tocopherol) = 1.49 iu.
•• Declared as 1.1mg d,l-α-tocopherol.
••• Declared as 0.95mg d,l-α-tocopheryl acetate.
ND Not Determined.
Prepared by:
FARLEY HEALTH PRODUCTS LTD.
1 Thane Rd, Nottingham NG2 3AA. March 1987.

SOURCES
a DHSS Reports on Health and Social Subjects Nos. 12 (1977), 18 (1980), 20 (1980).
b Macy, Kelly and Sloan, 1953 and Mettler, 1976.
c Manufacturers' information.
d Paul and Southgate, 1978 (103g = 100ml).
MANUFACTURERS AND PARENT COMPANIES
FHP Farley Health Products Ltd. (The Boots Company PLC UK.)
CG Cow and Gate Ltd. (NV Nutricia Holland)
W John Wyeth and Brother Ltd. (American Home Products) USA.
M Milupa Ltd. (Altana AG West Germany).

IMPORTANT NOTICE: Breast milk is the preferred food for babies. The OsterMilk range is intended to replace breast milk when breast-feeding is not possible or when a mother elects not to breast-feed. Infant formula should always be prepared according to the Feeding Guide and Mixing Instructions on the pack.

mineral content is reduced but iron salts are added and the energy value is restored by the addition of lactose. Vitamins A, D & C are added at appropriate stages. The chemical composition of such milks is more closely related to that of human milk than is the case with partially modified milks. Examples of such fully modified milks are Cow & Gate Premium, Osterfeed and SMA Goldcap. The complexity of their preparation tends to make them more expensive than less completely modified milks but the increased cost may be offset by government subsidies.

Storage

In order that milk feeds following their modification can be stored without deterioration during the period until they reach the customer, further processes are necessary during their preparation by the manufacturers.

Evaporated milks. Partial evaporation of water from milk leaves a concentrated solution which can be stored in vacuum packed tins for a long period. Tinned evaporated milk was the original type of infant feed which could be stored and is still popular in some parts of the world. Many evaporated milks are unmodified and therefore not suitable for young infants.

Once the tin is opened the evaporated milk is exposed to the same risk of infection and in the same way as is fresh milk and both have a limited duration of usefulness which can be extended by refrigeration.

Powdered milk. Reducing milk to the form of a dried powder diminishes its bulk very considerably and makes transport and storage more economical. Because of the presence of fat and a very small amount of moisture it is possible for dried milk to go rancid after very prolonged storage and expiry dates are indicated on packets. As this date is seldom approached in practice it is customary in this country to pack most dried milks in polythene bags within cardboard cartons thus reducing the cost to the consumer. The method employed in drying the milk has an effect on the technique used for reconstitution and some effect on its digestibility by the infant.

Drying processes

Roller drying. The first process to be used was introduced at the beginning of this century and involves passage of a thin film of partially evaporated and preheated milk over hot rollers. As the water evaporates the milk leaves the rollers as a thin sheet which is subsequently broken up into a fine powder. This method is now being superseded by spray drying.

Spray drying. In this process the partially evaporated milk after heating is sprayed either from a nozzle or from a revolving disk into a large chamber in which there is a continuous current of hot air. The resulting dried powder has a finer consistency than that produced by the roller-drying process. The Filtermat two-stage spray dryer is a further development which makes the resulting powder or granules easier to reconstitute.

Reconstitution

Dried milk powders are reconstituted by mixing the powder with clean uncontaminated water. Most manufacturers supply a measuring scoop in the packet and as these are not of standard size the scoop should be used only for the type of milk powder for which it was supplied. The milk powder must not be compressed into the scoop but should be scooped up lightly and any projecting beyond the rim of the scoop scraped off with a knife edge. Methods of mixing the powder and water and the temperature of the water necessary differ according to the make of powder and careful attention must be paid to the instructions on the packet. Roller-dried powders require a higher temperature of water and are more difficult to mix evenly.

Suitably modified cow's milk preparations correctly reconstituted in general require no further alteration before being used for infant feeding. Some feeds, however, may not contain added vitamins, iron etc., and care is needed when using preparations other than those mentioned earlier to check on the manufacturer's specification and advice about supplements. As will be explained in Chapter 9, low birth-weight infants who are growing very rapidly may require different formulae and additional supplements of iron and vitamins.

Hyperosmolality

If an infant is fed a diet which contains more minerals than the kidneys are capable of excreting with the water available there will be a rise in the blood level of those minerals and an increase in the osmotic pressure of the blood which may lead to water being withdrawn from the body cells with the possibility of damage as in the case of brain cells.

Renal solute load. This load may become excessive because of a highly concentrated feed or because of excessive loss of water from the body as occurs in diarrhoea. The combination of these is particularly dangerous. Only modified milks which have a lower mineral content and which reduce this danger should be used for feeding in the first few months of life. Care must be taken that the correct amount of water is used in their reconstitution.

Hypernatraemia. Sodium is the mineral which is most likely to cause an excessive solute load. Modified milks have a much lower content of sodium than unmodified milks. If excessive amounts of sodium are given the serum sodium rises, a condition called hypernatraemia.

Vitamins

All manufacturers are required to add vitamin D to milk feeds in specified amounts. Vitamin A is generally added with the vitamin D. After the milk has been dried or evaporated vitamin C is added to some preparations. Other vitamins and minerals are added to the modified cow's milk preparations. The vitamin and mineral content of dried or evaporated milks is stated on the container. Certain highly specialized feeds which are required only in the treatment of metabolic disorders may not have added vitamins or iron and supplements have to be provided.

Bottles and teats

Feeding with cow's milk involves the use of a delivery system which will be accepted by the infant and which protects him from the danger of aspiration of food or of infection from a contaminated bottle or teat. Design of bottles and teats has improved greatly in recent years and the commonly used wide-necked bottles are easier to clean and sterilize than the narrow-necked bottles previously used. Screw-on caps with the teat held in the reverse position (Fig. 8.10) allow feeds to be carried around after preparation without fear of spillage or contamination. Reversal of the teat to the normal feeding position is readily accomplished without touching the bulb of the teat. Disposable sterile bags held in an outer permanent frame to which the teat is attached are becoming more popular.

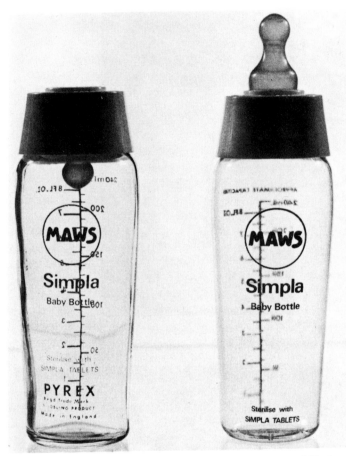

Fig. 8.10 Maw's Simpla baby bottle. (Photograph by courtesy of Henleys Medical Supplies Ltd.)

The sterile disposable inner bag is thrown away after each feed and absolves the mother of the necessity to sterilize the bottle (Fig. 8.11).

Prepared feeds

Recently a number of firms have marketed a range of feeds prepared and sterilized in the factory and issued in a sealed bottle containing 120 ml of feed (Figs. 8.12, 13 and 14). A separate sterile disposable teat is also supplied. By the use of such prepared feeds

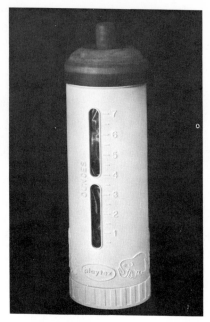

Fig. 8.11 Feeding bottle with disposable inner bag.

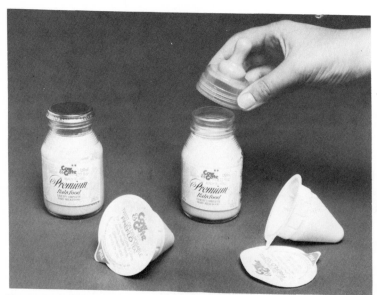

Fig. 8.12 Prepared feed and teat. (Photograph by courtesy of Cow & Gate Baby Foods.)

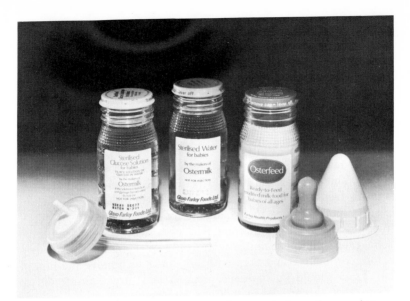

Fig. 8.13 Prepared feeds with sterile disposable teat and adaptor for use when tube feeding. (Photograph by courtesy of Farley Health Products Ltd.)

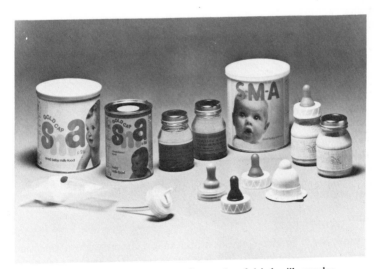

Fig. 8.14 Prepared feeds and corresponding packs of dried milk powder. (Photograph by courtesy of John Wyeth & Co.)

the work carried out in hospital milk kitchens is reduced. As the expense of providing or maintaining and staffing a large milk kitchen is no longer necessary many hospital authorities find that this method of feeding justifies the expense involved. At present it is unlikely that prepared feeds will become available at a price to attract the mother to use them at home.

Sterilization

Even in hospitals using factory-prepared feeds it is essential that medical and nursing staff should be knowledgeable about sterilization of feeds, bottles and teats and that they should be able to instruct mothers in methods suitable for use at home.

Cleaning is a very important part of this process and must be done thoroughly beginning with cold water to remove protein before coagulation and then with hot water to remove the film of fat. Teats should be thoroughly rinsed and turned inside out to ensure that all particles of milk are removed.

Sterilization by complete immersion of bottles and teats in a solution of sodium hypochlorite (Milton) or sodium dichloroisocyanurate (Maw's Simpla) for a period of 30 minutes is as effective as heat sterilization.

These methods are suitable for use at home and suitable containers are available commercially. Instructions for use are given by the manufacturers. It is important in any chemical method of sterilization to ensure that the bottle and teat are completely immersed and that all air has been expelled. Most mothers find that the convenience of chemical sterilization justifies the small extra cost involved. Sterilizing fluids such as sodium hypochlorite should be replaced every 24 hours. Manufacturers' instructions with regard to concentrations to be used must be observed. It is common practice to rinse bottles and teats after sterilization but this is not absolutely necessary provided that bottle and teat are emptied of sterilizing agent.

Preparation of feed

Water

In most areas in the UK tap water taken directly from the mains supply is virtually sterile and it is unnecessary to boil it before use. If water is obtained from a tank or if there is any doubt about its sterility it should be boiled before use for mixing feeds. In conditions of drought the public water supply may contain excessive quantities of nitrates which are potentially harmful. Under such circumstances alternative supplies of water should be used.

Bulk preparation of feeds so that the 24-hour requirements are prepared at one time is economical on staffing in hospital milk kitchens and may equally prove suitable to mother at home. Sterile feeds in sterile screw-top type bottles can be safely stored for up to 24 hours and refrigeration is preferable but not essential.

Temperature. If feeds are stored at room temperature there is no need to warm them further. Feeds stored in a refrigerator should be warmed to room temperature before being offered to a baby. There is a risk that in heating feeds mothers will bring them to temperatures which could harm baby's mouth. If heating is applied it is essential that the temperature of the milk be tested by shaking a drop on to the back of mother's hand to test whether it is unpleasantly hot. The use of microwave ovens to heat feeds can be dangerous and is not recommended.

Feeding technique

The technique of feeding a baby from the bottle is just as important as the technique of preparing the feed. As with the mother who breast feeds, relaxation is essential. This implies that mother has the feed prepared and ready to give before she settles in a comfortable position with her infant held securely but not tensely. The bottle must be held so that the teat is always full of milk and this must be checked frequently during a feed. As with the nipple it is important that the teat be allowed to pass well into baby's mouth so that he fixes on the teat in the same way that the breast-fed baby fixes on the nipple.

Rate of flow

Although too fast a flow for baby's comfort may occur with a well-worn teat, particularly if the hole has been enlarged, trouble is more likely to arise from too small a hole with a flow rate lower than that hoped for by the baby. This is most likely to occur with a new teat which is still firm. The hole can most readily be widened by jabbing a red hot needle tip into the hole and then washing away the burned material. It is wise to hold the other end of the needle in forceps or pliers or to push it into a cork before heating. A satisfactory hole allows milk to emerge from the bottle when inverted at a fast flow of drops but not as a continuous stream.

Time taken

Most babies will finish their feed within 15 minutes. If they are taking longer than this the rate of milk flow may be too low. Slow feeding is often accompanied by swallowing of excess air which may cause baby discomfort.

The teat. The consistency and shape of the teat are also of importance. Most babies take the bulb-ended type of teat well. Some, particularly small infants, prefer a soft teat while more vigorous infants do better with a firmer teat.

Breaking wind

Breaking wind is a time-honoured custom which allows mother and infant a break during the feed. Positioning of the infants so that the air rises to the fundus of the stomach makes it less likely that milk will be brought up when wind is broken. The other manoeuvres commonly applied such as rubbing or patting the back seem to be aimed at giving mother something to do and therefore may serve some purpose. It is very important for midwives and mothers to appreciate that a good burp by the infant is an indication of excess air swallowing rather than a source of pride to whoever is feeding the infant.

Frequency of feeds

As with breast feeding the frequency of feeds can in the first few days be left to the demands of the infant. In some hospitals, particularly those in which babies are kept separately from their mothers, this is not easy to achieve and an artificially fixed time interval between feeds is imposed more for the benefit of hospital staff than for the babies' well-being. Small babies may not be able to take sufficient volume at each feed to obtain their total requirement in the five or six feeds available on a four-hourly regimen. With a three-hourly regimen up to eight feeds in a day can be given and the total volume for each feed thereby reduced. There is no reason why, even in the most overcrowded and understaffed hospital, demand feeding by the infant cannot be instituted. Each infant has to be considered on his own merits and some may start with six or eight feeds at two- to three-hourly intervals and proceed to five feeds at four-hourly intervals as their capacity for taking an individual feed increases.

Volume

The volume of feed to be offered should be related to the average taken by babies of the particular age and weight concerned. Such average volumes must only be considered as a guideline and the appetite and activity of individual babies must always be considered. A breast-fed baby does not take the same volume at each feed and there appears to be no reason to expect the bottle-fed baby to be any more regular in his habits.

Baby's choice. The increasing use of prepared feeds in bottles containing 120 ml makes it easier to allow infants to choose how much they wish to take at individual feeds. If a check is required on the amount taken this can easily be calculated by subtracting the volume of milk left from the initial total of 120 ml using the markings on the bottle. Table 8.6 shows the volumes of feed taken by a group of 40 term babies during the first five days of life. Feeding continued until the infant appeared satisfied. For each day of life the table shows the mean or average volume taken by all of the babies together with the maximum and minimum taken by one infant on that day. The babies were all thriving satisfactorily in spite of the large differences in the volume of feed taken.

Average requirements. It is important that mothers as well as midwives and doctors should be aware of such variations and that a rigid pattern should not be imposed on all infants. At the same time it is useful to have guidelines so that the inexperienced mother can have some idea of what to expect her baby to take. As most mothers think of volumes of feed in relation to single feeds, the average daily intake of the infant expressed as ml per kg per 24 hours has to be divided by the number of feeds being given in the day to reach a measure of the individual feed. The figures shown in Table 8.6 can be taken as a guide for the first five days of life. By the seventh to tenth day of life term babies will generally be

Table 8.6 Daily intake of 40 term infants allowed to choose their own volume of feed. Day 1 refers to the first 24 hours after feeding commenced

| Day | Daily intake (ml/kg) | |
	Average	Range
1	63	30 to 103
2	89	50 to 130
3	115	77 to 153
4	127	80 to 170
5	136	90 to 183

taking 150 ml per kg per 24 hours in five feeds. For a baby of 3.5 kg this will be 100 ml per feed. In recording feeds it is useful to keep a record of the total daily intake.

Low birth weight infants

The feeding of low birth weight infants requires special consideration and is considered in more detail in Chapters 9 and 10. Fluid and energy requirements are higher than for mature infants but a longer period is required before the infant can accept the full volume which will often rise to 200 ml per kg body weight per day. Small infants may not be able to suck from the breast or bottle. Such infants are most safely fed by a nasogastric or nasojejunal tube. In order to avoid overdistension of the stomach feeds may have to be given in small volumes more frequently, for instance every hour or every two hours. In the smallest infants even this may not be tolerated and feeds can be given by slow infusion into the stomach or jejunum. A very few small or very ill infants may not tolerate this and intravenous feeding has to be used. When this involves total feeding by the intravenous route specialized knowledge is necessary, and this method should only be used by those fully conversant with the techniques and problems involved.

Reassessment of feeds

The feeding of infants requires periodic reassessment of the total feed given and the content of the feed. As the early very rapid rate of growth with its high energy requirement is followed by a slower rate of growth the need for food becomes relatively less great and mothers have to be taught this. Much of the overfeeding of infants later in the first year of life may stem from a reluctance to accept that the infant's requirements do not continue at the extremely high level of the newborn period. Such overfeeding may establish a pattern which persists into later childhood and adult life resulting in obesity.

As this book is confined to consideration of the care of the newly born the later feeding of infants will not be considered here.

EMOTIONAL RELATIONSHIP

One other aspect in which early feeding patterns may affect subsequent well-being is the emotional relationship which it establishes between a mother and her baby. Feeding is a social occasion in which mother and baby establish a very close contact which should be enjoyed by both. The baby not only enjoys the satisfaction of his hunger being satisfied but also obviously welcomes a feeling of warmth and security by being cradled in his mother's arms, and by being handled and spoken to. These stimuli are an important early requisite in the infant's communication and language development. Mothers also feel pleasure in feeding an infant who is feeding well.

Tensions can, however, easily arise either because mother is not relaxed in the first place or because baby is not thought to be feeding well and mother becomes anxious and strained. Over-anxiety by parents or attendants, frequent handling of the baby at every whimper, attempts to give feeds when they are not wanted all create an atmosphere of tension which distresses the infant as much as his attendants and which may persist into later life as a factor in preventing normal emotional development.

Satisfaction

For a satisfactory relationship to be established mother and baby must be confident, relaxed and satisfied with the method of feeding and the type of feed being used. This brings us back to a phrase used at the beginning of this chapter — any method of feeding which provides the basis for normal growth and development and which keeps the infant and mother happy is acceptable.

FURTHER READING

Atkinson, S. A., Bryar, M. H. & Anderson, G. H. (1978) Human milk: difference in nitrogen concentration in milk from mothers of term and premature infants. *Journal of Pediatrics*, **93**, 67.

American Academy of Pediatrics (1980) Human milk banking *Pediatrics*, **65**, 854.

Bjorksten, B., Burman, L. G., Chateau, P. De. Frederikson, B., Gothefors, L. & Hernell, O. (1980) Collecting and banking human milk: to heat or not to heat. *British Medical Journal*, **281**, 756.

Brock, J. H. (1980) Lactoferrin in human milk: its role in iron absorption and protection against enteric infection in the newborn infant. *Archives of Disease in Childhood*, **55**, 413.

Butler, J. E. (1979) Immunologic aspects of breast feeding, anti-infectious activity of breast milk. *Seminars in Perinatology*, **3**, 255.

Cockburn, F. (1983) Milk composition — the infant human diet. *Proceedings of the Nutrition Society*, **42**, 361.

Cussen, G. H. (1980) Breast feeding and neonatal morbidity. In *Topics in Perinatal Medicine*, ed. Wharton, B. A. London: Pitman.

Jelliffe, D. B. Jelliffe, E. F. P. (1978) *Human Milk in the Modern World*. Oxford: Oxford University Press.

Lucas, A. (1983) Human milk and infant feeding. In: *Perinatal Medicine*, eds Boyd, R., Battaglia, F. C. London: Butterworth.

Lucas, A. (1986) Infant feeding. In: *Textbook of Neonatology*, ed. Roberton, N. R. C. Edinburgh: Churchill Livingstone.

Ogra, P. L. & Dayton, D. H. (1979) *Immunology of Breast Milk*. New York: Raven Press.

Pullan, C. R., Toms, G. L., Martin, A. J., Gardner, P. S., Webb, J. K. G. & Appleton, D. R. (1980) Breast feeding and respiratory syncytial virus infection. *British Medical Journal*, **281**, 1034.

Saarinen, U. M., Kajosaari, M., Backman, A. & Siimes, M. A. (1979) Prolonged breast feeding as prophylaxis for atopic disease. *Lancet*, **ii**, 164.

Schanler, R. J. & Oh, W. (1980) Composition of breast milk obtained from mothers of premature infants as compared to breast milk obtained from donors. *Journal of Pediatrics*, **96**, 679.

9

Low birth weight infants

Delivery at term, that is from 37 to less than 42 completed weeks (259 days up to and including 293 days) of pregnancy, increases the chances of an infant's survival. Delivery before or after term increases the risk of perinatal death. Although the danger of early delivery has always been recognized, no means of assessing the degree of risk of what was generally called prematurity was available until agreement was reached on the definition of prematurity.

Definitions

In earlier editions of this book, in accordance with an international agreement, the word premature was used to describe all babies weighing 2500 g or less at birth. Although it is permissible to talk about the premature birth of a baby the phrase 'premature baby' should no longer be used.

Low birth weight

Low birth weight (LBW) is the phrase used to describe all infants weighing less than 2500 g (up to and including 2499 g). This group of infants is at a major disadvantage compared with the much larger group weighing over 2500 g.

Very low birth weight. Very low birth weight (VLBW) is the phrase used to describe all infants weighing less than 1500 g (up to and including 1499 g). The effects of preterm delivery and low birth weight on survival are shown in Table 2.4 (page 24). It is evident that the mortality increased with reducing maturity and birth weight. Such infants generally require the facilities available in intensive care nurseries and where these are available survival rates of 90% (i.e. mortality rates of less than 100 per 1000 births) are being reported for infants weighing 1001 to 1500 g. If an infant shows signs of life after complete expulsion from his mother he is classified as liveborn irrespective of his birth weight and should be included in any analysis of birth weight specific data.

Significance. VLBW infants account for about 10% of the number of LBW infants but for about 60% of the perinatal deaths in LBW infants. Although this book does not attempt to go into the details of intensive care, differences in the management and treatment of the VLBW infant will be mentioned where applicable. The problem of low birth weight and more particularly of very low birth weight is the most important challenge confronting those responsible for the care of the newly born infant.

Preterm infants

A preterm infant is one delivered before 259 days (37 weeks) as based on the menstrual age of the pregnancy (Fig. 9.1). A birth is preterm if it occurs up to and including the 258th day of gestation. A new day commences at midnight. Thus a pregnancy at 37 weeks (259 days) on 4th July is classified as preterm if the baby is born on 3rd July at 11.59 pm (23.59 hours).

Postnatal examination. Methods of assessing the infant's state of development at delivery which allow an estimate to be made of the stage of pregnancy at which birth took place are described later.

Weight. Most preterm infants are of low birth weight and weigh less than 2500 g at birth.

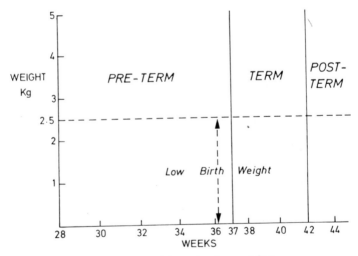

Fig. 9.1 Classification by menstrual (gestational) age of fetus.

Weight for gestational age

Birth weight is not an acceptable measure of maturity because low birth weight may be caused either by preterm delivery or by slow fetal growth (Table 9.1). A further definition is therefore required taking into account menstrual age. Infants less than the 10th percentile of the weight distribution for their particular menstrual (gestational) age are termed light-for-dates and infants over the 90th percentile are termed heavy-for-dates (Fig. 9.2).

Table 9.1   Outline of causes of low birth weight

Preterm delivery
  Maternal ill-health
  Complications of pregnancy
  Fetal abnormality
Slow fetal growth
  Malnutrition in utero
  Poor placental function
  Fetal poisoning (alcohol and smoking)
Hypoplasia
  Constitutional
  Chromosome abnormality
  Fetal poisoning (alcohol and smoking)
Combination of above

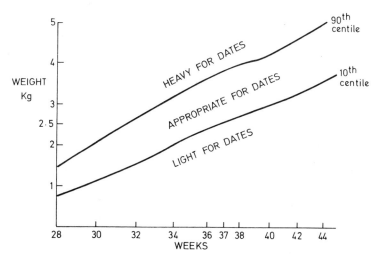

Fig. 9.2 Weight for menstrual (gestational) age of fetus.

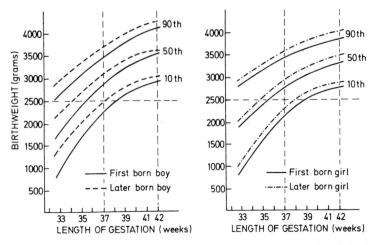

Fig. 9.3 Weight percentiles for gestational age, sex and birth order (*British Births 1970*)

Light-for-dates. Figure 9.3 shows a percentile distribution of weight at different gestational ages. It will be seen that some appropriate-for-dates infants born at term will be 2500 g or less at birth.

Small-for-dates. The phrase small-for-dates (small for gestational age) is used when measures other than weight, e.g. length, chest circumferences and head circumferences are below the 10th percentile. Infants who are below the 10th percentiles for their gestational age at birth have often been noted at earlier stages of pregnancy to be small and their smallness is associated with failure of adequate growth through much of pregnancy. Possible reasons for this have already been discussed in Chapter 4. In general they can be classified as malnourished or hypoplastic.

Usefulness of classification. Figure 9.4 shows examples of how this classification applies to infants of varying birth weight and gestational age. As will be discussed later in this chapter this division of infants into the various categories mentioned is useful as a guide to the problems they are likely to face in the neonatal period and as an indication of their longer-term prognosis. In particular we must learn to recognize those infants who have failed to grow adequately in utero as they have problems of a different nature from those LBW babies who are adequately nourished but who were delivered before term.

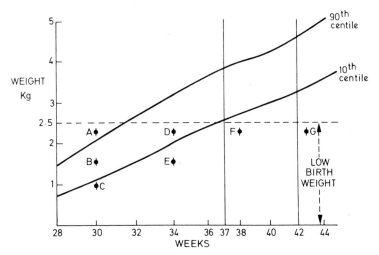

Fig. 9.4 Classification of low birth weight infants:
A   Preterm, heavy- for-dates
B & D   Preterm, appropriate-for-dates
C & E   Preterm, light-for-dates
F   Term, light-for-dates
G   Post-term, light-for-dates

Postnatal assessment of maturity

As a check on the information available from antenatal examinations it is useful to have methods of assessment of maturity which are based on examination of the infant at birth. Before we consider the particular problem facing preterm and light-for-dates babies we shall, therefore, consider methods of assessment of maturity after delivery.

The first examination to be described is based on that described by Dubowitz, Dubowitz and Goldberg (1970). It can be carried out at any time during the first five days of life provided that there is no evidence of intrapartum asphyxia or birth injury. The method is easily learned and with practice the examination can be completed in about 10 minutes.

The assessment is based on a series of external characteristics and a number of neurological signs based on posture and primitive reflexes. Each sign is given a score.

External characteristics

The external signs and the scoring system used are shown in Table

Table 9.2 Scoring system for external criteria

External sign	Score*				
	0	1	2	3	4
Oedema	Obvious oedema of hands and feet; pitting over tibia	No obvious oedema of hands and feet; pitting over tibia	No oedema		
Skin texture	Very thin gelatinous	Thin and smooth	Smooth; medium thickness. Rash or superficial peeling	Slight thickening. Superficial cracking and peeling especially of hands and feet	Thick and parchment-like; superficial or deep cracking
Skin colour	Dark red	Uniformly pink	Pale pink; variable over body	Pale; only pink over ears, lips, palms, or soles	
Skin opacity (trunk)	Numerous veins and venules clearly seen, especially over abdomen	Veins and tributaries seen	A few large vessels clearly seen over abdomen	A few large vessels seen indistinctly over abdomen	No blood vessels seen
Lanugo (over back)	No lanugo	Abundant; long and thick over whole back	Hair thinning especially over lower back	Small amount of lanugo and bald area	At least half of back devoid of lanugo
Plantar creases	No skin creases	Faint red marks over anterior half of sole	Definite red marks over > anterior $\frac{1}{2}$; indentations over < anterior $\frac{1}{3}$	Indentations over > anterior $\frac{1}{3}$	Definite deep indentations over > anterior $\frac{1}{3}$

Nipple formation	Nipple barely visible; no areola	Nipple well defined; areola smooth and flat, diameter < 0.75 cm	Areola stippled, edge not raised, diameter < 0.75 cm	Areola stippled, edge raised, diameter > 0.75 cm
Breast size	No breast tissue palpable	Breast tissue on one or both sides, < 0.5 cm diameter	Breast tissue both sides; one or both 0.5–1.0 cm	Breast tissue both sides; one or both > 1 cm
Ear form	Pinna flat and shapeless, little or no incurving of edge	Incurving of part of edge of pinna	Partial incurving whole of upper pinna	Well-defined incurving whole of upper pinna
Ear firmness	Pinna soft, easily folded, no recoil	Pinna soft, easily folded, slow recoil	Cartilage to edge of pinna, but soft in places, ready recoil	Pinna firm, cartilage to edge; instant recoil
Genitals Male	Neither testis in scrotum	At least one testis high in scrotum	At least one testis right down	
Female (with hips half abducted)	Labia majora widely separated, labia minora protruding	Labia majora almost cover labia minora	Labia majora completely cover labia minora	

* If score differs on two sides, take the mean.

From Dubowitz, L. M. S., Dubowitz, V. & Goldberg, C. (1970). Clinical assessment of gestational age in the newborn infant, *Journal of Pediatrics*, 77, 1–10; adapted from Farr and associates (1966) *Developmental Medicine and Child Neurology*, 8, 507.

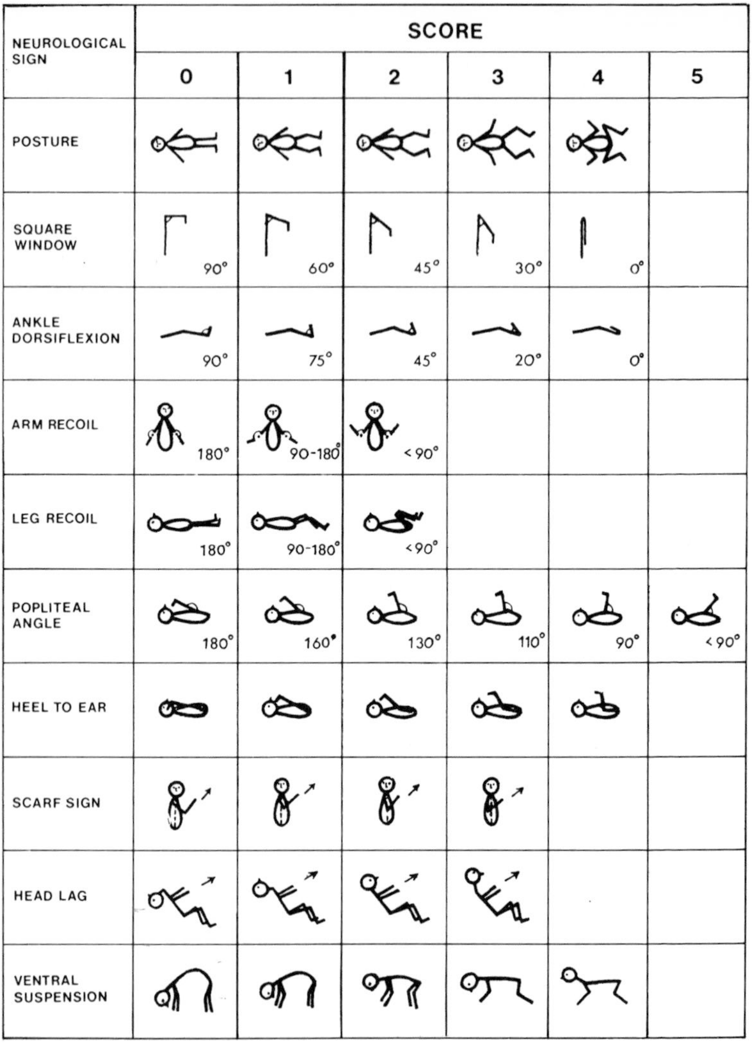

NEUROLOGICAL SIGN	SCORE					
	0	1	2	3	4	5
POSTURE						
SQUARE WINDOW	90°	60°	45°	30°	0°	
ANKLE DORSIFLEXION	90°	75°	45°	20°	0°	
ARM RECOIL	180°	90-180°	<90°			
LEG RECOIL	180°	90-180°	<90°			
POPLITEAL ANGLE	180°	160°	130°	110°	90°	<90°
HEEL TO EAR						
SCARF SIGN						
HEAD LAG						
VENTRAL SUSPENSION						

Fig. 9.5 Scoring system for neurological signs.
(Figures 9.5 and 9.6 are reproduced by kind permission of the authors and C. V. Mosby Company from Dubowitz, L. M. S., Dubowitz, V. & Goldberg, C. (1970). Clinical assessment of gestational age in the newborn infant, *Journal of Pediatrics*, 77, 1–10.)

9.2. Some of these signs are less easy to score than others but in general little difficulty is found. As each sign is explained in the table no further comment will be made here.

Neurological signs

The signs used and the scores given are demonstrated diagrammatically in Figure 9.5. The legend describes the techniques of assessment of the neurological criteria.

Final score

The maximum score of 70 is equally divided between the external characteristics and the neurological signs. The score achieved by an infant is plotted on a graph (Fig. 9.6) which correlates the score with gestational age.

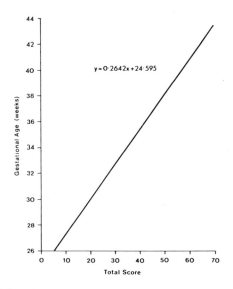

$y = 0.2642x + 24.595$

Fig. 9.6 Graph for calculation of gestational age from total score.

Rapid method of assessment

A simpler more rapid method of assessment which can be carried out even on the very ill baby has been described by Parkin, Hey and Clowes (1976). Their scoring system is based on skin colour, skin texture, breast development and ear firmness (Table 9.4) which enables the gestational age (Table 9.3) to be estimated to within ± 15 days (95% confidence limits) at any time during the first 48 hours of life.

Table 9.3 Calculation of mean gestational ages from the total scores of skin texture, skin colour, breast size and ear firmness

Score	Gestational age Weeks
1	27
2	30
3	33
4	$34\frac{1}{2}$
5	36
6	37
7	$38\frac{1}{2}$
8	$39\frac{1}{2}$
9	40
10	41
11	$41\frac{1}{2}$
12	42

THE PRETERM INFANT

The significance of low birth weight has been discussed earlier in this chapter. Preterm delivery is a major cause of low birth weight and is associated with a greatly increased risk of mortality and morbidity. The degree of risk increases progressively the longer before term that an infant is born. Improved methods of management have increased the chance and quality of survival of even very low birth weight infants but the risk of complications remains sufficiently high to justify every effort being taken to prevent preterm delivery.

Prevention of preterm delivery

Prevention of preterm delivery requires knowledge about the factors which predispose to the onset of labour before term. As knowledge of the factors responsible for the onset of labour at term is incomplete it is not surprising that we are also ignorant about many of the reasons why women go into labour before term.

Factors predisposing to preterm delivery

Some factors are recognized as carrying a high risk of inducing premature labour and these are listed in Table 9.5.

Table 9.4 Scoring system for rapid assessment

	0	1	2	3	4
Skin texture. Tested by picking up a fold of abdominal skin between finger and thumb, and by inspection.	Very thin with a gelatinous feel	Thin and smooth	Smooth and of a medium thickness, irritation rash and superficial peeling may be present	Slight thickening and stiff feeling with superficial cracking and peeling especially evident on the hands and feet	Thick and parchment like with superficial or deep cracking
Skin colour. Estimated by inspection when the baby is quiet	Dark red	Uniformly pink	Pale pink, though the colour may vary over different parts of the body, some parts may be very pale	Pale; nowhere really pink except on the ears, lips, palms and soles	
Breast size. Measured by picking up the breast tissue between finger and thumb.	No breast tissue palpable	Breast tissue palpable on one or both sides, neither being more than 0.5 cm in diameter	Breast tissue palpable on both sides, one or both being 0.5–1 cm in diameter	Breast tissue palpable on both sides, one or both being more than 1 cm in diameter	
Ear firmness. Tested by palpation and folding of the upper pinna	Pinna feels soft and is easily folded into bizarre positions without springing back into position spontaneously	Pinna feels soft along the edge and is easily folded but returns slowly to the correct position spontaneously	Cartilage can be felt to the edge of the pinna though it is thin in places and the pinna springs back readily after being folded	Pinna firm with definite cartilage extending to the periphery, and springs back immediately into position after being folded	

Table 9.5   Factors carrying a high risk of preterm delivery

MATERNAL
  General
    Age: below 20 years
    Height: less than 155 cm
    Poor socioeconomic status
    Heavy workload
    Poor nutrition
    Unmarried
  Obstetric
    Primiparity
    Pre-eclampsia
    Antepartum haemorrhage
    Chronic ill-health
    Smoking
    Previous history of preterm delivery
FETAL
  Multiple pregnancy
  Congenital abnormalities
  Slow intrauterine growth

Preventive measures

Improvement in socioeconomic status. As will be seen some of the factors such as poor social circumstances, poor nutrition and small stature are not amenable to short-term medical treatment. They still constitute a considerable problem in the UK but are a major cause of preterm delivery in developing countries. Raising the general standard of living in a community lowers the incidence of preterm delivery and political or economic efforts to achieve this end are likely to produce a reduction in preterm delivery more readily than advances in medical knowledge.

Antenatal care. Regular and careful supervision during the antenatal period improves the chance of early recognition and treatment of complications of pregnancy which may lead to preterm delivery. Education of the mother in general health care and in the recognition of early warning signs of developing problems will all help to allow improved antenatal care.

Obstetric care. If a mother goes into labour before term every effort should be made to get her to a maternity unit with an intensive-care baby unit for delivery and care of her baby. Mothers must be told in the antenatal clinic of the action they should take should they suspect that labour is starting. The greatly increased risk of delivery of a small preterm infant at home must be stressed. The mother's uterus is the ideal transport incubator for bringing such as infant to hospital.

By the use of beta-agonists such as ritodrine which act as uterine relaxants there is evidence that in many mothers with premature onset of labour delivery can be delayed. Treatment must be carefully supervised and monitored and should be carried out only in a suitably equipped and staffed hospital. This is a further reason for early admission to hospital of mothers who go into labour prematurely.

The method by which a preterm infant is to be delivered must be decided in the light of knowledge of the risk involved with spontaneous vaginal delivery. For instance it may be preferable to deliver primiparous breech presentations by Caesarean section and to use forceps to assist the preterm infant being delivered with the head presenting.

Resuscitation

Midwifery, obstetric, anaesthetic and paediatric staff may be involved in the care of the infant at delivery. It is essential that all those likely to be involved should have been trained in resuscitative procedures and be aware of the need to maintain the infant's body heat. Resuscitative measures are discussed in Chapter 20. When the need for resuscitation is anticipated before delivery an experienced member of the paediatric team should be present in the delivery room. If an emergency arises in the absence of paediatric staff the individual on the spot who is best qualified should be responsible for the vital process of resuscitation.

Warmth

Early cooling can be avoided by drying the infant's skin and by carrying out resuscitation under a suitably designed infant warmer of which a number of varying designs is commercially available.

Transfer to nursery. When the baby is transferred from the labour ward to another hospital, or even to another ward in the same hospital, there is always the danger of hypothermia and such journeys should always take place in a portable incubator. A heated portable incubator, ready for immediate use, should be retained in the labour ward (Fig. 9.7). In the absence of a portable incubator the baby should be wrapped in a warm dry towel or a blanket or enclosed in an aluminium swaddler while being moved (Fig. 20.10).

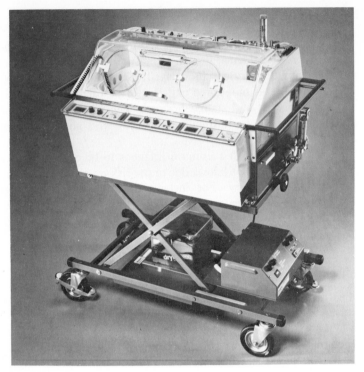

Fig. 9.7 Transport incubator. (Photograph by courtesy of Vickers Medical.)

Specially equipped ambulances are available in some areas to transport preterm infants from home or the smaller district hospitals to the designated regional intensive care unit.

Indications for special care nursery. Not all LBW infants require the facilities of an intensive- or special-care baby unit. It is probable, however, that many infants of 2000 g or less will require extra attention and will be admitted in the first place to special care wards for observation. Any infant over 2000 g who is showing evidence of respiratory difficulty or who is not maintaining his temperature readily should also be in the special care unit until fit for return to mother.

General characteristics of the preterm baby

Appearance

The preterm infant's head and abdomen are large and his thorax

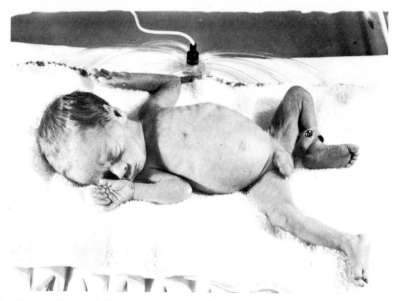

Fig. 9.8 Preterm infant showing large head and abdomen.

small (Fig. 9.8). The skin is soft in texture and pink in colour. The forehead may be wrinkled, and frequently in the very small baby the veins of the head show prominently. In the female the labia minora are visible and not hidden by the labia majora as in the term infant. The testes have often not descended into the scrotum in the preterm male infant. A generalized lack of subcutaneous tissue results in prominence of the body skeleton.

Activity

The preterm baby is commonly described as being inactive and as sleeping throughout the day except when disturbed for feeding. In point of fact there are few preterm babies who are absolutely still even in sleep. If a preterm baby is observed in an incubator his breathing will be seen to be rhythmical but not wholly regular. His abdominal muscles are constantly moving. Every now and again a limb will flex and relax. At one time he may be seen lying on his back, his arms lazily outstretched and at another lying easily on his side, his lower limbs gently flexed at hips and knees. Occasionally a very small infant shows remarkable activity during the first day or two of life after which his behaviour resembles that of other larger preterm babies. In the course of time increasing bodily vigour affords unmistakable evidence of growing strength.

Changes after birth

Weight. After birth there is usually loss of weight. For a variable period extending over a number of days there is a progressive slight loss of subcutaneous tissue, usually evident in the face, trunk and limbs. Reversal of the trend is gradual and dependent upon the ability to achieve adequate nutritional intakes. Commonly the presence of oedema hides the loss of subcutaneous tissue and gives spuriously high body weights.

Muscle tone. As tissue tone improves, muscle groups become more clearly defined. This is first evident in the calf muscles. The nasolabial and other skin folds become more prominent about the same time. Later, but only slowly, the musculature and related tissues increase in bulk, until eventually the face becomes chubby.

Respiration. For some time after birth, respiration is often irregularly erratic in rate, rhythm and amplitude. A more constant pattern slowly evolves, but breathing remains essentially abdominal in character.

Changes in activity. In the course of time activity increases in vigour, and this is reflected in the increasing strength of the cry and in the growing determination with which nourishment is taken. As body tone increases, the infant periodically indulges in a slow, deliberate stretching of the entire body reminiscent of an adult awakening from a satisfying sleep. Yawning is characteristic and sneezing common.

Jaundice. As compared with that in the term infant jaundice is often both more pronounced and more prolonged (Chapter 15). Jaundice in the small preterm baby must always be kept under close observation and kernicterus prevented by early treatment (Chapter 15).

Nursing care

The most significant factor in the survival of a LBW infant is the standard of nursing care provided to meet his requirements. Advances in the understanding of physiological processes and the provision of complicated electronic equipment help to improve the service which the nurse provides but do not replace it. This aspect of the care of the preterm infant is so important that a separate chapter (Chapter 10) is devoted to it.

Feeding

Importance

During the third trimester of pregnancy the fetus begins to 'store' nutrient materials such as fat (subcutaneous and brown fat) and the carbohydrate glycogen. Infants born prematurely and particularly those born during the second trimester have very limited supplies of energy as shown in Table 9.6. There are also very limited quantities of fat soluble vitamins and minerals in VLBW infants. Unless nutrient materials are supplied within an hour or two of birth the tissues of the VLBW infant will begin to break down and the infant will be in a catabolic condition. A major concern of all involved in caring for the preterm infant is the prevention of tissue catabolism and this is achieved by early feeding with a balanced diet. The diet required to prevent tissue destruction and to promote growth will depend not only on the size of the infant at birth but also on tissue and organ maturity and on the infant's ability to tolerate the feed. Feeding is essential for the further growth of all infants and is of particular importance to the preterm infant. This is because the very high intrauterine rate of growth and development can only be achieved after birth with a high intake of the factors essential for growth. Among other things these include fluid, energy sources and amino acids. Most preterm infants cannot accept their full requirements of all these factors immediately after birth and feeding has to be adjusted very carefully to make sure that the infant receives as much as he can tolerate of an appropriate food until he is able to take sufficient to re-establish a normal rate of growth.

Table 9.6 Body compositions of preterm and term infants at birth

Gestational age (wk)	22	26	29	40
Weight (g)	500	1000	1500	3500
Water (g)	433	850	1240	2380
Fat (g)	6	23	60	525
CHO (g)	2	5	15	34
Protein (g)	36	85	125	390
Total energy (kcal)	225	670	1295	6455
MJ	0.95	2.82	5.44	27.1

Changed policy. Earlier and more liberal feeding of preterm infants is now a generally accepted policy. Previously the risks attached to early feeding, which included the possibility of aspiration after vomiting a feed, were considered too great to justify feeding before the third or fourth day. Now it is clear that the harm caused by delayed feeding, with the resultant metabolic acidosis, hypoglycaemia, jaundice and serious brain damage, is greater than the risks of early feeding, which, with a good standard of supervision, are relatively low.

Early feeding

The policy of early feeding has resulted in an improvement in growth and later neurological development. There has also been a fall in such problems as hypoglycaemia and jaundice.

The first feed. The first feed should be given as early as possible in keeping with the infant's condition and before three hours of age.

Method

Infants of over 35 weeks' gestation who weigh more then 2000 g will generally have little difficulty in feeding from the breast or from a bottle.

Infants of about 32 to 35 weeks' gestation may be able to take some feeds by bottle particularly during the first day or two, but as they become quickly tired by bottle feeding they must be supervised very carefully and tube-fed before they become exhausted.

Tube feeding will be required at some stage for most infants of less than 35 weeks' gestation and for some more mature infants. The risks of this method have been greatly reduced since the introduction of disposable feeding tubes which can be left in place for longer periods. Complications of tube feeding do still occur and must always be borne in mind. They include faulty passage of a tube into the trachea with a major risk of the infant's death if a feed is given before the mistake has been recognized. In the smallest and illest babies gastric distension may prove a problem and result in aspiration after vomiting. This risk can be diminished by nasojejunal or transpyloric feeding. Weight gain is rapid as the entire feed is retained. Leaving a nasogastric tube in place for long periods leads to the risk of ulceration of the nose or pharynx and of perforation of the stomach. Repeated withdrawal of a tube increases the risk of aspiration. Most of these dangers can be reduced by good nursing technique. The nursing aspects of tube feeding are dealt with in Chapter 10.

Frequency. As discussed in Chapter 8 the frequency of feeding will depend upon the volume of feed which the infant can tolerate at an individual feed. This volume of tolerance will increase progressively but as the infant's total volume requirements may not be reached for two to three weeks after birth small and frequent feeds are likely to be required by most preterm infants. For the smallest, of the order of 1000 g, a continuous intragastric infusion is required. Others will require half-hourly, hourly, two-hourly or three-hourly feeds according to the volume which they can tolerate. The interval between feeds is progressively increased as the volume tolerated per feed increases. Most mothers find it difficult to give more than eight feeds a day when their baby returns home, and the feeding regimen should be arranged to bring the total number of feeds down to this by the time of baby's discharge.

Volumes. Guidelines only can be given as to the total volume of feed to be given in the 24 hours. Much will depend upon the infant's capacity to tolerate these volumes and this capacity may vary from day to day with changes in the infant's condition. Preterm infants have a greater fluid and energy requirement than term infants. Total 24 hour volumes on the first day should be of the order of 30 to 50 ml per kg.

For example an infant of 30 weeks gestation weighing 1.5 kg at birth could be offered continuous intragastric tube feeding of 3 ml an hour for the first 24 hours increasing to 4 ml an hour on day 2. Thereafter volumes should increase as indicated in Fig. 9.9 according to the infant's well-being and tolerance. As the volume tolerated increases, the total volume is increased. Individual infants may tolerate bolus feeds at one- or two-hourly intervals later in the first week of life, whereas others may have to be maintained on continuous infusion for some weeks. The skill and art of the neonatal nurse is critical in the evaluation of each infant's requirements and when this transition can be safely accomplished.

If at any stage vomiting, abdominal distension or other sign of distress occurs the programme has to be readjusted so that baby receives more frequent smaller feeds which allow the same total daily intake without causing problems.

Milk

Composition. Giving an infant a suitable volume of feed is only an indication of satisfactory nutrition if the feed is of a satisfactory composition. As stated in Chapter 8 human breast milk can be accepted as having a model content for the feeding of human

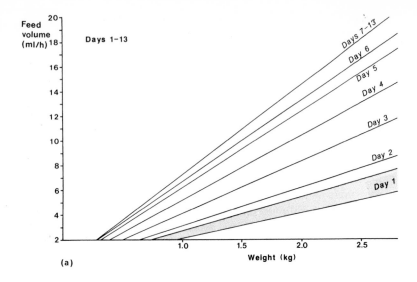

(a)

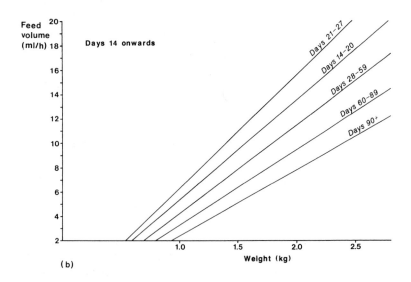

(b)

Fig. 9.9 (a) A guide to the hourly volume (ml/hr) of food required by LBW infants during the first two weeks of life. On day 1 the line below the stippled area gives the volumes recommended for appropriately grown preterm infants. The line above the stippled area gives the volumes recommended for light-for-dates infants. (b) A guide to the hourly volume (ml/hr) of feed required by LBW infants from day 14 onwards.

infants. No completely satisfactory substitute has been marketed but many preterm infants can thrive satisfactorily on the modification of cow's milk.

Breast milk. Experience suggests that breast milk is important for all babies including VLBW babies. Whilst fresh milk from the infant's own mother is preferable, pooled human milk fulfils an important nutrient and some protective function. The freezing and pasteurization of expressed breast milk may cause destruction of the antimicrobial properties of human breast milk and therefore reduce the protective benefits of feeding with breast milk (Chapter 8).

Modified cow's milk. Where human milk either from the infant's own mother or from a breast-milk bank is not available modified cow's milk may be used for feeding LBW infants. Unmodified cow's milks are not suitable and should never be used (Chapter 8). Suitable modified cow's milk preparation and their compositions are shown in Table 9.7.

Energy. Satisfactory weight gain is generally achieved and maintained on a daily intake of 460 to 500 kJ per kg per day (110 to 130 kcal per kg). Human breast milk has 280 kJ per dl (67 kcal per 100 ml) and it is advisable when feeding the VLBW infant to use the higher energy content feeds together with fresh human milk. It is our practice to give mother's fresh colostrum/milk during the first week and then to add artificial formulae to replace up to 50% of the total volume intake indicated in Fig. 9.9.

Protein. Mature human breast milk contains approximately 1.5 g protein per 100 ml. A preterm infant requires a minimum protein intake of 2 g per kg per day and cannot tolerate more than 6 g per kg per day. A preterm infant fed on breast milk must therefore take 150 ml per kg per day before his minimum protein requirements are satisfied.

Minerals. The mineral content of breast milk (0.2%) is lower than that of unmodified cow's milk (0.7%). Although increasing the solute load adds problems to the feeding of preterm infants, the increased quantities of sodium, calcium, phosphorus and other minerals are necessary to ensure adequate growth and bone mineralization.

It must be remembered that enteral feeding of the preterm infants is an unphysiological procedure. Trying to mimic the nutrition which the immature infant would have received in utero via the placenta, using the immature gut and associated organs to

Table 9.7 Nutritional comparison of preterm infant formulae available in the UK. Comparison per 100 ml.

		OSTERPREM (Farley Health Products)	NENATAL[a] (Cow & Gate)	PREAPTAMIL[a] (Milupa)	PREMATALAC[a] (Cow & Gate)	SMA LOW[a] BIRTH WEIGHT (Wyeth)	MATURE HUMAN MILK DHSS[b]	MATURE HUMAN MILK Macy et al[c]
Macronutrients								
Protein†	g	2.0	1.8	2.1	2.4	2.0	1.34	1.45
Fat	g	4.9	4.5	3.6	5.0	4.4	4.2	3.8
		(veg oils + milk fat)	(veg oils + milk fat + MCT)	(veg oils + milk fat)	(veg oils + milk fat)	(Beef oleo + veg oils + MCT)		
Saturated	%	39.5	48	46.9	47.5	48.9	50.1	52
Unsaturated	%	60.5	52	53.1	52.5	50.9	48.5	48
Carbohydrate*** (as disaccharide)								
Lactose	g	7.0	7.0	8.3	6.3	8.2	7.0	7.0
Maltodextrin	g	6.0	2.3	8.3	6.3	4.1	—	—
Glucose	g	1.0	2.6	—	—	4.1	—	—
	g	—	2.1			—		
Energy	kcal	80	76	74	79	80	70	68
	kJ	334	318	308	330	334	293	285
Minerals								
Sodium	mg	45	20	35	60	32	15	15
Potassium	mg	65	60	80	95	75	60	55
Chloride	mg	60	40	43	80	53	43	43
Calcium	mg	70	100	60	67	75	35	33
Magnesium	mg	5	15	7	11	7	2.8	4
Phosphorus	mg	35	50	45	53	40	15	15
Trace elements								
Iron	µg	40	800	700	650	670	76	150
Copper	µg	120	80	10	50	70	39	40
Manganese	µg	3	—	10	10	20	ND	0.7
Zinc	µg	1000	800	100	400	500	295	530
Iodine	µg	7	20	—	4	8.3	7	7

		133	107	132	169	128	88	91
Potential renal solute load*	mOsm/l							
Vitamins								
Vitamin A	μg	100	80	150	80	96	60	53
Vitamin D	μg	8.0	3.0	1.1	1.1	1.3	0.01	0.01
Vitamin E	mg**	10.0	4.0	1.25	1.0	1.0	0.35	0.56
Vitamin K	μg	7	—	—	3.2	7.0	ND	1.7
Vitamin B1	μg	95	90	100	70	80	16	16
Vitamin B2	μg	180	150	100	100	130	31	42.6
Niacin/Niacinamide	μg	1000	900	1250	850	630	230	172
Vitamin B6	μg	100	70	100	80	50	6	11
Vitamin B12	μg	0.2	0.2	0.28	0.12	0.2	0.01	Trace
Folic Acid	μg	50.0	13	12.5	3.5	10.0	5.2	0.18
Pantothenic Acid/ Calcium Pantothenate	μg	500	500	1250	250	360	260	196
Biotin	μg	2.0	1.0	3.85	3.1	1.8	0.76	0.4
Vitamin C	mg	28.0	12	12.5	6.5	7.0	3.8	4.3
Other								
Choline	mg	5.6	25	—	5.6	16.5	ND	9.0
Inositol	mg	3.2	130	—	—	—	ND	39.0
Taurine	mg	5.1	—	—	—	—	4.8	ND
Carnitine	mg	1.0	—	—	—	—	ND	ND
Osmolality	mOsm/kg	300	340	350	342	268		

* Method of Ziegler and Fomon, 1971; Calculated values
† Total Nitrogen × 6.38
** 1 mg vitamin E = 1.5 iu
*** Some manufacturers quote carbohydrate as monosaccharide; in these cases, the values have been converted to disaccharide.

Sources
a Manufacturers' information (1980 and 1981)
b DHSS Reports on Health and Social Subjects
  Nos 12 (1977) and 18 (1980).
c Macy, Kelly and Sloan, 1953 and Mettler, 1976
ND Not determined

Manufacturers and Parent Companies
Farley Health Products Ltd. (The BOOTS Company PLC UK)
Cow & Gate Ltd. (NV Nutricia, Holland)
John Wyeth and Brother Ltd. (American Home Products, U.S.A.)
Milupa Ltd. (Altana AG, West Germany)

Published by kind permission of Dr Ian Barr and **FARLEY HEALTH PRODUCTS** (The Boots Company PLC UK) digest and absorb milks of varying composition, is no easy task. The successes achieved are a remarkable testament to man's ingenuity and to the inherent survival capacity of the human infant.

Parenteral feeding

The ability of infants to tolerate gastric feeds may be so limited that they cannot be given an adequate intake by this method. This is most likely to occur in infants who have respiratory or other problems. In such circumstances fluid must be given parenterally. For short periods simple solutions such as dextrose/mineral solutions may suffice, but in the volume required they cannot alone provide sufficient energy for temperature regulation and growth. Much has yet to be learned about the total intravenous feeding of small preterm infants with amino acid and lipid preparations and as an adjunct to enteral nutrition. The reader is referred to the further reading list for more information.

Since the more extensive use of feeding by constant infusion of breast milk and special preterm formulae into the stomach or jejunum the need for parenteral feeding of very small but healthy infants has been greatly reduced.

A feed chart should be kept for each infant showing the time, the type of feed, the volume given, the method by which it was given and how the infant reacted. In addition the total volume of feed given in each 24-hour period should be calculated and recorded. It is very useful to have this total volume recorded daily so that the infant's weight can be checked against the volume of intake.

As most infants who are not breast fed will be receiving a standard feed it is essential that the composition of that feed — its energy, protein, vitamin and mineral content — should be known to those in charge of feeding so that a check on these factors can be kept.

Supplements

As explained in Chapter 8 the vitamin and iron content of both human and cow's milk is not generally sufficient to supply the requirements of the preterm infant during his most rapid period of growth. Vitamin supplements should be given from ten days of age and continued during the first year of life. In the authors' unit the supplements given to preterm infants are from oral preparations readily available in the UK. In other countries different commercial preparations are used. Our current policy is as follows: from day 10 all LBW infants receive a half of a Ketovite* tablet crushed and added to the feed together with 0.4 ml Childrens Vitamin Drops BPC. This provides vitamin A (2000 IU), vitamin D (800 IU), vitamin C (70 mg), folic acid (125 μg) and other B group vitamins. Additional vitamin E 25 mg/day is given orally as tocopherol succinate for the first six weeks of life. For further information see page 473.

Opinions differ as to the need for iron supplementation for breast-fed infants and there may be a disadvantage in introducing supplementary iron too early. It is suggested that supplements of iron should be commenced at the age of one month (30 mg Fe/day) and continued during the first year of life. Such supplements are given to prevent the late anaemia of prematurity (Chapter 18).

Complications of preterm delivery

The complications associated with preterm delivery are really a reflection of the structural and functional immaturity of the individual organs of the baby as compared with their counterparts in an infant who has gone to term. The cerebral and brain-stem centres share in this immaturity of development and theoretically it can be argued that neurological immaturity contributes in varying degree to most of the handicaps experienced by the preterm baby. Although the implications of immature development of the peripheral, sympathetic, parasympathetic and central nervous systems are not fully understood, knowledge concerning other factors giving rise to handicap are more precise.

The principal handicaps in question relate to temperature control, respiratory, renal and alimentary function. Additional to these are the immature infant's liability to haemorrhage, anaemia, jaundice, infection and hypoglycaemia.

Hypothermia

Core temperature. Throughout this chapter reference is frequently made to the need to prevent loss of heat from preterm infants so

---

* Paines and Byrne Ltd, Greenford, Middlesex.

that body temperature can be maintained. The most significant body temperature is that which applies to the internal organs and which is referred to as core or central temperature. Skin, or superficial, temperature is dependent on a number of factors which may change rapidly. Core temperature changes more slowly and, particularly in small preterm infants, is affected by skin temperature. In a satisfactory environment (Table 9.8) core temperature will remain stable within a small range of normal and skin temperature will not differ by more than 0.5 °C from core temperature. An environment which satisfies these conditions is called a neutral thermal environment and is the environment which we should aim at creating for all low birth-weight infants (Chapter 5). The precise conditions required for a neutral thermal environment may be slightly different for each infant and therefore the situation has to be assessed separately for each baby.

Table 9.8 Suggested incubator temperatures for unclothed infants

Weight of infant (kg)	Temperature of incubator (°C)
1	35
2	34
3	33

Heat loss. The means by which infants produce and lose heat have already been discussed in Chapter 5. Preterm infants are able to produce heat by metabolic activity including the burning of brown fat. Unless they are in a suitable environment, however, their ability to produce heat is readily overburdened by the ease with which they lose heat. Heat loss takes place from the skin by radiation, convection, conduction and evaporation of moisture; heat is also lost from the lungs and airways, and the urine and faeces. The relatively larger surface area increases skin loss and the lack of subcutaneous fat means that the deeper tissues are less well insulated from the effect of fall in skin temperature. Hypoxia is accompanied by reduced metabolic activity and a fall in body temperature.

Neonatal cold injury. Loss of heat greater than that which can be replaced by the infant leads to hypothermia. Initially this is evident as lowering of skin temperature and later as a fall in core temperature. If the fall in skin temperature can be corrected

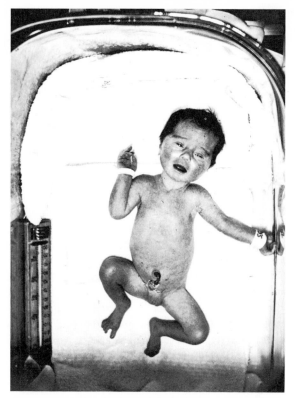

Fig. 9.10 Neonatal cold injury with sclerema (hardening) of subcutaneous tissues.

rapidly the fall in central temperature can be prevented. Severe hypothermia with progressive fall in core temperature is a serious complication and may be irreversible. Before the dangers of hypothermia were fully appreciated infants developed what was called neonatal cold injury in which the subcutaneous tissues particularly of the cheeks, buttocks and limbs became increasingly firm until movement was prevented (Fig. 9.10). Such infants often had very low blood sugars, bowel movement ceased, and internal haemorrhages occurred. Death was common. Treatment in the later stages was seldom successful and the only useful line of management is prevention of heat loss and the recognition of early stages of fall in skin temperature.

The significance with regard to nursing techniques and medical procedures is discussed in Chapters 10 and 20.

Respiratory distress

Embarrassment of respiratory function may manifest itself in rapid shallow respirations, attacks of cyanosis, increased subcostal recession, movement of the alae nasi, or periods of apnoea. The underlying problem may be in the respiratory system but is not necessarily so. Since the diaphragm is the main muscle involved and the thoracic cage is soft, any obstruction to the airway will produce marked subcostal, intercostal and suprasternal indrawing. The diminished cough reflex creates difficulty in clearing mucus or other matter blocking the trachea or bronchus. Extra muscular effort is required and the infant may become exhausted. Inefficient oxygen exchange may occur in the alveoli because of inadequacy of the pulmonary vascular circulation. Any depression of central nervous function reduces muscle activity including respiration. This in turn may be due to a wide variety of conditions including hypoxia and haemorrhage.

Idiopathic respiratory distress syndrome (RDS) will be discussed in greater detail in Chapter 16. RDS is a major cause of death in immature infants. The disorder is related to immaturity of the lungs, being rare in term infants, and occurring with increasing frequency and severity at decreasing gestational ages. Sixty per cent of VLBW infants develop respiratory distress syndrome of varying severity. With the introduction of modern methods of intensive care mortality figures have fallen steadily. Factors which probably predispose to respiratory distress syndrome are intrauterine hypoxia and antepartum haemorrhage. Other possible factors are maternal diabetes and Caesarean delivery. Though the aetiology of the condition is not fully understood, it seems clear that absence from the lungs of surfactant (Chapter 16) plays an important part. There is also increased pulmonary vascular resistance and reduced pulmonary blood flow, leading to right-to-left shunting of blood, arterial hypoxaemia, and cyanosis.

Apnoeic attacks occur in 70–80% of VLBW infants and may be associated with RDS, infection, hypoxaemia, intracranial haemorrhage, hypoglycaemia and patent ductus arteriosus but frequently there is no obvious cause. Increasing the oxygen concentration of inspired air or giving theophylline (see Chapter 16) may diminish the frequency of apnoeic attacks. Continuous positive airways pressure applied through nasal cannulae or face mask may reduce the frequency of apnoeic episodes. Intermittent positive pressure ventilation is indicated for prolonged or recurrent apnoea. Respir-

atory depression and apnoeic attacks resulting from maternal analgesia with pethidine may be relieved by the intramuscular injection
of naloxone 0.02 mg per kg.

Hypoglycaemia, which is common in light-for-dates babies, also
occurs in preterm babies during the first 72 hours of life, but may
develop in any baby under stress as, for example, in the respiratory
distress syndrome, congestive cardiac failure, following exchange
blood transfusion and in association with perinatal asphyxia.
Hypoglycaemia may also be found in babies of diabetic mothers
and also in infants heavier than the 90th percentile. As mentioned
previously, early feeding of preterm babies has been adopted to
overcome the problem of hypoglycaemia.

In view of the high incidence of hypoglycaemia in the LBW
infants, especially in VLBW infants, measurement of blood glucose
levels using Dextrostix or BM Test Glycemie 20/800 readings
should be obtained two- to three-hourly for the first 12 hours and
then every four hours thereafter depending on the results. Treatment of hypoglycaemia is discussed in Chapter 16.

Renal dysfunction

The kidneys play an essential part in the maintenance of the body's
water and mineral content. Although the preterm infant's body
contains relatively more water than does that of the term infant
(Table 9.6) this extra water does not protect the immature infant
from readily becoming dehydrated. The capacity for preterm
infants to concentrate and dilute their urine and to modify their
mineral salt excretion is somewhat limited but by no means absent
(Chapter 5). There is therefore a narrower range of tolerance of
water and mineral load.

Dietary load. The important lesson to be learned is that great
care has to be taken in assessing the fluid and electrolyte state of
preterm infants. Evidence of oedema or dehydration indicates that
the range of the kidney's tolerance has been exceeded. By a better
understanding of an infant's requirements for fluid and minerals
and by arranging management accordingly it should be possible to
avoid these signs of failure to respect the considerable but limited
ability of the preterm infant's kidneys to deal with the load
presented to it. By ensuring good central and peripheral circulation
and encouraging growth by providing a balanced nutrient intake
the load on the immature glomeruli and tubules can be kept to a
minimum.

Digestive problems

In the matter of alimentary function the preterm infant is subject to both mechanical and secretory handicaps. Immature development of the submucosal and myenteric nerve plexuses and the muscular layer of the alimentary tract makes for ineffective neuromuscular control, which may account for regurgitation of feeds, passage of loose stools and possibly functional intestinal obstruction. In addition there are many neuropeptide hormones such as gastrin, cholecystokinin and vasoactive intestinal peptide produced in the gastrointestinal tract and which influence gastrointestinal motility and digestive secretions. Identical peptide hormones are found in the thalamus and other areas of the brain and their interrelationship with appetite, nutrition and growth are the subject of much current investigation.

The physical effort involved in sucking may prove too exhausting and tube feeding may be necessary. The ability of a preterm infant to digest and absorb food within a few hours of birth is evident from the success achieved with early feeding.

Limit of tolerance. It is clear, however, that there is a limit of tolerance which applies both as to the volume given at one feed and the amount of the individual constituents of the diet. Much attention has been paid in the past to the fat and protein content of the preterm infant's feed. It is now also recognized that until the enzyme systems of the small intestine are fully developed there is a limit to the infant's tolerance for carbohydrates such as lactose.

Functional intestinal obstruction produces the signs of an intestinal obstruction without an organic obstruction to the bowel being demonstrable. The abdomen becomes distended (Fig. 9.11) and bile-stained fluid is aspirated from the stomach or is vomited. There is delay in the passage of meconium. The condition often clears spontaneously within 24 to 48 hours, sometimes after the passage of a mucus plug (Fig. 9.12). A gastrografin enema given under careful supervision will help to exclude Hirschsprung's disease (Chapter 19) or other organic abnormality and frequently hastens the passage of meconium and the return of normal bowel function.

Necrotizing enterocolitis is also associated with signs of intestinal obstruction but is a much more serious condition with a considerable mortality. Signs of obstruction are present and the infant is seriously ill. Radiological examination may show gas present in the intestinal wall. Haemorrhagic necrosis of the bowel wall may lead

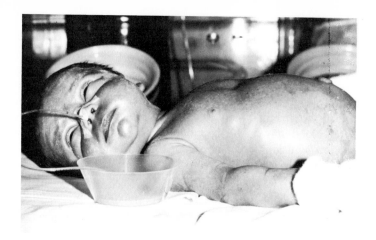

Fig. 9.11 Abdominal distension due to functional intestinal obstruction.

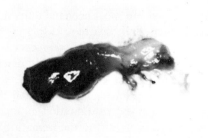

Fig. 9.12 Mucus plug passed by baby shown in Fig. 9.11 with relief of functional obstruction.

to perforation. Treatment is by gastric aspiration, intravenous fluids and systemic antibiotics. Laparotomy will be indicated if signs of perforation develop. As stated previously, breast feeding affords a degree of protection against the development of necrotizing enterocolitis.

Haemorrhage

The various factors responsible for bleeding will be fully discussed in Chapter 18. Two factors in particular favour bleeding — pronounced fragility and abnormal permeability of the capillaries together with delay or failure of blood clot formation.

Cerebral haemorrhage. Intraventricular haemorrhage, which occurs most commonly in male infants of less than 35 weeks' gestation, may be associated with fragile and poorly supported vessels in the germinal matrix of the brain, hypoxia and disordered cerebral blood flow. The commonest clinical signs are apnoeic attacks, convulsions, or unexplained deterioration. Mortality is high and in those who survive a ventricular haemorrhage a not-infrequent complication is obstructive hydrocephalus signalled by a rapid increase in head size, vomiting and possibly convulsions (Chapter 13).

Infection

The susceptibility of the pattern baby to infection is far greater even than that of the term infant. Infection has already been touched on earlier in this chapter and is discussed at length in Chapter 14.

Gram-negative infection. In most neonatal units in the UK Gram-negative organisms such as *E. coli* have displaced staphylococci as the commonest pathogens. Group B streptococcus is a particular hazard for the preterm infant and in some nurseries is now the major infecting organism and cause of mortality and morbidity from infection. *Pseudomonas aeruginosa* — which flourishes in wet apparatus such as incubators, resuscitation equipment and ventilators — is another serious hazard to the immature baby. Since the signs of infection in the newborn are often non-specific, such infections should be suspected whenever a preterm baby becomes ill or has apnoeic attacks without any other obvious cause. In these circumstances it is wise to obtain cultures of blood, cerebrospinal fluid and urine, to obtain nose, throat and umbilical swabs, and, without waiting for the results of the cultures, to start treatment with systemic antibiotics. Monilial infections are more common in preterm than in term infants especially those given antibiotics and such infections may readily invade the bloodstream when there are indwelling cannulae or catheters.

Jaundice

Functional immaturity of the liver with defective conjugation of bilirubin accounts for the high levels of unconjugated bilirubin in the preterm baby. There is an increasing risk of kernicterus, causing death or permanent brain damage with the possible eventual development of microcephaly, deafness, athetoid cerebral palsy and mental handicap as the serum bilirubin level rises (Chapter 15). Kernicterus is more likely to occur if the baby is hypoxic or acidotic. In seriously ill babies kernicterus may occur at lower serum bilirubin levels. Exchange blood transfusion should be carried out if the serum bilirubin approaches a dangerous level.

Prevention. Clinical experience has taught that infants are less likely to develop a high bilirubin level if they are given adequate nutrition. By exposing susceptible infants to a source of blue light dangerous levels of hyperbilirubinaemia can generally be prevented (Chapter 15).

Prognosis of preterm delivery

It is extremely difficult to compare mortality statistics of VLBW infants from different neonatal units and different parts of the world because of the ambiguity surrounding the use of the word 'viability'. However, if all infants of 500 g and above with a heart beat or respiratory gasp at birth are considered liveborn, as is proposed by WHO, then the figures will be directly comparable. Over the last 20 years the mortality of infants weighing 1001 to 1500 g has fallen considerably and is now in the region of 15%.

The more recent introduction of neonatal intensive care has also improved the prognosis for those weighing 501 to 1000 g due to the better management of respiratory problems especially respiratory distress syndrome. In the best centres survival rates of 50% and more occur with low levels of handicap in the survivors.

Low birth weight babies who are of appropriate weight-for-dates should continue to develop normally after birth so long as their nutritional requirements are met and they are protected from the hazards associated with preterm delivery. Even so, children who were born too soon do show some impairment of performance when they reach school age but not to the extent recorded in earlier studies which reported cerebral palsy, blindness and deafness in up to 30% of surviving preterm infants. These handicapping conditions and the associated mental retardation have been greatly reduced as a consequence of the early relief of birth asphyxia, the maintenance of body heat and the introduction of correct feeding. Recent follow-up studies have reported major handicap in less than 10% of surviving infants.

Follow-up. Low birth weight babies should be seen regularly in the follow-up clinic for developmental examinations including assessment of hearing and vision, so that any neurodevelopmental deficits can be detected and treated as soon as possible. To enable direct comparison of follow-up studies of VLBW infants and to avoid future confusion it has been suggested that the number of children with major handicaps (cerebral palsy, low IQ, severe deafness and impaired vision) and minor handicaps (conditions bordering on normality) should be expressed as a proportion of all VLBW livebirths (handicap rate) and that the ratio of normal to handicapped survivors (handicap ratio) should be reported separately. The importance of the long-term follow-up for preterm babies is discussed in Chapter 21.

Ethical considerations. It is important that the new technologies are not used to prolong the process of dying. With improved management of respiratory problems brain-damaged infants, who previously would have died, are surviving. Because of the increased risks of mental and physical handicap in the very immature infant neonatal intensive care methods must be kept under constant review.

GROWTH RETARDED INFANTS

The light-for-dates (LFD) infant and the preterm infant have in common the problems associated with lack of nutritional reserve such as hypoglycaemia and hypothermia. However, the brain and other body organs of the LFD infant will be at a maturity commensurate with the gestational age so that given that there are no major congenital abnormalities these LFD infants will thrive if given adequate nutrition.

Intrauterine growth retardation

Causes of slow intrauterine growth are shown in Table 9.9. It will be noted that there is a close similarity between this table and Table 9.5 which shows factors carrying a high risk of preterm onset of labour.

General characteristics of the light-for-dates infant

Light-for-dates infants may be delivered before, at or after term, the only criterion being that they lie below the 10th percentile for

Table 9.9 Causes of intrauterine growth failure

MATERNAL
  General
    Poor socioeconomic conditions
      Malnutrition
      Heavy workload
        Unmarried
    Height: less than 155 cm
    Living at high altitudes
    Racial and constitutional
    History of previous light-for-dates infants
    Maternal metabolic disorder
  Obstetric
    Complications of pregnancy (e.g. preeclampsia)
    Poor placental function
    Alcohol consumption
    Smoking
    Poor antenatal care
    Parity first or third onwards
FETAL
    Multiple pregnancy
    Congenital abnormalities
    Chromosomal abnormality
    Congenital infection

weight for their gestational age. Some of these infants will have been malnourished late in pregnancy and are often of normal length but underweight for that length (Fig. 9.13). When fetal growth retardation is detected from before 28 weeks by fetal ultrasound it is likely that at birth the infant's weight and body size (length and OFC) will be small, i.e. small for date. Such small-for-dates

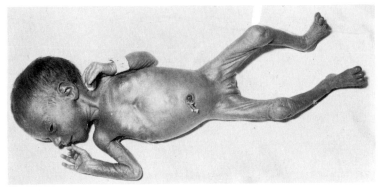

Fig. 9.13 Light-for-dates malnourished infant showing lack of subcutaneous fat and dry skin.

Table 9.10 Contrasting features of appropriate-for-dates preterm and light-for-dates malnourished infants

Feature	Preterm	Light-for-dates
Definition	Born before 37 weeks' gestation	Birth-weight below 10th percentile for gestational age
Vernix	Present in variable amounts	Little or absent
Skin	Red and transparent	Dry, folds of lax skin
Subcutaneous tissue	Sparse	Sparse
Skull	Bones soft and pliable	Bones less pliable
Facies	Doll-like	Mature
Abdomen	Prominent	Usually flat or scaphoid
Cord	Thick and fleshy	Thin, flabby and stained
Cry	Feeble	Mature
Muscle tone	Hyptonic, frog-like position	Variable. Usually active
Complications	Hypothermia	Hypoglycaemia
	Respiratory distress syndrome	Hypocalcaemia
	Infection	Hypothermia
	Cerebral haemorrhage	
	Jaundice	

(SFD) infants may have congenital abnormalities including chromosomal abnormalities such as trisomies 15, 18 and 21.

The contrasting features of preterm appropriate-for-dates and light-for-dates malnourished infants are shown in Table 9.10.

Appearance of malnourished infant

The skin is dry, coarse and inelastic, and shows signs of cracking or desquamation especially over the abdomen and on the dorsa of the feet and hands (Figs. 9.14, 9.15). In the severe case the face

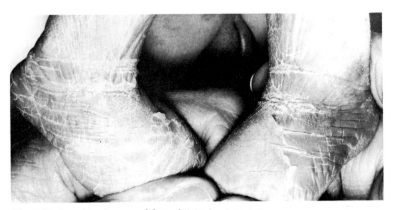

Fig. 9.14 Dry skin dorsum of feet of light-for-dates infant.

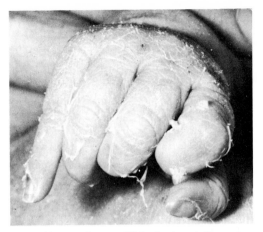

Fig. 9.15 Dry scaly skin over fingers of light-for-dates infant.

is wizened and the expression surprisingly mature and alert. Variations in the clinical picture have been related to the duration of the detrimental influences.

Other occasional findings include a scaphoid abdomen, and (in babies with a preceding history of fetal distress) green or yellow discoloration of the umbilical cord and nails. Should signs of persistent respiratory distress develop within a few hours of birth the possibility of meconium aspiration or group B streptococcal pneumonia must be considered.

Feeding

The LFD baby will usually be able to suck and swallow satisfactorily. Early and adequate feeding is especially important in the LFD baby to correct metabolic acidosis, prevent hypoglycaemia and lessen the degree of physiological jaundice. Human milk is an entirely satisfactory food and produces adequate growth during the first year of life. The introduction of early mixed feeding is therefore both unnecessary and undesirable.

Complications associated with the light-for-dates baby

Hypoglycaemia

The LFD baby is particularly subject to hypoglycaemia during the first 48 hours of life as a direct consequence of insufficient stores of energy-producing glycogen. Other important factors which contribute to the hypoglycaemia are the high consumption of glucose by the relatively large brain and disordered insulin secretion as may occur in the infants of diabetic mothers (Chapter 17).

Asymptomatic. Blood-glucose levels are considerably lower in the first weeks of life than later, but in the LFD baby particularly they may reach dangerously low levels, usually on the second and third days of life. Although hypoglycaemia is defined as a true blood-glucose level below 1.2 mmol per 1 (20 mg per 100 ml) many babies have a lower blood-glucose level without ever exhibiting any abnormal signs or symptoms and probably do not develop any long-term neurological damage.

Symptomatic. On the other hand, hypoglycaemia accompanied by unresponsiveness, periods of lethargy, failure to suck, apnoeic and cyanotic attacks and fits is associated with a considerable risk of permanent brain damage and intellectual retardation. Such symptomatic hypoglycaemia should not only be actively treated but also prevented and detected before symptoms occur.

Diagnosis. Dextrostix may be used as a screening test for hypoglycaemia, low readings being checked in the laboratory on a whole blood sample for true blood-glucose levels. Readings should be obtained two- to three-hourly during the first 12 hours of life. In the presence of abnormal signs measurements of blood glucose should be made every four hours until the infant's blood glucose returns to normal.

Treatment. Hypoxia and chilling predispose to hypoglycaemia in the LFD baby so resuscitation must be prompt and carried out in a warm environment. Early feeding of LFD babies will prevent the development of hypoglycaemia in most cases. Ideally the feed should be of breast milk starting with 60 ml per kg in the first 24 hours and increasing up to 150 ml per kg by the fourth day. If the mother is unable to meet the baby's demand and human breast-milk is unobtainable then complementary feeds should be given. Additional benefits of early feeding include rapid correction of metabolic acidosis and the lessening of physiological jaundice.

Symptomatic hypoglycaemia should be a very rare occurrence so long as the instructions on prevention and early detection have been followed. When it does occur an immediate intravenous injection of glucose (1 g per kg body-weight) should be given followed by an infusion of 10% glucose at a rate of 75 ml per kg per day. The management of the baby with asymptomatic hypoglycaemia is to ensure adequate intake of milk.

Hypothermia

Due to the sparseness of subcutaneous fat and lack of brown adipose tissue the LFD infant loses heat readily. Chilling is more likely to occur in the presence of hypoxia, more especially if the birth weight is less than 2000 g. It follows that an essential part of nursing care is to maintain the body heat of LFD babies.

Other problems

Infection, functional intestinal obstruction and enterocolitis affect the LFD baby in the same way as the preterm baby.

Hypothermia and hypoglycaemia may be further complicated by pulmonary haemorrhage. Better temperature control and correction of hypoglycaemia have reduced the incidence of this complication.

Congenital malformations, chromosomal abnormalities and intra-uterine viral infections are frequently the cause of intrauterine growth failure so the LFD baby should be carefully examined for evidence of hidden malformations or intrauterine infections.

Prognosis

If the malnourished infant's growth has been seriously impaired before delivery it is likely that his subsequent physical development will be similarly affected and not corrected by improvements in paediatric care. This deleterious effect on future development may be compounded if the complications of being born too small are not quickly diagnosed and treated. Thus early delivery of the malnourished fetus and the greater care employed to prevent the harmful effects of hypoglycaemia have reduced the incidence of neurological handicap, including cerebral palsy, mental retardation, fits and learning difficulties, in the LFD infant. However, like those infants who are born too soon those who are born too small show some impairment of performance when they reach school age, but those born too small are at a greater disadvantage and appear less likely to benefit from recent advances in neonatal care.

Health services for the low birth weight infant

Not only the treatment of the ill low birth weight baby but also the care of the healthy low birth weight baby is very demanding in terms of medical and nursing staff, skill and equipment. The staffing of special-care and of intensive therapy nurseries has already been discussed in Chapters 2 and 6. Not all maternity departments will be able to achieve these levels of staffing and will not therefore be able to provide the high standards of care required by the very low birth weight infant. In each district policy decisions with regard to services for low birth weight infants will be required so that mothers going into labour before term can be delivered in a hospital where suitable facilities are available for the care of her infant.

Our prime objective must be the prevention of preterm delivery. Where preventive efforts are not successful the best service available must be provided for the infant in order to diminish the many hazards associated with preterm delivery.

FURTHER READING

Auld, P. A. M. (Ed.) (1980) Neonatal intensive care. *Clinics in Perinatology,* **7** no. 1.

Cockburn, F. (1985) Parenteral nutrition in low birth weight infants. *British Journal of Parenteral Therapy,* **6**, 68–74.

Davies, D. P., Haxby, V., Herbert, S. & McNeish, A. S. (1979) When should pre-term babies be sent home from neonatal units? *Lancet,* **i**, 914–915.

Dweck, H. S. (Ed.) (1977) The tiny baby. *Clinics in Perinatology,* **4** no. 2.

Finberg, L. (1980) One milk for all — not ever likely and certainly not yet. *Journal of Pediatrics,* **96**, 240–241.

Horwood, S. P., Boyle, M. H., Torrance, C. W. & Sinclair, J. C. (1982) Mortality and morbidity of 500 to 1499 g birthweight infants liveborn to residents of a defined geographic region before and after neonatal intensive care. *Paediatrics,* **69**, 613–620.

James, W. H. (1980) Gestational age in twins. *Archives of Disease in Childhood,* **55**, 281–284.

Jones, Rosamond A. K., Cummins, Mary & Davies, Pamela A. (1979) Infants of very low birth weight. *Lancet,* **i**, 1332–1335.

Lancet (1980) The fate of the baby under 1501 g at birth. **i**, 461–463.

Lancet (1980) Is bronchopulmonary dysplasia the cost of survival for some preterm infants? **i**, 690–691.

Lemons, P., Stuart, M. & Lemons, J. A. (1986) Breast feeding the premature infant. *Clinics in Perinatology,* **13:1**, 111.

Neilson, J. P., Whitfield, C. R. & Aitchison, T. (1980) Screening for the small for dates fetus: a two stage ultrasonic examination schedule *British Medical Journal,* **i**, 1203–1206.

Schanler, R. J. & Oh, W. (1980) Composition of breast milk obtained from mothers of premature infants as compared to breast milk obtained from donors. *Journal of Pediatrics,* **96**, 679–681.

Sell, E. J. (1986) Outcome of very very low birth weight infants. *Clinics in Perinatology,* **13:2**, 451–459.

Yu, V. Y. H. & Hollingsworth, E. (1979) Improving prognosis for infants weighing 1000 g or less at birth. *Archives of Disease in Childhood,* **55**, 422–426.

Yu, V. Y. H., James, P., Hendry, P. & MacMahon, R. A. (1979) Total
parenteral nutrition in very low birthweight infants: a controlled trial. *Archives
of Disease in Childhood*, **54**, 653–661.
Yu, V. Y. H., Loke, H. L., Bajuk, B., Syzomonowicz, W., Orgill, A. A. &
Astbury, J. (1986) Prognosis for infants born at 23 to 28 weeks gestation.
British Medical Journal, **293**, 1200–1203.

10

Nursing care of low birth weight infants

Special care nurseries

In spite of advances in medical science and the provision of sophisticated equipment the survival of the LBW baby still depends on the skill and attention of those providing his nursing care. Further training is required for those who undertake this highly specialized form of nursing, and a high staff to patient ratio is necessary to provide the intensive care called for the successful rearing of LBW infants. Nursing care can be made easier by the provision of suitable equipment housed in accommodation designed for the purpose. As discussed in Chapter 2 the maternity departments of district hospitals should each have a special care nursery designed or adapted for its specific function. A more limited number of regional intensive therapy nurseries are now available to deal with infants requiring highly specialized treatment.

Staffing. It will therefore be necessary for a considerable number of nurses or midwives to receive special training in the care of the newborn. The training of staff and the number of staff required have already been discussed in Chapter 2.

Design. Policy decisions about the design of nurseries may seem remote from the day-to-day nursing and medical care of the newborn. It is essential, however, that nurseries be designed and constructed with nursing procedures and facilities for parents and staff in mind. This involves an overall plan which should allow separation of dirty and clean traffic. The infants requiring most intensive care should be nearest to the nursing station and clearly visible. Adequate space must be allowed without causing unnecessary movement. Floors, walls, windows and surfaces must be easily cleaned. Facilities for the washing and drying of hands must be available in every room. Piped air, oxygen and suction should be available.

Temperature. The temperature of each nursery should be controllable within the range 25–30 °C. As adequate ventilation is also essential an air-conditioning system is generally necessary to provide a satisfactory degree of control of the environment. Extra humidity is most readily provided within incubators. In a well-designed nursery it is possible to provide accommodation at different temperatures to suit the requirement of individual infants. The smallest babies although in incubators should be in rooms kept at 30 °C. This temperature should also be maintained in any room where procedures involving the undressing of infants are undertaken. Larger infants can be nursed in cots at a room temperature of 25 °C. Before discharge home the infants should be nursed in cooler rooms with a temperature within the range of 20–25 °C so that they become accustomed to a temperature which can be achieved with extra heating in most homes.

It is essential that parents are involved in the care of their baby. This 'Family Centred Care' can be provided in any Special Care Baby Unit. Visiting by parents, siblings and grandparents should be encouraged. A room where families can sit and relax is helpful; playthings for children can be provided and, if possible, tea and coffee making facilities. An information area with posters, leaflets and photographs of equipment, together with photographs of families and their infants who have been in the Unit, can help to dispel anxiety.

A vital part of nursing care is the promotion of parent-baby attachment. Birth of a LBW baby is a traumatic and distressing experience for parents. Nursing staff must understand and recognize their needs. The parents may mourn the loss of a normal baby and show different emotions, anger, guilt, anxiety or even indifference. Parents of small babies may take longer to accept them and may be reluctant to form an attachment. Prospective parents should be welcome to visit the Unit and have their questions answered. A booklet giving information and describing the Unit can be helpful. Parents should see and hold their baby before he is transferred to the Special Care Baby Unit. They should be given a photograph of their child. They need to visit the Unit as soon as possible and the nurse should encourage them to at least touch, stroke and talk to their baby. Their questions need to be answered and explanations given on the management of their baby's care and the equipment that will be used. Parental consent for treatment should be obtained. As soon as possible parents should be given the opportunity to hold their baby. A mother may not feel close until she has experienced this loving moment.

Eye-to-eye contact is important. Helping the nurse to care for their baby and feeling involved helps the parents. Mothers should be encouraged to express their milk when the infant is for any reason unable to suckle naturally. This milk, preferably freshly obtained, can with suitable nursing supervision be given through a nasogastric tube by the infant's mother. Dressing the baby in individual clothes can be a positive contribution to the care. Constant reassurance, support and encouragement by nursing and medical staff must be given. Many units now have support groups for parents. They can discuss their anxieties and problems with each other and members of staff. It can be distressing for a mother when she is discharged from hospital before her baby. Most mothers feel sad and express concern about leaving their baby. Good communication is essential. The telephone number of the unit should be provided and help given with transport arrangements when necessary to ensure regular visiting. When the time for baby's discharge approaches the needs of each individual family should be reassessed. Mother and baby rooms should be available where the mother can give total care to her baby for several days prior to discharge. This allows for many difficulties to be overcome.

Transitional or shared care with the mother may be used to nurse well LBW babies or larger infants with minor problems. This prevents separation at a sensitive period in the bonding process. Babies are nursed at the mother's bedside. Breast feeding may be more successful and babies may be discharged earlier. The babies may be under the supervision of the Special Care Baby Unit staff.

Equipment

Much of the nursing care of infants involves the use of special equipment such as incubators, monitors, infusion pumps, ventilators and other intricate apparatus. The nursing staff must be trained in the use of such equipment. Instruction must include a description of the function of the machine and the limitations of its action, the correct method of usage, the responsibility of the nurse and the doctor with regard to the initial settings and subsequent changes and the action to be taken if the machine appears to be faulty. All doctors and nurses should be aware of the emergency electricity supply available should the main source fail. Similarly if all power should fail written instructions should be available as to the actions to be taken. There should always be at least one fully trained nurse on duty who is conversant with all the equipment available, where is it kept and how it should be connected to electricity, oxygen or air supply. Where the possibility exists that special equipment will be required this should be thoroughly checked in good time so that it is known to be in working order before it is required. The nursing staff should also be trained in the methods to be used in cleansing and sterilizing special equipment and in precautions to be taken to avoid contamination of equipment.

Equipment should be evaluated for its reliability, ease of use as well as its relative cost before deciding on its purchase. Nursing staff should be involved in the evaluation to determine any advantages and disadvantages in the equipment. Running and maintenance costs should be considered as this can be very expensive. A medical technician may be employed to service the equipment.

Incubators

It is interesting at this juncture to take a look into the past at the development of the incubator and the early methods of provision of warmth which is so essential to a LBW baby's survival. There are some reports in early writings of special attempts to preserve warmth in small babies; a Swiss monk of the tenth century reports on a premature baby being wrapped in animal fat to keep him warm. There is also a report of a baby who survived to become a famous historian, being born in 1577 and at birth no bigger than the palm of his father's hand. He was noted to be perfectly formed, so his father gave instructions to keep him in an oven, and he was reared in this way!

The forerunner of the modern incubator was first used in Bordeaux in 1857. It was a double-lined cradle with a water jacket into which hot water was poured to maintain the correct temperature. A similar apparatus was used in Moscow in 1878. The first closed incubator was introduced by Farmer in 1881. It was a closed wooden box with air holes in the lid. A lower compartment contained water heated by gas, spirit or oil, with the water kept circulating. Modifications were made, the most important being an alarm bell which rang when the temperature rose too high. A thermostatic device which maintained a constant temperature was incorporated in the incubator which was in use at the City of London Lying-in Hospital in 1884. The use of incubators was very

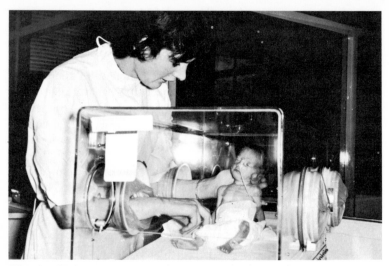

Fig. 10.1 Mother handling her preterm infant in an incubator.

popular in France, and various charitable centres were opened for the care of LBW babies which the public could visit on payment of a fee to see the babies in their incubators, as in fact more than one baby might share the same incubator. The practice of administering oxygen to premature babies was increased after the Second World War and produced many new designs of incubators to provide warmth and the administration of oxygen at the same time.

Modern incubators

Various designs of incubators are now available and some are very expensive items of equipment. They are not indispensable but they are of great value in nursing care. The baby can be nursed in an environment where temperature, humidity and oxygen content is easily regulated. The oxygen concentration can be monitored. Observation of the baby is much more satisfactory as he can be nursed without clothing. The respiratory pattern can be carefully studied and any change of colour noted immediately.

Servocontrol. Incubators provided with a temperature servocontrol mechanism are now widely used. The infant's temperature is measured by a thermocouple attached to the skin. The temperature is read on a calibrated dial which gives a constant reading. At the same time the result is fed into a servocontrol mechanism which controls the heater of the incubator. The mechanism can be set to

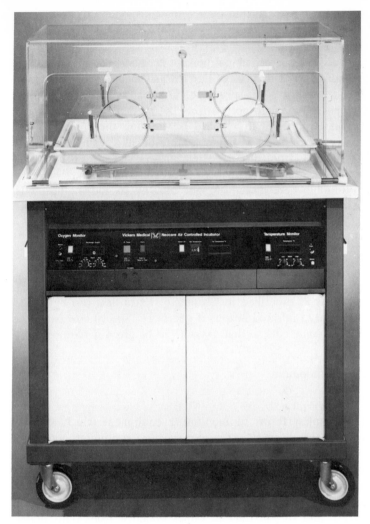

Fig. 10.2 Air-controlled incubator with temperature and oxygen monitors. (Photograph by courtesy of Vickers Medical.)

maintain the infant's skin temperature within a narrow range, the midpoint of which can be altered to suit the infant's requirements. Incubators without a servocontrol mechanism can be set to maintain a constant air temperature at a predetermined level (Fig. 10.2).

Humidity. Control of humidity is much less precise but in most incubators there is a certain degree of control of the moisture content of the circulating air. In modern incubators the heated air is circulated by a fan, but in older models no fan was provided and convection currents were relied upon to maintain a circulation of air.

Access. Incubators cannot be kept permanently closed and access is required for a number of nursing and medical procedures. Suitable access ports are provided. It must not be forgotten that frequent use of such ports affects the efficiency of the incubator.

Heat loss can be minimized by keeping the rooms in which incubators are used at a temperature of 30 °C. This also reduces the heat loss from the incubator surfaces and prevents misting of the inner surface of the hood. Incubators must never be used in a position where direct sunlight can, by its radiant heat effect, overheat the infant, even though the incubator air temperature is not elevated.

Cots

In nurseries heated to 30 °C many LBW babies can be nursed in open cots as described in Chapter 6. Extra heat can be provided by overhead infrared heaters if necessary. Special covers are available for some cots so that oxygen can be given if required.

Other equipment

Monitors

The simplest forms of monitoring equipment which should be available in all special care nurseries are continuous temperature recorders, apnoea monitors and oxygen analysers. Highly complex and therefore expensive sets of monitoring equipment are available commercially. Such apparatus can give a continuous recording of the ECG, heart rate, respiratory rate, blood pressure and the oxygen and carbon dioxide values obtained from transcutaneous monitors. The high cost of such monitors will probably limit their use to intensive therapy nurseries.

Apnoea monitors are available in a number of forms, all of which produce an audible alarm after the infant has ceased to breathe for a preset period. They are relatively cheap and a most useful aid to nursing observation (Fig. 10.3).

Infusion pumps

High precision syringe pumps are available which will deliver fluids

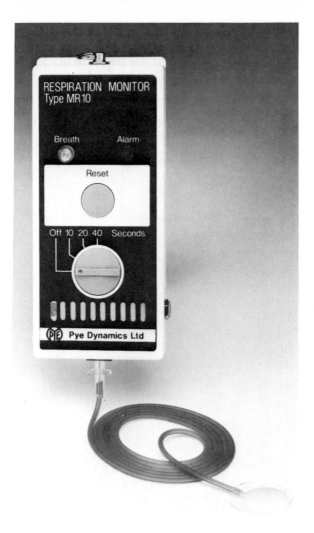

Fig. 10.3 Respiration Monitor. (Photograph by courtesy of Pye Dynamics Ltd.)

at rates down to 0.1 ml per hour. These have made intragastric, intrajejunal or intravenous feeding of VLBW infants much easier and more successful.

Ventilators

Simple ventilators which are essentially mechanical means of

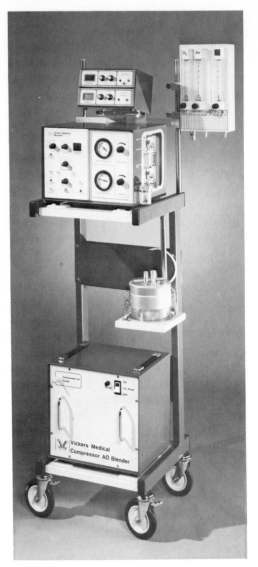

Fig. 10.4 Neonatal ventilator system. (Photograph by courtesy of Vickers Medical.)

providing intermittent positive pressure or limited total pressure are easy to operate and relatively cheap (Fig. 10.4). Although they are not sufficient for dealing with complicated respiratory problems they are suitable for maintaining respiration in the infant with recurrent temporary apnoea and are widely used in special care nurseries. The more highly sophisticated ventilators are better reserved for intensive therapy nurseries.

ORGANIZATION OF NURSERIES

The successful running of special care nurseries requires the introduction of an agreed policy with regard to almost all aspects of nursing and medical care. Such policies must be kept constantly under review and the effect of changes in policy assessed for short- and long-term effects. It follows that a careful record must be kept of the date of introduction of any particular policy and it is useful to note the reason why previous policy was changed. A book stating current policy with regard to standard procedures for such items as reception and immediate care, prevention of infection, maintenance of respiration, maintenance of body temperature, feeding, skin and toilet care, nursing care in special circumstances, preparation for discharge, death of an infant, should be easily available for all staff to consult. It can most conveniently be in the form of a loose-leaf folder which can be readily altered. Space should be left for suggestions as to improvement in procedure.

It is important that parents be allowed to record their impressions as they can often make most useful suggestions. The care that the baby and his family receive is affected by the attitude and actions of the staff. Good team work is essential and assists in improving the quality of care. In-service training programmes for new staff members and continuing education of existing staff are important and may help in the reduction of stress.

Some of the items mentioned in the preceding paragraph are worthy of more detailed discussion.

Prevention of infection

This subject is discussed in greater detail in Chapter 14. Encouragement of breast feeding contributes greatly to the prevention of infection.

Isolation facilities. Facilities should be available within or nearby any special care nursery for the separate nursing in isolation of any infants considered likely to have a clinical infection. Nurses working in the isolation section should not have duties within the general special care nursery.

Staff

Medical, nursing and ancillary staff entering the nursery should be free from infection. Earlier in this chapter the importance of parents entering the unit was discussed. Parents too must be carefully briefed on the prevention of infection. No one with a cold, sore throat, skin infection or diarrhoea should be allowed into the unit.

Although some special care units expect all staff entering the unit to change into gowns, other units have not found this necessary or practicable.

Provided that those staff with respiratory tract infections are excluded from nurseries there is insufficient evidence to justify the continued use of face masks for routine medical and nursing procedures.

Hand washing is the most important basic procedure in the prevention of cross-infection and must be carried out with meticulous care. Wash basins must be provided in each nursery with elbow taps together with a supply of paper towels to be used once only and discarded. All buckets or receptacles for soiled linen or paper should have foot-operated pedals. The hands and the forearms should be thoroughly washed with a liquid soap containing an antiseptic such as chlorhexidine (Hibiscrub), a povidone iodine scrub (Betadine) or vigasam soap (Gammaphene) under running water.

Hand-washing must be carried out before any procedure in the unit and prior to handling each baby and immediately afterwards.

Domestic cleanliness. Domestic staff must be allocated to the special care nursery only and have no other duties outside that area. A cool short-sleeved uniform should be provided. In-service education of domestic staff on the importance of their work being carried out with meticulous care is essential. Modern suction cleaning equipment for floors has greatly reduced the danger of flying dust. All surfaces, furniture and equipment must be damp-dusted with a disposable cleaning cloth. Walls and ceilings must be washed down frequently. Hand basins and water taps require thorough cleaning as they may harbour *Pseudomonas aeruginosa*, which can cause serious infections in the new-born.

It is excellent practice if possible to empty one cubicle or area in the special care nursery in rotation and thoroughly air and clean both it and the furniture. This procedure could be carried out so that the whole nursery (depending on its size) is thoroughly cleaned frequently.

Soiled linen must be handled as little as possible by nursing staff and should be collected in a disposable bag and removed from the nursery area immediately. It should never be allowed to lie on the floor. There is now a wide range of disposable items on the market such as napkins, sheets and baby gowns, all of which are rapidly improving and in the future may completely replace the washable linen.

Cots and mattresses should be thoroughly cleaned when a baby has been discharged home.

Incubators can be a source of infection if not thoroughly cleaned. The makers give detailed instructions regarding dismantling of various parts for cleaning. These should be studied carefully and adequate time allowed to carry out the recommended procedures. As faecal organisms may contaminate the humidity tanks it is advisable to change the distilled water daily. The use of antiseptic solutions may eventually damage the lining of the incubator tanks. In many units incubators are run dry and where humidity is required this is provided by a separate humidification system.

Incubator ports can be a channel through which infection may enter the incubator. Some units use one side for 'clean procedures' such as feeding and the other side for 'dirty procedures' such as changing napkins. Filters on the air inlet must be changed according to the makers' instructions.

Any extra tubing for the ventilator, suction, resuscitation and extra humidity etc. which is not disposable should be autoclaved or treated by immersion in an antiseptic solution according to the policy of the Control of Infection Committee (Chapter 14). When all cleaning procedures are completed swabs must be taken from the inside of the incubator and water taken for bacteriological examination and the incubator should not be put into use until the reports prove that there is no infection present. Some units have not found this necessary and will follow this procedure only after nursing an infant with a confirmed infection. Because of the risk of infection to a baby who requires prolonged nursing care in an incubator the baby should be transferred to a clean incubator each week.

Feeds. Where feeds are being prepared, special precautions against the risk of infection have to be taken. This has already been discussed in Chapter 8.

Immediate care

As stated earlier at least one incubator fully prepared and warmed should always be available for the reception of infants from the delivery rooms or elsewhere. On admission to the special care nursery the infant's name should be checked against the name on the records provided and information about the pregnancy and delivery recorded. Meanwhile the infant's immediate requirements are being assessed and a decision made as to whether incubator nursing is required. This decision will depend upon the infant's maturity, weight, temperature and general condition.

The following observations are made:

Temperature

Colour, noting pallor, cyanosis or jaundice

Respiration with particular reference to rate, depth and regularity

Heart rate

Activity, observing movements and strength of cry

Time of passage of urine

Time of passage of meconium

Umbilical cord is checked for control of bleeding

Abnormal signs such as convulsions are reported

The incubator temperature is recorded

The oxygen content is measured and recorded.

Respiratory pattern. Any infant who shows evidence of respiratory distress, whether this be excessive chest movement, indrawing, grunting, cyanosis or apnoea, should be reported immediately. The baby is nursed with an apnoea monitor attached. This will give an audible warning if the baby stops breathing for a set period — usually 10–15 seconds. This alerts nursing and medical staff and appropriate resuscitation can be carried out immediately. Close observation of the colour, rate, regularity and depth of breathing is essential. Warm humidified oxygen is given if the baby is cyanosed and the oxygen concentration should be monitored closely.

Maintenance of body temperature

This is one of the greatest problems in nursing LBW babies who lose heat readily and have limited powers of heat production. The baby's temperature should be maintained in the Thermoneutral range. Extreme care must be taken to ensure that LBW babies do not become cold. Their rectal temperature should lie in the range 36.5–37.5 °C, with an abdominal skin temperature of 36.5–37.5 °C. Use hats and bootees to reduce heat loss and dress the baby when his condition is stable. Each baby must have his own low-reading thermometer giving readings down to 25 °C. Every care must be taken during nursing procedures to prevent heat loss by avoiding unnecessary exposure and preventing excessive air movements.

Feeding

The type of feeds and amounts given have already been dealt with in Chapters 8 and 9. The method of feeding is important as LBW babies may have poor sucking and swallowing reflexes. The cardiac sphincter is poorly developed and regurgitation of food occurs readily. The cough reflex is feeble and inhalation of the feed may occur. Large feeds must be avoided and the baby handled after feeding as little as possible.

The lower the gestational age the weaker the intestinal activity and abdominal distension may occur following feeds and give rise to cyanotic attacks. The method of feeding employed depends on the baby's condition and gestational age.

Breast feeding. Most babies who weigh 1500 g and over and who are in good general condition will cope well with breast feeding. Breast feeding must be carefully supervised and care must be taken not to allow the baby to become exhausted by prolonged attempts to feed. For babies who cannot feed directly at the breast, mother's milk can be given either by bottle or by nasogastric tube. Enthusiasm and encouragement go a long way in achieving successful breast feeding.

Bottle feeding. Bottle feeding can be used to give human milk or a modified cow's milk. It is essential to ensure that the teat is soft and has a hole large enough to permit a steady flow of drops when the bottle is inverted. The feed may be warmed or it may be given at room temperature.

The baby should be wrapped and held with the spine and head well supported. Care must be taken to ensure that the teat is always filled with milk to ensure that air is not being sucked in by the baby. A finger under the chin assists the baby to suck. In the middle and at the end of the feed the baby is supported in a sitting position with the spine extended and 'winded'. Following the feed the baby is left lying on his right side and the incubator tray or cot left tilted head up for 20 to 30 minutes. The prone position is favoured by many following feeds as it has been shown that the stomach empties more quickly in this position and with less interference to respiration. Careful attention to detail is essential during bottle feeding of a LBW baby.

Intragastric tube feeding. In babies of low gestational age and those whose general condition is poor, tube feeding is used to ensure an adequate intake and to prevent exhaustion. This method of feeding must only be carried out by nurses who have had experience in nursing LWB babies. Nurses in training and when appropriate the baby's own parents will require to be supervised by an experienced nurse. If carried out with meticulous care it is a safe and most suitable method of feeding. The baby receives the feed with no physical effort and minimal handling.

The technique most widely practised is to use a sterile disposable infant feeding tube which is left in situ and only requires to be changed to the other nostril every two to three days. Sterile disposable infant feedings sets are readily available.

The head of the cot is raised. In order to determine how far a tube should be inserted, before the tube is removed from its sterile wrapping, it is measured against the baby. Holding the tip at the xiphisternum and extending the tube upwards to the lobe of the ear and then forward to the bridge of the baby's nose, the tube is then marked at this site.

After washing her hands, the midwife passes the tube gently along the floor of the nostril and down into the oesophagus until the mark previously made is at the baby's nostrils. The mouth is inspected to ensure that the tube has gone into the oesophagus. The tube is fixed to baby's skin with a narrow strip of micropore tape. A small amount of gastric juice is aspirated and tested with litmus paper. If the reaction is acid, the tube can be assumed to be in the stomach. The barrel of a syringe is then attached to the tube and a feed is poured in and the rate of flow regulated by raising or lowering the syringe. When the whole feed has been run into the tube, 1 ml of sterile water is injected to clear it and a small spigot may be inserted to seal the open end.

The baby must be very carefully observed throughout the feed for any colour change or apnoea, and following the feed for any regurgitation which so easily could be inhaled.

The baby's cot is left with the head tipped up for 20 to 30 minutes following feeds and the baby nursed on his right side or prone. All aseptic precautions must be carefully observed with the equipment used and during the administration of a feed.

The amount of feed actually taken must be recorded on the baby's chart. Vitamins and iron preparations may be added to the feeds (Chapter 8).

Jejunal feeding. If intragastric feeding proves difficult because of distension and vomiting some centres advocate the passage of a tube through the pylorus into the jejunum. This procedure is not always easy and may create new problems.

Nasojejunal/transpyloric feeding

Possible indications:

1 Healthy VLBW (i.e. <1500 g) infants who are liable to apnoeic attacks.

2 Sick preterm or term infants with recurrent apnoea or problems with regurgitation (? or respiratory distress).

3 Following upper G.I. tract surgery via a transanastomotic tube.

Contraindications:

1 Ileus, whether functional due to prematurity, or secondary to illness elsewhere.

2 History of necrotising enterocolitis.

Method:

1 Passing the tube

  i Use silastic nasojejunal tubes only.

  ii Measure the length of tube required: from the glabella to the outstretched heel is equal to the distance from the nostril to the third part of the duodenum (except in babies weighing <1000 g: in these use chin to outstretched heel).

  iii Mark this point on the tube with a black silk tie.

  iv Pass the tube via the nostril to the stomach.

  Lie the baby on his right side in semi-prone position. Advance the tube 1–2 cm per hour until the black silk marker is reached.

  OR

  Pass the tube via the nostril to the stomach.

  Lie the baby on his right side in the semi-prone position and advance the tube progressively over about 10 minutes until the black silk marker is reached.

  v X-ray the abdomen to confirm the position of the tip of

the tube. For 'nasojejunal' feeding aim for the 3rd–4th part of the duodenum, i.e. just over the left edge of the spine. For 'transpyloric' feeding aim to have the tip on the right of the abdomen, clearly away from the stomach gas bubble and through the pylorus. Transpyloric gives a more physiological mixing of milk with bile and pancreatic secretions but the chance of regurgitation of milk and/or the tube is increased.

vi Secure the tube by applying at 2 × 1 cm piece of Stom-adhesive to the cheek and sticking the silastic tube to this with Micropore.

vii Replace the tube electively every two weeks.

2 Feeding

Use a pump to give a continuous milk infusion.

Start at 1–2 ml/hour.

Increase can be faster than by nasogastric feeding, so that full requirements are reached after 24–48 hours.

3 Aspiration

Pass an orogastric tube and aspirate every 3–4 hours — replace if 2 ml or less. If milk is aspirated the n–j tube may have been regurgitated into the stomach.

General handling and daily care

The nursing care of LBW babies demands the highest standard possible. The ultimate survival of the baby depends largely upon the standard of nursing care, constant observation and the keeping of accurate detailed records.

Minimal handling is essential especially in the babies of lower gestational age. Cleansing, changing, and weighing of the baby must be carried out prior to feeding to avoid the possibility of regurgitation. All procedures must be carried out in the cot or incubator and each baby must have his own equipment for his exclusive use.

Toilet. The skin may be cleaned using water and cotton wool swabs. The skin folds (axillae, groins, neck and behind the ears) must be given special attention as abrasion of the skin surfaces by particles of debris may very easily occur. The napkin area also requires very careful cleasing. This treatment can be carried out daily until the baby is able to tolerate a daily bath.

The eyes should be examined daily. If clean they are left alone.

The mouth must be inspected at each feeding time. The preterm baby is prone to oral thrush infection which must be recognized and treated as soon as possible.

The cord is treated as already described in Chapter 6. The baby being nursed in an incubator is at additional risk from infection.

Weighing. Frequency of weighing varies with the policy of units. The smallest babies can be weighed on electronic scales. The scales should be brought to the cot and the baby weighed lying on a sheet of disposable tissue which is changed between each baby. The weight usually falls (or remains stationary) during the first seven to ten days of life. Thereafter the weight should slowly rise and the birth weight may be regained in two or three weeks.

Nursing care in special circumstances

Oxygen therapy. Oxygen is a potent agent which may have toxic effects in VLBW infants. It has been linked with both retinal and pulmonary damage. For this reason it should be used with extreme care and its concentration continuously analysed when in use.

Oxygen may have to be given in high concentration but this should be used for as short a period of time as possible. There are various oxygen analysers available for measuring the oxygen content of the inspired air. The concentration should be monitored continuously while the baby is receiving additional oxygen. A more accurate method of controlling oxygen therapy is by monitoring the level of the infant's arterial oxygen tension (Chapter 20).

During phototherapy. The value of phototherapy in reducing hyperbilirubinaemia is now well established (Chapter 15). The baby is nursed naked under the phototherapy unit. The eyes are covered with a sterile cotton mask to reduce the potential risks associated with exposure to continuous high intensity light exposure. There is frequently temperature instability so that careful temperature control is essential. Fluid intake may have to be increased to replace fluid lost from skin and loose stools which is a common associated feature. The length of treatment is governed by the infant's serum bilirubin concentration.

Preparation for discharge

Nursing staff in special care nurseries tend to become very attached to infants under their care. They must remember that they are acting on behalf of the infant's mother and that part of their duty is to teach mother to gain confidence in her ability to look after her baby at first in hospital then at home. Preparation for discharge of a LBW infant who may need to remain in a special care nursery for two or three months must begin well before the baby is expected to be ready for discharge. Continuity of advice can be helped by having a specialist health visitor or community neonatal sister who will visit mother and baby in hospital and later at home. She will liaise with the family doctor and the practice health visitor, check home conditions, and be responsible for arranging subsequent supervision. Mother will have been encouraged to handle and care for her baby from birth. She will have gained confidence and be able to take over the regular management including feeding but will benefit from further experience by admission to the 'mothers' room' of the special care baby unit for a day or two. Problems which occur can be overcome prior to discharge.

Follow-up

It is only when assessing the progress of infants who have been cared for in special-care nurseries that the success or failure of the policies of management can be assessed (Chapter 21).

FURTHER READING

Harvey, D. (1987) Parent-Infant Relationships. Perinatal Practice, vol. 4. Chichester: Wiley Medical.
Klaus, M. H. & Fanaroff, A. A. (1979) *Care of the high-risk neonate*, 2nd edn. Philadelphia: Saunders.
Lancet (1979) Separation and special care Baby Units, i, 590.
Myles, M. F. (1985) *A Textbook for Midwives*, 10th edn. Edinburgh: Churchill Livingstone.
Strickland, M., Spector, S., Hamlin-Cook, P., Hanna, C., Moore, C., Bellig, L. & Fiorato, A. (1980) Nurse training and staffing in the neonatal intensive care unit. *Clinics in Perinatology*, 7, 173.

11

Congenital abnormalities

In describing the development of the normal fetus in Chapter 4 mention was made of hereditary and environmental factors which might interfere with development of the fetus, and the value of genetic counselling was discussed. In this chapter attention will be concentrated on abnormalities of development which allow fetal life to progress until the age of potential viability and which are evident as abnormalities of form or function detectable at birth.

Fetal death

It must be remembered, however, that the most seriously malformed products of gestation cause embryonic and fetal death at an early stage of pregnancy and are generally unrecognized when they are aborted. The remaining abnormal fetuses, whether live-born or stillborn, have congenital abnormalities caused by a host of genetic and environmental factors, some known and others as yet unrecognized. This group is now of greater relative importance as a cause of perinatal mortality and morbidity as birth trauma, infection and other causes of perinatal death come under control.

Incidence

Recognition. Assessment of the incidence of congenital abnormalities is simplest when confined to major well-recognized abnormalities such as anencephaly or spina bifida which are clearly visible at birth. A firm diagnosis of cardiac, renal or cerebral abnormality is seldom possible at birth and it may be weeks or years before an abnormality is confirmed. With less serious forms of abnormality in which function may not be affected, as in the case of birthmarks, embarrassment may be the principal handicap.

Opinions differ as to whether such conditions should be classified as abnormalities.

Range. Variations in frequency of examination, in interpretation of signs and the period of follow-up as well as the skill of the physician concerned account for much of the range of incidence of congenital abnormalities quoted in different surveys. Where the incidence of specifically defined abnormalities is studied and these errors are excluded, considerable differences in incidence are still found in different parts of the world and in different parts of one country. Such studies of the epidemiology of congenital abnormalities can provide evidence as to aetiological factors.

Notified congential malformations

The report 'On the State of the Public Health' published annually includes figures of the incidence of notified congenital malformations. The figures for some of the years 1970 to 1980 for England and Wales are shown in Table 11.1. It will be seen that around 12 000 infants a year are notified as suffering from congenital malformations. This is likely to be a gross underestimate. The study of British births in one week in 1970 during which reports were completed on all infants suggested a much higher incidence of malformation at 52.1 per 1000 than the 21.4 per 1000 total births notified in 1980. This discrepancy reflects a difference in definition and in the method used for collection of data rather than a true change in incidence of that magnitude.

Changing incidence. There does, however, appear to be some change in the incidence of notified congenital malformations of a smaller degree as shown in Table 11.1. Although there has been a reduction in the total number the incidence has increased. Congenital abnormalities remain a major cause of perinatal death and result in handicap to many surviving infants.

Table 11.1 Change in incidence of notified congenital malformation (England and Wales)

Year	Congenital malformation	Incidence per 1000 L and S.B.
1970	14019	17.64
1974	12730	19.67
1976	12384	20.99
1978	12197	21.50
1980	14134	21.38

Causative factors

Prevention is clearly the most acceptable form of management. This requires prior knowledge of the causative factors involved. These are many and frequently interaction between two or more such factors appears to be necessary. Table 11.2 lists some of the principal situations known to be associated with increased risk of congenital abnormality.

Table 11.2   Causes of congenital abnormality

GENETIC
  Inherited
  Mutations
ENVIRONMENTAL IN UTERO
  Viral Infections
    e.g. rubella
  Nutritional
  Alcohol
  X-rays
  Chemicals
  Drugs
  Mechanical
    Pressure effects
    Constricting bands
UNKNOWN

Genetic

Inherited factors. The part played by inherited factors such as abnormal genes in the causation of congenital abnormality recognizable at birth is relatively small. Many inherited genetic disorders are of a metabolic nature and only become evident later in infancy or require special investigation for their detection at birth. Some inherited skeletal abnormalities such as achondroplasia and cardiac abnormalities can be recognized at birth or even in prenatal life by X-ray or ultrasound examination of the fetus.

Mutations. Chromosomal abnormalities, the majority of which are mutants, are an uncommon cause of congenital abnormality. Infants with a chromosomal abnormality may show no physical abnormality at birth but the autosomal trisomies are associated with recognizable abnormality the commonest of which is Down's syndrome.

Environmental

Of the adverse environmental factors liable to cause deformity of the fetus many are only harmful during the period of organogenesis during the first trimester of pregnancy. Knowledge about the part played by viral infections is slowly increasing. A number of studies have now been carried out on the part played by drugs (Table 11.3a and b). Studies of the effect of various deficiencies in the maternal diet before or during pregnancy are not yet conclusive but do suggest that maternal nutrition may play a part in the causation of some congenital abnormalities including neural tube defects. Excessive consumption of alcohol by the mother during early pregnancy may produce malformations of the fetus called the Fetal Alcohol Syndrome. Oligohydramnios results in excessive pressure of the uterine wall on the growing fetus and may result in deformities of the limbs such as talipes (Fig. 11.1). More localized pressure changes from amniotic bands can cause local constriction around a limb which occasionally results in intrauterine amputation (Figs 11.2 and 11.3).

Table 11.3a Drugs or other agents which may cause fetal abnormalities if taken by the mother

Drug/agent	Organs affected
Alcohol	Eyes, cranium, face, skeleton, brain; stunted
Aminopterin	Cranium, face, skin, ears; death
Amphetamines	Heart, lip, skeleton, urogenital
Anaesthetics	Skeletal and face suggested — very rare; affects theatre staff
Androgens and synthetic progestogens	Masculinized females
Antiemetics	All probably harmless save diphenhydramine
Antithyroid drugs	Thyroid, brain
Aspirin	Probably nil
Busulphan	Eyes, palate; stunted
Chlorambucil	Urogenital
Chloroquine	Deafness and choroidoretinitis possible
Cigarette smoking	Reduced birth weight
Corticosteroids	Probably nil
Cyclophosphamide	Palate
Diazepam	Cleft lip and palate possible
Diethylstilboestrol	In first trimester predisposes to vaginal carcinoma and adenosis (after 15 years)
Iodine excess or deficiency	Goitre, hypothyroidism, brain

Table 11.3a (cont'd)

Drug/agent	Organs affected
Lithium	Heart, great vessels
Methotrexate	Skeletal
Paramethadione	Heart, palate, face, brain
Phenytoin and barbiturates	Lips, skull, skeleton, ear, heart
Progestogens	Masculinization of the female
Quinine	Hypoplasia of optic nerve and deafness in high doses
Radiation	Neural tube, skeleton; microcephaly
Streptomycin	Deafness
Tetracycline	Teeth discoloured and enamel hypoplasia
Thalidomide	Skeleton, heart, ears, eyes
Troxidone (trimethadione)	Heart, palate, face, brain
Vitamin A deficiency	Brain, eyes, palate, skeleton
Vitamin D excess	Infantile hypercalcaemia possible
Folic acid deficiency	Brain, neural tube
Warfarin	Nose, skeleton, eyes, brain; nasal hypoplasia, chondrodysplasia punctata in first trimester optic atrophy, microcephaly, mental retardation in second and third trimester.

Table 11.3b Teratogenicity of various drugs and other agents

Teratogenic	Probably teratogenic	Possibly teratogenic
Alcoholism, chronic	Amphetamines	Amantadine
Aminopterin	Anaesthetics	Antacids
Androgens	Aspirin	Chloridiazepoxide
Antithyroid drugs	Busulphan	Clomiphene
Azauridine	Chlorambucil	Cyclamate
Barbiturates	Chloroquine	Ethionamide
Iodine	Cyclophosphamide	Iron
Iodine lack	Diazepam	Lithium
Methotrexate	Folic acid deficiency	Lysergic acid
Phenytoin	Paramethadione	Meprobamate
Progestogens, synthetic	Quinine	Nicotinamide
Progestogen/oestrogen	Smoking	Phenmetrazine
Radiation, excessive	Troxidone (trimethadione)	Pyrimethamine
Stilboestrol		Sulphonamide
Tetracyclines		Tolbutamide
Thalidomide		Tricyclic drugs
Vitamin D deficiency		Vitamin A excess
Warfarin		

Adapted from Gray, O. P. & Cockburn, F. (1984) *Children: a handbook for children's doctors*. London: Pitman.

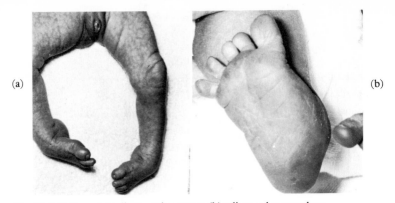

Fig. 11.1 Talipes: (a) talipes equino-varus; (b) talipes calcaneo-valgus.

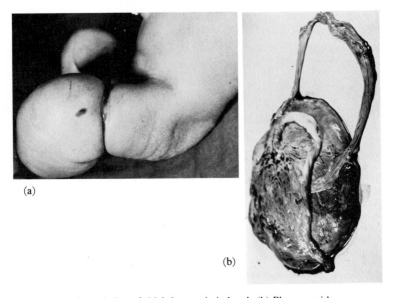

Fig. 11.2 (a) Constriction of thigh by amniotic band; (b) Placenta with costricting amniotic band.

Unknown. As shown above, a variety of causes of congenital abnormality are known but in the majority of cases no cause can be recognised.

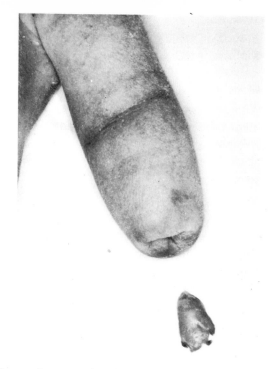

Fig. 11.3 Intrauterine amputation of hand.

Prevention

Of the causes listed in Table 11.2 and 11.3 some are capable of control by doctors and midwives with the co-operation of the mother.

Rubella immunization. Education with regard to the risk from rubella and the benefit of protective immunization could lead to generations in whom this problem has been eliminated. For the mother who was not immunized naturally or artificially before pregnancy immunization can be offered shortly after delivery. Immunization must not be carried out during pregnancy and pregnancy should be avoided for three months after immunization.

Drugs. Supervision of drugs being presented to pregnant women so that no drug is given without good reason limits the risk from drug-induced abnormalities.

X-rays. Limitation of non-urgent abdominal X-rays in women of child-bearing age to the period of up to 12 days from the first day of the last menstrual period is designed to prevent unnecessary exposure of the fertilized ovum to X-radiation at a time when pregnancy is unsuspected. Avoidance of exposure to X-rays during the first three months of pregnancy is essential.

Genetic counselling

In families with a known high risk of abnormal offspring genetic counselling may help the family to decide whether they wish to have further children. If they do not, contraceptive advice should be given.

Therapeutic termination. Where there has been proven exposure to harmful factors in early pregnancy or where there is a high risk of hereditary abnormality consideration has to be given to the justification for therapeutic termination of pregnancy.

Prenatal diagnosis. In some situations examination of chorionic villus biopsy material, the amniotic fluid, ultrasonography or direct inspection of the fetus using an endoscope passed into the amniotic cavity may be necessary before a decision can be reached (Chapter 4).

Sterilization

The ultimate preventive management is contraceptive advice or sterilization and this has to be accepted as the only suitable means of management in some situations of high risk.

ABNORMAL DEVELOPMENT

As in over half the cases of congenital abnormality we are not able to identify a cause and therefore to take preventive action we are still likely to be faced with problems of management of infants born with an abnormality. Most of these have resulted from a disturbance in embryological development. An understanding of the faults which occur in the early development of the embryo helps in the understanding of the deformities present at birth. In general terms abnormalities arise because of:

Failure of development, e.g. amelia, microcephaly
Failure to unite, e.g. cleft lip, spina bifida
Failure to divide, e.g. syndactyly
Failure to canalize, e.g. intestinal atresias
Failure to migrate, e.g. malrotation of bowel
Failure to atrophy, e.g. branchial clefts.
Excess division, e.g. polydactyly

The embryological basis

The mouth and face

The lips are developed from three processes — a midline central nasal process and the two wings of a branchial arch (the maxillary processes) which grow out on each side from dorsal attachments to the head to meet the nasal process ventrally in the midline. When fusion does not take place a cleft lip results (Fig. 11.4). The failure to fuse usually occurs between a maxillary process and the fronto-nasal process, resulting in a lateral cleft lip. This may consist of a complete cleft extending up to the nostril or of only a slight notched depression of the lip margin. It may be unilateral or bilateral.

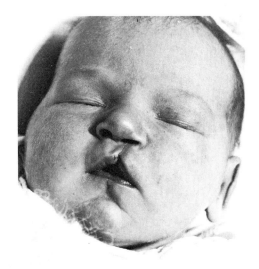

Fig. 11.4 Cleft lip.

Cleft palate is another example of failure to fuse. The palate originates as two palatal processes from the same branchial arch as the lips and from other mesoderm processes (the nasal septum and the premaxilla) extending downwards, from the primitive head. Fusion begins between the premaxilla and the anterior edges of the palatal processes, and extends posteriorly along the opposed edges of those processes. Depending upon the exact nature of the failure to fuse, cleft palate can assume one of a variety of forms. Cleft palate may exist alone or be associated with cleft lip (unilateral or bilateral) (Fig. 11.5).

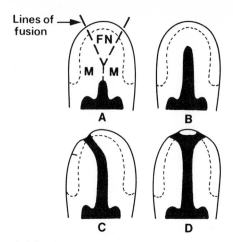

Fig. 11.5 Forms of cleft palate and hare lip. A = midline defect of soft palate, B = midline defect of soft and hard palate, C = unilateral cleft lip and palate, D = bilateral cleft lip and palate, FN = fronto-nasal process, M = maxillary processes.

Micrognathia is smallness of the mandible, which is another structure derived from a branchial arch. It is an example of failure to develop.

Branchial arch abnormalities. Cleft lip, cleft palate and micrognathia each represent a departure from normal in the embryological development of the first branchial arch. Other anomalies now generally considered to be variants of the same basic developmental error include mandibulofacial dysostosis (*Treacher-Collins syndrome*) (Fig. 11.6), mandibular hypoplasia and glossoptosis (*Pierre-Robin syndrome*), mandibular dysostosis, hypertelorism, and deformities of the external and middle ear (Fig. 11.7). The disorders mentioned above are collectively termed *the first arch syndrome* as they probably arise from inadequacy of blood supply to the first branchial arch.

Gastrointestinal tract

The oesophagus. As the neck grows in length corresponding development of the oesophagus may be interrupted, giving rise to stenosis. Abnormal development may occur also during the time that the trachea is evolving from a pharyngeal pouch. A portion of the oesophagus may be completely absent or represented by a fibrous cord — atresia being present in either event. The anomaly

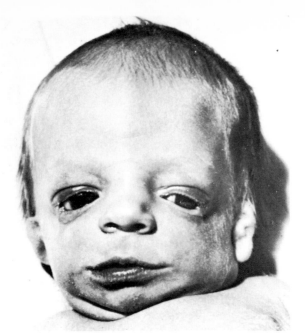

Fig. 11.6 Mandibulofacial dysostosis (Treacher-Collins syndrome).

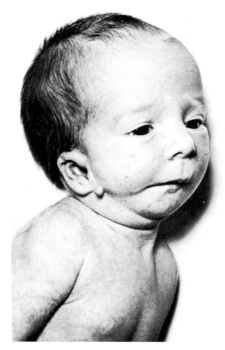

Fig. 11.7 First arch syndrome showing unilateral deformity of the mandible and ear.

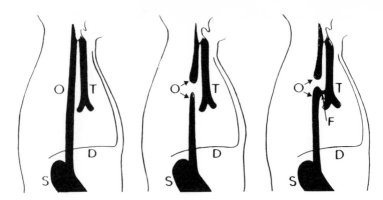

Fig. 11.8 Oesophageal atresia. The figure on the left shows the anatomy
in a normal baby. The other figures show two types of oesophageal atresia.
O = oesophagus, S = stomach, D = diaphragm, F = fistula, T = trachea.

is rare, but the most likely form to be encountered consists of a
distally blind upper pouch and a lower pouch communicating with
the trachea (by a persistent fistula) at one end and with the stomach
at the other (Fig. 11.8). A fourth type of anomaly which can be
difficult to diagnose is where the oesophagus is uninterrupted but
a communication exists between the oesophagus and trachea (H-
type fistula). The affected infant is subject to recurrent episodes
of aspiration pneumonia and the diagnosis requires expert radiological examination.

Diaphragm. Errors in the development of the diaphragm may
occur as failures of migration or fusion. Diaphragmatic anomalies
are rare. When they occur they usually consist of persistence of one
of the lateral openings which is a feature of early development. The
deficiency is almost always on the left side and enables the intestines to herniate (diaphragmatic hernia) through the opening with
the risk of strangulation.

The midgut. Any part of the midgut may be stenosed or
occluded. Duodenal atresia is the form most commonly encountered and is usually the result of local failure of the primitive gut
to canalize.

Departure from the normal progressive rotation of the gut may
result in the development of abnormal adhesions, the suspension
of large and small intestine by a single short pedicle, or in the
midgut having a notably narrow mesenteric attachment. These are
all circumstances which favour the occurrence of acute intestinal
obstruction due to volvulus.

Meckel's diverticulum is an uncommon anomaly related to early development of the intestine. It represents the part of the vitelline duct which opens into the ileum. The diverticulum may persist as a projection from the ileum, as a fibrous cord attached internally to the umbilicus, or as a sinus opening externally at the umbilicus (Fig. 11.9).

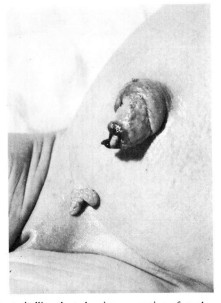

Fig. 11.9 Persistent vitelline duct showing evacuation of stool.

The hindgut

Abnormalities of the anus and rectum may take several forms. An imperforate anus results when the anal membrane remains intact. Incomplete 'rupture' of the membrane accounts for partial atresia or anal stenosis. Rectovesical and rectourethral fistulae are attributable to failure of the cloaca to become completely separated into its alimentary and urogenital sections. Rectovesical fistulae are very rare in females but rectovaginal fistulae are encountered (Fig. 11.10).

Abnominal wall

Impaired development of the abdominal wall may result in the fetal

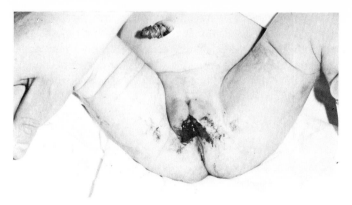

Fig. 11.10 Rectovaginal fistula with meconium being passed through the vagina.

membranes and intestines, which normally extend temporarily into the base of the umbilical cord, not being able to return to the abdominal cavity. Should this persist, exomphalos develops and the infant is born with abdominal viscera herniated through the abdominal wall and enclosed by peritoneum and amniotic membrane.

Genitourinary tract

The kidneys may be the site of polycystic disease which results from an abnormality of development of the nephrons. Abnormal fusions can give rise to a single horseshoe kidney.

The bladder. Developmentally the bladder is derived from a number of structures. Extroversion of the bladder (ectopia vesicae) (Fig. 11.11) is an anomaly consisting of imperfect closure of the anterior abdominal wall, absence of the anterior wall of the bladder, and failure of pubic fusion anteriorly. The reason for the occurrence of the anomaly is not known, but the fact that the umbilicus is invariably situated in an unusually low position indicates that the disturbance of development has taken place early in fetal life.

Patent urachus is a persistent sinus extending from the bladder and opening to the exterior at the umbilicus which occurs if the urachus does not undergo complete obliteration. Alternatively a cyst may develop in the line of the urachus.

The penis. At an early stage of the development of the penis a groove flanked by raised margins appears on the undersurface of

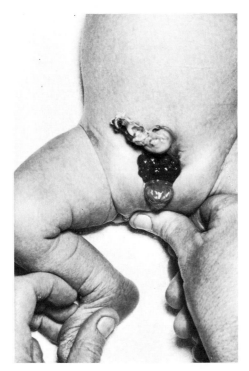

Fig. 11.11 Ectopia vesicae with epispadias and low position of umbilicus.

the organ. The groove deepens and the overhanging margins meet, converting the groove into a patent tube. Closure of the ventral wall of the penis proceeds from behind forwards. Hypospadias results when ventral fusion is incomplete (Fig. 11.12). The nature of the

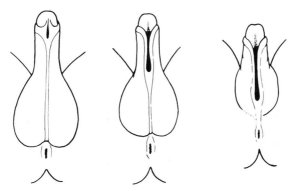

Fig. 11.12 Degrees of hypospadias.

hypospadias depends on the site of imperfect fusion, and may simulate the appearance of the external genitalia in the female.

The testes and inguinal canals. The testes form in the abdominal cavity and normally before birth they pass through the inguinal canals to reach the scrotum. In their descent into the scrotum the testes are contained in a sac of peritoneum. The sac becomes sealed off immediately above the testes and at the external inguinal ring, the intervening portion becoming obliterated. The process of obliteration may not take place. If, as a result, the sac still communicates with the abdominal cavity, a hernia may develop — gut entering the sac. If, on the other hand, despite sealing off of the sac from the abdominal cavity, the sac does not become obliterated, fluid may collect in it, forming a hydrocele (Fig. 11.13).

Exceptionally descent of the testes into the scrotum may be incomplete. The testis may remain in the abdominal cavity or inguinal canal (Fig. 11.14) or after passing through the inguinal canal it may take up an abnormal position (ectopic testis) in the upper thigh or lower abdominal wall (Fig. 11.15).

The spinal cord and column

The spinal cord develops from the neural tube, and the vertebral column from the mesodermal segments lying adjacent to the tube. Each vertebra is formed as a result of fusion of three processes. Of these, one represents the body of the vertebra and the other two the lateral halves of the neural arch and vertebral spine. Anomalies

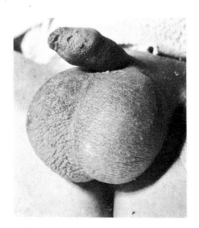

Fig. 11.13 Bilateral hydrocele.

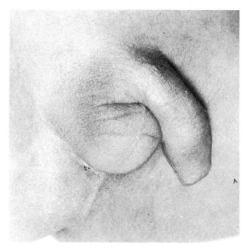

Fig. 11.14 Undescended right testicle.

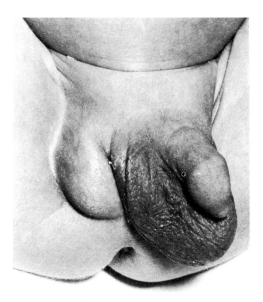

Fig. 11.15 Ectopic right testicle.

of the cord and column result from imperfect separation of the neural tube from the main ectodermal mass and from imperfect fusion of the two lateral sections of the neural arches.

Spina bifida is a defect in the vertebral column. The contents of the column may be visible and may herniate through the defect. When the herniated structures consist of meninges only, the condition is known as meningocele.

Myelomeningocele. When nerve tissues are included in the sac, the condition is described as myelomeningocele. Occasionally there is no hernia despite defect of the vertebral column (spina bifida occulta). A localized depression of the skin or a hairy mole may be present over the site of the anomaly. Spina bifida may occur anywhere in the spine but is found most commonly in the lumbo-sacral region (Fig. 11.16).

Pilonidal sinus. At first the neural tube remains open at its caudal end, closure taking place with the fusion of the ectodermal layer of skin in the midline. The distal end of the tube is converted into a delicate filament which remains attached distally in the region of the coccyx. A midline depression of the skin in the neigh-bourhood of the coccyx (pilonidal depression) sometimes indicates the point of attachment. Failure of the caudal end of the neural

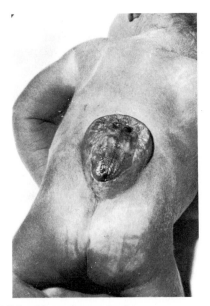

Fig. 11.16 Spina bifida with meningomyelocele.

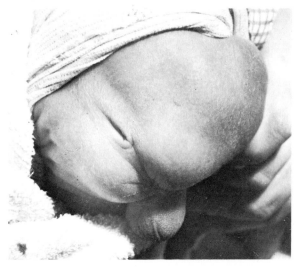

Fig. 11.17 Pilonidal sinus.

tube to become closed gives rise to a sinus (pilonidal sinus) which opens to the exterior (Fig. 11.17).

The brain

The head end of the neural tube undergoes considerable elaboration to form the brain. Developmental errors analogous to those described in connection with the cord may also involve the brain.

Anencephaly. Failure of the cephalic end of the cord to close gives rise to the condition known as anencephaly in which development of the vault of the skull and cerebral hemispheres is minimal.

Microcephaly. Characterized by pronounced smallness of the skull and by an anterior fontanelle closed or almost closed at the time of birth, microcephaly results from failure of the cerebral hemispheres to grow during intrauterine life (Fig. 11.18).

Hydrocephalus. Another condition which is sometimes but not always the result of errors of development is hydrocephalus. Normally the cerebrospinal fluid is secreted by the choroid plexuses into the ventricles of the brain. The fluid circulates in the ventricular system and in the subarachnoid space of the spinal cord, but its main flow is directed over the surface of the brain where it is absorbed into the venous sinuses. Any structural maldevelopment

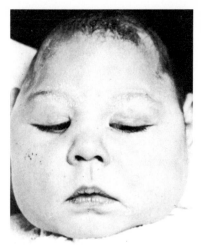

Fig. 11.18 Microcephaly.

which interferes with the normal circulation or absorption involves the risk of excessive accumulation of cerebrospinal fluid within the skull and dilatation of the ventricles characteristic of hydrocephalus. The structural anomaly may be primarily developmental or secondary to intracranial infection or trauma in utero. Interference with absorption gives rise to communicating hydrocephalus, and interference with flow from the ventricles to obstructive hydrocephalus. Meningomyelocele is frequently associated with hydrocephalus resulting in lacunar skull. In these cases the spinal anomaly is accompanied by herniation of brain substance into the spinal canal (Arnold-Chiari malformation). The protruding brain substance is subjected to abnormal pressures which interfere with the circulation of the cerebrospinal fluid, leading to the subsequent development of hydrocephalus (Fig. 11.19).

Encephalocoele is a protrusion of the meninges through a midline defect in the occipital bone. Parts of the brain may be present in the sac with resulting microcephaly.

The heart and great vessels

Arrest or interference with the normal development of the heart occurs at various stages of intrauterine life. The fifth to eighth week of fetal existence corresponds to a particularly important phase in the evolution of the heart and great vessels.

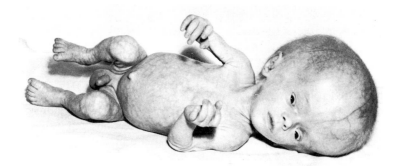

Fig. 11.19 Hydrocephalus.

Septal defects. Development of the septa separating the chambers of the heart may be arrested before closure is complete. As a result, normal circulation within the heart may be interfered with and mixing of deoxygenated and freshly oxygenated blood occurs.

Transposition. Disturbance of the normal process of rotation of the embryonic heart and great vessels may result in the eventual malposition of of certain structures. Thus the pulmonary artery may arise from the left instead of the right ventricle (transposition of the great vessels). In this event oxygenated blood is returned to the lungs while the poorly oxygenated blood in the right ventricle leaves the heart by the aorta to supply the body. Life is possible only if there is a shunt at septal level or patency of the ductus arteriosus.

Valve stenosis. Other deformities which occur include narrowing of the rings of the aortic and pulmonary valves and failure of the aorta and pulmonary arteries to develop normally in size.

Patent ductus arteriosus. Normally the ductus arteriosus undergoes spontaneous closure shortly after birth and becomes gradually converted into a fibrous cord. Where this does not occur, the ductus arteriosus remains patent — a remnant of a structure essential for intrauterine existence but unnecessary for healthy survival after birth.

Single chamber. A heart consisting of only one, two or three instead of the usual four chambers is sometimes seen at post-mortem examination on a stillborn child or infant dying shortly after birth. In such as infant disturbance of cardiac development has occurred at an even earlier stage in embryonic existence than in cases of septal defect or of transposition of the vessels.

The urgency of diagnosis

The urgency of diagnosis and treatment in infants with congenital abnormality depends upon the degree of risk associated with that abnormality. Those that produce the most marked abnormality of form may not be as urgent a problem as those with major abnormality of function. The following section therefore deals with congenital abnormalities liable to cause early neonatal death irrespective of their anatomical site. Subsequent sections will deal with abnormalities by the body system principally involved.

ABNORMALITIES LIABLE TO CAUSE EARLY NEONATAL DEATH

Atresia of the larynx is fortunately very rare but if recognized at birth, because of the extreme but ineffective inspiratory efforts, can be treated by immediate puncture of the web or by tracheotomy. Survival is rare because of associated maldevelopment of the lungs.

Laryngeal webs and *laryngeal stenosis* are also rare and produce immediate stridor when respiration begins. Tracheotomy may be required.

Choanal atresia when bilateral is a complete obstruction between the nose and the pharynx. Breathing is possible only through the open mouth (Fig. 11.20). If the mouth is closed, as during feeding,

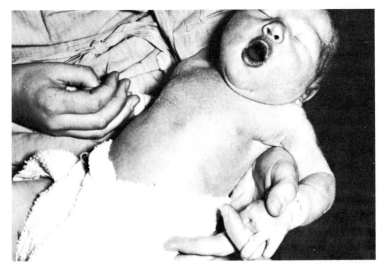

Fig. 11.20 Choanal atresia with mouth breathing.

breathing is not possible and there is marked indrawing of the chest and cyanosis until the baby opens his mouth. There may be difficulty in establishing respiration or symptoms may be delayed if the infant learns to open his mouth frequently. Treatment is surgical by perforation of the obstructing plate. The symptoms are less marked in unilateral choanal atresia.

Glossoptosis in which the tongue rolls backward into the posterior pharynx obstructing the larynx is also a cause of respiratory obstruction. This is most likely to occur where there is hypomandibulosis and cleft palate as in the *Pierre-Robin syndrome* (Fig. 11.21). Immediate treatment is by holding the baby's face and head down and pulling the tongue forward. This position should then be maintained. A suitable method using a stockinette bandage to suspend the head is shown in Figure 11.22.

Macroglossia (a large tongue) may similarly obstruct the airway and require surgical treatment (Fig. 11.23).

Oesophageal atresia

Oesophageal atresia may be recognized before birth. As the fetus cannot swallow amniotic fluid hydramnios occurs and oesophageal atresia should always be excluded by passing a large (9FG) diameter oro-gastric tube into the stomach in all pregnancies compli-

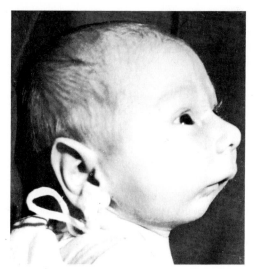

Fig. 11.21 Hypomandibulosis (Pierre-Robin syndrome)

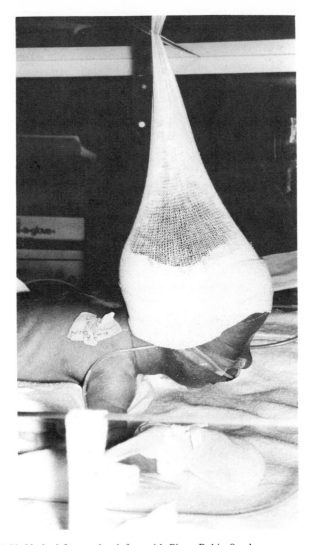

Fig. 11.22 Method for nursing infant with Pierre-Robin Syndrome.

cated by maternal hydramnios. After birth the upper oesophageal pouch, which commonly ends at the level of the cricoid cartilage, fills with saliva and mucus. Respiration becomes bubbly and aspiration of oral fluid produces respiratory obstruction and cyanosis. The types of tracheo-oesophageal fistula associated with oesophageal atresia were shown in Figure 11.8. Where no air reaches the

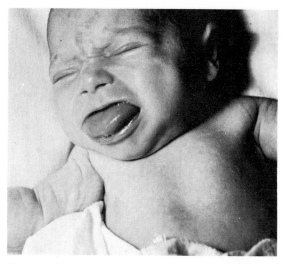

Fig. 11.23 Macroglossia.

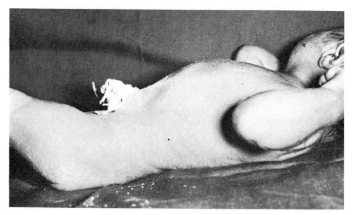

Fig. 11.24 Flat abdomen with no air in the stomach or bowel. (Due to oesophageal atresia *without* an oesophagotracheal fistula.)

stomach the abdomen will remain flat (Fig. 11.24). The diagnosis can be confirmed by passing a radio-opaque and suitably large catheter into the upper pouch and taking an X-ray of the neck (Fig. 11.25). Immediate treatment is continuous aspiration of the upper oesophageal pouch to prevent overflow of mucus and the withholding of feeds. If the gap between the upper and lower

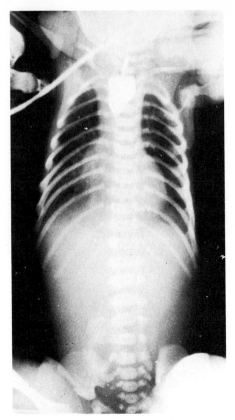

Fig. 11.25 Radio-opaque material outlining upper oesophageal pouch in baby shown in Figure 11.24. Note the absence of air below the diaphragm.

oesophageal segments allows, primary anastomosis of the proximal and distal ends should be performed. Where this is not possible it is usual to exit the proximal oesophageal pouch to the neck and to create a gastrostomy to allow feeding. At the same time any fistulae are closed to prevent aspiration pneumonia. The final corrective operation will be performed in later infancy. The prognosis is best in those infants diagnosed and treated early before chest complications develop.

Diaphragmatic hernia

Diaphragmatic hernia most commonly occurs through the left diaphragm where the left pleuroperitoneal canal has failed to close

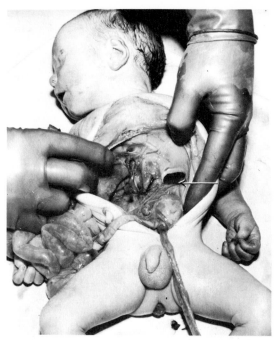

Fig. 11.26 Diaphragmatic hernia. The arrow indicates the abnormal opening in the diaphragm through which the intestine passed into the thorax. The intestine, seen on the left, has been withdrawn.

(Fig. 11.26). Abdominal viscera are present in the thorax and there is frequently underdevelopment of the lung. Symptoms of marked respiratory distress may occur from the moment of birth or be delayed for hours after birth. The symptoms occur earliest where there is most displacement of lung. The left chest may appear overfilled and the abdomen flat. Diagnosis is confirmed by X-ray, which shows air-containing bowel shadows in the chest (Fig. 11.27). The treatment is surgical. If this is not immediately available endotracheal intubation and artificial ventilation may be required to maintain life until surgical treatment can be undertaken. With rapid recognition and treatment more than 50% of affected infants should survive.

OTHER ABNORMALITIES

The majority of congenital abnormalities do not present quite such an urgent problem of diagnosis and treatment as those just

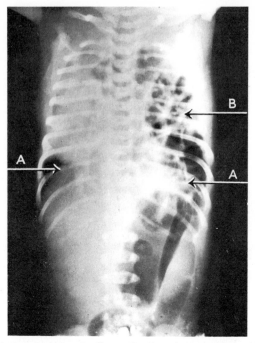

Fig. 11.27 Diaphragmatic hernia. X-ray of patient shown in Figure 11.26 before withdrawal of the intestine. A, diaphragm; B, intestine in the left chest.

discussed. It therefore seems more appropriate that these should be described under the heading of the anatomical region or the physiological system principally involved.

Face, mouth and neck

Many conditions such as Down's syndrome, achondroplasia, and some of the chromosomal abnormalities have characteristic facies which are a combination of a number of distinct features. These will be described under the heading of the principal system of the body involved. Apart from the recognized syndromes there are many infants with odd faces whom our American colleagues call funny-looking kids (or FLK syndrome) who cannot be allotted to any particular syndrome. Some of these infants will also have abnormalities such as cleft lip or palate, and when each of the individual abnormalities of the face, mouth and neck are mentioned it must be remembered that many of these abnormalities occur as one component of multiple abnormalities in the one infant.

Cleft lip may be uni- or bilateral and can occur on its own or in combination with cleft palate. Isolated cleft lip is commoner in boys and is often familial. Unless the failure of fusion is extensive there is little interference with sucking and breast feeding is possible (Fig. 11.28). The lip is repaired surgically at about two months of age. Mothers can be reassured by being shown photographs of the excellent results of good surgery.

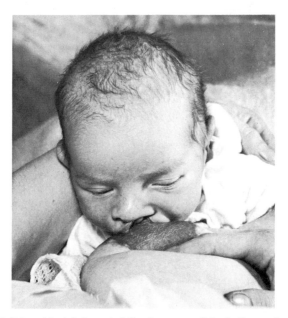

Fig. 11.28 Baby with cleft lip and cleft palate successfully feeding at the breast.

Cleft lip and palate occur in several forms. In the most extensive form (Fig. 11.29) with bilateral clefts and distortion of the premaxilla the result is unsightly. As other abnormalities are frequently present a full and careful examination of the whole infant is essential. Moulding of the maxilla into a more satisfactory shape can be achieved by plates specially prepared by orthodontists. This makes subsequent surgical repair simpler and more effective. It is useful to be able to show mothers with an affected infant the successful results of treatment of another infant with paired before and after photographs such as those shown in Figure 11.30. Even with severe abnormalities feeding by normal bottle and teat is often possible particularly with an orthodontic plate in position. Middle ear infec-

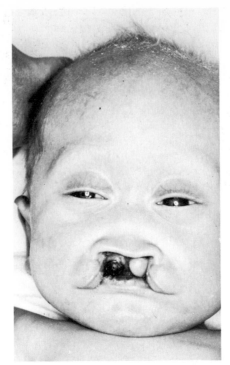

Fig. 11.29 Bilateral cleft lip and cleft palate with rotation of the premaxilla.

tion is a constant risk and the ears should be examined regularly. Less extensive clefts may not require orthodontic preparatory treatment before surgery. It is advisable for infants with cleft palates to be examined and reviewed regularly by a team of paediatric physician and surgeon, orthodontic surgeon and ear, nose and throat surgeon — to decide the most appropriate therapy. This may require referral to a regional centre.

Other abnormalities of the facial bones give rise to characteristic facies by which some syndromes including those of the first arch syndrome are recognized. The Pierre-Robin syndrome has already been considered. Mandibulofacial dysostosis (Fig. 11.6) is less frequently a cause of difficulty with breathing and feeding but these may occur because of the tongue falling back (glossoptosis). The immediate treatment is as for Pierre-Robin syndrome. Later complications including hearing problems and repeated tests for hearing should be arranged.

True tongue tie is a very rare condition. This condition has been

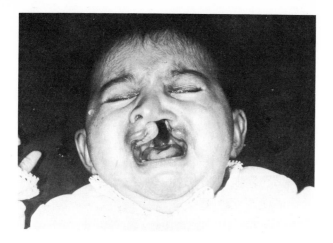

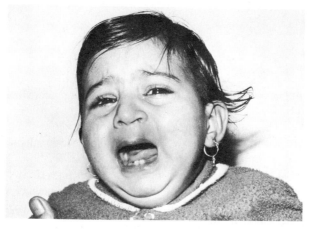

Fig. 11.30 Cleft lip and palate in an Asian child before and after operative correction.

overdiagnosed in the past because of failure to recognize that the frenum passing from the tongue to the floor of the mouth is normally short in the newborn. In the healthy infant there is no indication for cutting the frenum at this age. The tongue becomes more mobile as the infant grows. Only in infants with severe limitation of tongue movement and inability to suck is division of the frenum indicated.

Teeth may be present at birth or erupt shortly afterwards. They are generally loose and either fall out or are readily removed.

Epulis is a projection from the gum (Fig. 11.31) most commonly

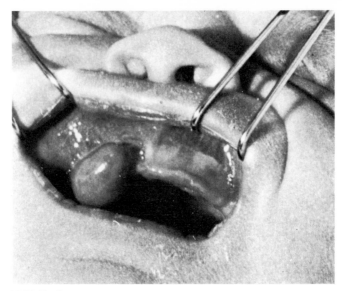

Fig. 11.31 Epulis.

of the upper jaw. It may interfere with feeding and should be removed.

Ranula is a cystic swelling caused by obstruction of the sublingual duct. Most resolve without treatment but occasionally surgery is required if the cyst persists and interferes with feeding.

Branchial arch anomalies may present as skin tags (Fig. 11.32), cysts or sinuses. They may be found in the preauricular region or along the anterior border of the sternomastoid muscle. Surgical removal is generally required.

Cystic hygromas are most common in the neck (Fig. 11.33) although they may occur elsewhere (Fig. 11.34). They consist of a mass of proliferating lymph vessels and may cause pressure symptoms. Treatment is by surgical removal.

Goitre is rare in the newborn. Thyroid function may be normal as in simple goitre, decreased as in goitrous cretinism or increased as in the infant of a thyrotoxic mother.

The eye

Absence of the eye (anophthalmia) or a small eye (microphthalmia) are not always obvious at birth but should be looked for if the eye sockets are not normally filled.

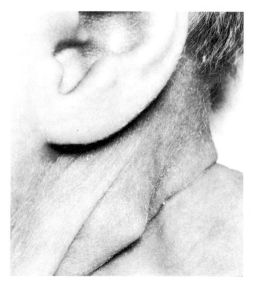

Fig. 11.32 Branchial cyst.

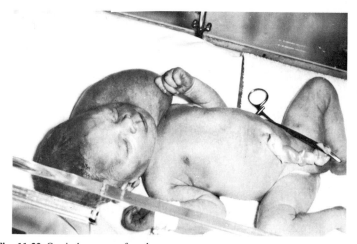

Fig. 11.33 Cystic hygroma of neck.

Congenital glaucoma, enlargement of the eye, follows obstruction to drainage of the aqueous humour. Similar enlargement from other causes such as injury or infection is termed buphthalmos. Treatment depends on the cause and the opinion of an ophthalmologist should be sought (Fig. 11.35).

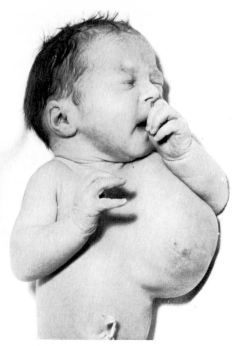

Fig. 11.34 Cystic hygroma of axilla.

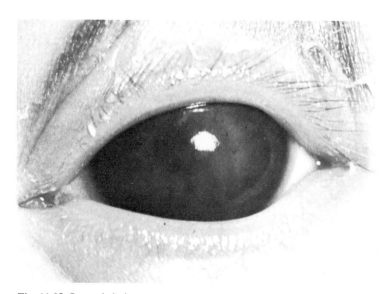

Fig. 11.35 Congenital glaucoma.

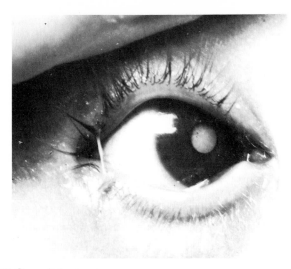

Fig. 11.36 Congenital cataract.

Congenital cataract may be evident at birth or become obvious during the following weeks. The cause in many cases is hereditary. Others follow maternal rubella in the first trimester of pregnancy or are associated with galactosaemia (Fig. 11.36).

The eyelids are occasionally partially fused at birth. In marked cases surgical separation is required (Fig. 11.37). Rarely the eyelids

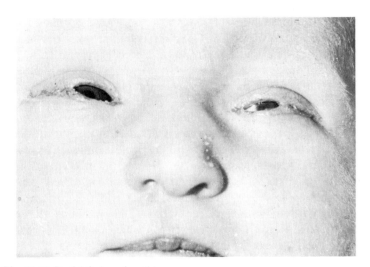

Fig. 11.37 Partial fusion of eyelids.

are everted after birth. This condition settles spontaneously. Obstruction of the nasolacrimal duct is sometimes misdiagnosed as prolonged conjunctivitis. Although there may be a slight yellow discharge there is no evidence of inflammation and tears can be seen trickling from the eye. Most ducts clear spontaneously and no treatment other than hygiene is required in the neonatal period.

Dermoid cysts are occasionally found overlying portions of both cornea and conjunctiva. They are more commonly found at the outer end of the upper eyelid.

Retinoblastoma, which may be present at birth, is a potentially fatal tumour of the retina of the eye in which death can be prevented by early diagnosis and treatment. A greyish-yellow reflex is evident behind the pupil which may be dilated. Both eyes must be examined. In any case of doubt an ophthalmologist's opinion must be sought. Treatment is drastic by enucleation of one or both eyes. If this is not acceptable radiotherapy together with cryotherapy and photocoagulation is available as an alternative. As the condition is inherited as a dominant character, genetic advice should be given.

Central nervous system

Neural tube defects

Neural tube defects, which include, anencephaly, myelomeningocele and hydrocephalus, constitute the largest single group of congenital abnormalities in most surveys. There is, however, a considerable geographical and seasonal variation in incidence; as mentioned earlier 'epidemics' of these defects appear to occur and it has been suggested that these may be related to environmental causes. Antenatal diagnosis by screening mother's serum for alphafetoprotein with subsequent confirmation of suspected cases by amniocentesis or ultrasonography leading to therapeutic termination of pregnancy in affected cases is already reducing the incidence of neural tube defects in centres where such techniques are available. Neural tube defects are more common in mothers of lower socioeconomic status. It is thought that there could be a genetic predisposition to neural tube defect which will become manifest given certain environmental conditions. The possibility that this could be due to nutritional deficiencies which could be corrected by pre- and periconceptional supplementation of the diet with folate and B vitamins is being investigated.

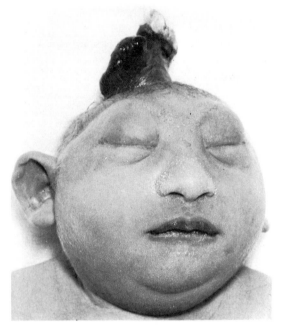

Fig. 11.38 Anencephaly.

Anencephaly is the commonest of the neural tube defects. Because of the major malformation of the skull and brain affected infants are stillborn or die shortly after birth (Fig. 11.38).

Spina bifida and myelomeningocele is less rapidly fatal and therefore constitutes the larger clinical problem. Eighty per cent of infants with myelomeningocele develop hydrocephalus.

The spinal defect most commonly occurs in the lumbar region (Fig. 11.16) but may occur elsewhere in the spinal column (Fig. 11.39). There is considerable variation in the degree of associated abnormality of the vertebral bodies. The presenting signs are generally the presence of the sac which if intact may protrude but if it has been punctured will lie flattened over the depression between the sides of the spina bifida. The sac may be a simple myelocele with no nervous tissue or a meningo-myelocele in which the spinal cord is exposed and enters the sac. Skin may cover the smaller sacs. If the sac has burst it should be covered with a non-adhesive sterile dressing. The assessment of the degree of neurological involvement is not simple and examination at birth can be

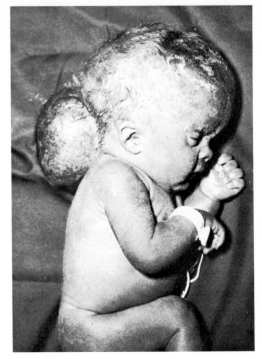

Fig. 11.39 Cervical spina bifida and meningocele.

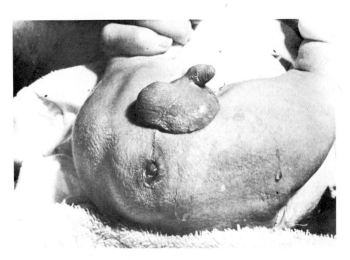

Fig. 11.40 Patulous anus and dribble incontinence of urine because of lack of sphincter control in an infant with spina bifida.

misleading. One or both lower limbs are commonly paralysed and there is often loss of sphincter control (Fig. 11.40).

Opinions differ as to the need for immediate surgical treatment to cover an exposed sac with skin. Without this treatment even very severely affected infants may survive and subsequent management is made more difficult. Surgical treatment while limiting the risk of infection and of further deterioration in neurological function is not of course curative and may precipitate the onset of hydrocephalus and the need for further operations.

Hydrocephalus may have been recognized during delivery but more commonly is evident later as widely spread skull sutures even although the occipito-frontal circumference (o.f.c.) is normal. Repeated measurement of o.f.c. will show a rapid increase in size and the classical, clinical, ultrasonic and radiological features of hydrocephalus will become more obvious (Figs 11.41 and 11.42). Treatment is by the surgical introduction of a controlled drainage system to reduce the intracranial pressure.

The longer term complications of spina bifida are principally renal and orthopaedic. Many question whether the quality of life achieved by the procedures required to correct these abnormalities justifies the considerable expenditure of skill and time involved, particularly when society at the same time allows large numbers of healthy fetuses to be aborted.

Policy in relation to spina bifida therefore varies from centre to

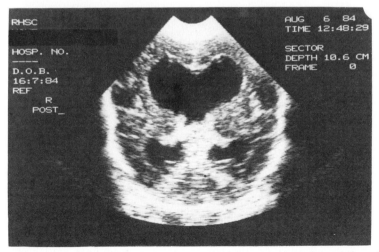

Fig. 11.41 Ultrasound of head showing dilated ventricles (with kind permission of Dr Mark Ziervogel).

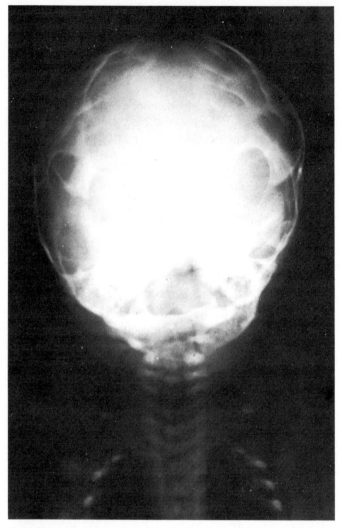

Fig. 11.42 X-ray of skull in hydrocephalus. (Lacunar skull.)

centre. If all the staff concerned are not aware of or disagree with local policy parents may be given conflicting advice and it is important that this should be avoided. Referral to a regional assessment centre where available allows more detailed neurological and other assessment. Policy with regard to an individual infant can then be decided on the basis of objective findings taking into account the parents' wishes.

Microcephaly is not amenable to treatment unless the small skull size is due to premature fusion of the cranial sutures (craniosynostosis) in which case surgical treatment is possible. Other forms of central nervous system (CNS) abnormality are seldom obvious as such at birth but may present in the first month of life as abnormalities of behaviour such as convulsions. In obstetrics units making routine ultrasound examinations of the fetus, an increasing number of intracranial and other abnormalities are being identified prenatally.

Some CNS abnormalities may be suspected because of associated physical abnormality as in Down's syndrome (mongolism) which is considered later. A limited number of potential causes of mental abnormality can be recognized by specific testing for bio-chemical abnormality as in the case of phenylketonuria and hypothyroidism.

Cardiovascular system (CVS)

With the development of new techniques of investigation and surgical treatment it is now possible to save the lives of some infants with serious cardiac abnormalities who would otherwise have died shortly after birth. It is therefore more important now to recognize such conditions early and to have a planned policy of investigation. Cardiac abnormalities occur in 1–2% of liveborn infants. About half of these will die within the first weeks or months of life. This is therefore a serious and relatively common form of congenital abnormality.

Plan of management. The detailed investigation of the more serious anomalies is complicated and will not be referred to here. It is essential however that doctors and midwives dealing with the newborn should be able to recognize the earliest signs which might indicate a cardiac abnormality and arrange for further investigation and treatment without delay. How this is done will vary according to the facilities available in any particular unit. In all units an agreed plan of action is vital and this will generally involve consultation with cardiologists skilled in the management of such problems in the new-born.

Commoner abnormalities in CVS

Although there is a large number of individual abnormalities which can occur in the cardiovascular system nine of these account for about 85% of the total. These nine are shown in Table 11.4

Table 11.4   The common types of congenital cardiac abnormality

Anatomical abnormality	Functional disorder
Hypoplastic left heart syndrome Transposition of the great vessels Fallot's tetralogy	Hypoxaemia
Aortic stenosis Pulmonary stenosis Coarctation of the aorta	Obstruction and pressure overload
Ventricular septal defect Atrial septal defect Patent ductus arteriosus	Shunting and circulatory overload

grouped according to their principal interference with function. The remaining 15% of cardiac abnormalities include a wide range of abnormalities which are individually rare and for further details about these reference should be made to textbooks of paediatric cardiology.

Cyanotic group

The abnormalities shown in Table 11.4 are compatible with varying lengths of life if not corrected by surgery. The first group is characterized by early onset of cyanosis — the earlier the onset the worse the prognosis.

Hypoplastic left heart syndrome which includes hypoplasia of the left ventricle, aortic valve and aortic arch is the commonest cause of cardiac death in the neonatal period.

Transposition of the great vessels is the second most common cause of death. The anatomy is very variable and complex. In the commonest form the aorta arises from the right ventricle and the pulmonary artery from the left ventricle, life being made possible by a shunt at ventricular or atrial level and by patency of the ductus arteriosus. This shunt can be increased in some cases by atrial septostomy using a balloon catheter (Rashkind procedure). By this means life may be preserved until the infant is large enough for corrective surgery.

Fallot's tetralogy is pulmonary stenosis associated with ventricular septal defect, overriding of the right ventricle by the aortic valve and hypertrophy of the right ventricle. Although cyanosis is a common finding in older children it is less commonly found in the neonatal period unless the pulmonary stenosis is of severe degree.

Obstructive group

Valve stenosis. Obstructive lesions as in severe stenosis of the pulmonary or aortic valves or coarctation of the aorta throw an extra burden on the associated ventricle and heart failure may follow. Cyanosis is an early feature in severe pulmonary stenosis. Diagnosis may first be suspected by the presence of a cardiac murmur on first day examination.

Coarctation. Absent or delayed femoral pulses point to the likelihood of coarctation of the aorta. Heart failure frequently develops within the first week or two.

Surgical treatment is possible for each of these conditions following medical treatment for the heart failure.

Ductus dependent stenosis. Where either the pulmonary or the systemic circulation is dependent on blood flow through a ductus arteriosus it is essential that the ductus remain patent. Prostaglandin E2 has been used successfully to keep the ductus open until surgery can be performed.

Shunt lesions

Patent ductus arteriosus, ventricular septal defect and atrial septal defect are generally first discovered because of the presence of a cardiac murmur. This may not be present on the first day examination but may be detected later in the first week of life. The shunt increases pulmonary blood flow to a varying extent according to its size and heart failure is commonest where there is the largest increase in flow.

Reversal of the shunt from a left to right to a right to left shunt will cause cyanosis. This is most likely to occur where there is increased resistance to pulmonary blood flow and increase in pulmonary artery pressure.

Persistent fetal circulation. The high pulmonary vascular resistance of fetal life may persist for a varying length of time after delivery causing a right to left shunt through the ductus arteriosus producing cyanosis. Ultrasound examination or cardiac catheterization may be required to exclude a more complicated structural abnormality.

Cardiac failure

During the first month of life cardiac failure is a common complication of congenital cardiac abnormality. The commonest of the abnormalities likely to precipitate failure are coarctation of the aorta, transposition of the great vessels, patent ductus arteriosus and aortic atresia. Other acquired abnormalities such as myocarditis, endocardial fibroelastosis or profound anaemia, as in hydrops fetalis, also cause heart failure.

Clinical manifestations. An abnormal weight gain, increase in pulse and respiratory rates and difficulty in feeding are the first clinical signs of failure likely to be noticed. Each or all may be attributed to other causes, and the presence of cardiac failure may not be recognized until signs such as dyspnoea, moderate cyanosis and hepato-splenomegaly occur. Peripheral oedema is a late sign and cardiac failure should be diagnosed and treated before it is present. Pulmonary signs are variable and not a reliable indication of the presence or absence of failure.

Medical management. The treatment of cardiac failure in infants in the first month of life differs only in detail from management at later ages. Dosages of the drugs used must be calculated carefully by the doctors concerned and the nursing staff must pay particular attention to the measurement of the doses given.

Frusemide by intramuscular injection 1.0 mg per kg per dose can be used in the early stages of treatment to promote diuresis and repeated in four to six hours if indicated. Regular weighing and checks of plasma potassium and sodium are required to assess the effectiveness of diuretic therapy and prevent hypokalaemia.

Occasionally digoxin therapy is helpful. The digitalizing dose of digoxin is of the order of 50 to 60 μg per kg of body weight and is normally given in three or four doses over a period of 12 to 24 hours according to the severity of the signs of failure and the rapidity of the infant's response. The initial doses may be given intramuscularly or intravenously. A daily maintenance dose of 20–25% of the digitalizing dose divided into two doses can generally be given by mouth. Treatment with digoxin should be withheld if the heart rate falls below 100 per minute.

In addition to drug therapy the infant should be propped up and nursed in oxygen. Tube feeding may be required and careful monitoring of the fluid and nutrient intake is necessary to maintain a balance between calorie intake and fluid overload.

Investigation

Of the nine abnormalities listed in Table 11.4 three are responsible for almost half of the neonatal deaths due to cardiac abnormality.

The three are hypoplastic left heart syndrome, coarctation of the aorta and transposition of the great vessels. Surgical treatment is available for the last two. It is important therefore that accurate clinical observations are made and where a potentially lethal heart abnormality is suspect investigation in a suitably equipped centre is called for. This will generally include ultrasound and Doppler examination and or cardiac catheterization. These should be carried out on all infants who have been in cardiac failure or who have been persistently cyanosed because of a cardiac cause. The number of infants requiring such investigation in any one maternity unit is small and it is only by the referral of infants to a regional centre that we can hope for an improvement in the present high mortality from serious cardiac abnormalities. Where this policy is in force there is already evidence of improvement in the situation.

Alimentary system

Consideration has already been given to diaphragmatic hernia and oesophageal atresia which are a threat to life because of interference with respiration.

Duodenal atresia or severe stenosis presents as vomiting occurring shortly after the first feed. There is an increased incidence of these disorders in children with Down's syndrome. Bile may or may not be present according to the site of the stricture. The lower abdomen is flat as opposed to the distended upper abdomen. X-ray of the abdomen shows the characteristic double bubble sign (Fig. 11.43). Treatment is surgical.

Intestinal atresia may occur at any level. The further down the bowel the site of the obstruction the later will be the onset of symptoms of vomiting which becomes bile-stained and then faecal in type. Obstruction of the small intestine may be due to atresia, stenosis, duplication, volvulus and malrotation or meconium ileus.

Anal atresia should be recognized at the first examination (Fig. 11.44) but other abnormalities in this region are not so easily diagnosed but are noted as delay in passage of meconium, passage of meconium from an abnormal site (Fig. 11.45) or difficulty in inserting a rectal thermometer. Treatment of bowel obstruction at any level in the neonate is almost always surgical.

Meconium ileus is obstruction of the intestine by thick viscid meconium and is the earliest manifestation of cystic fibrosis with absence of pancreatic trypsin. The meconium contains unaltered albumin which can be recognized in a suspension of meconium by

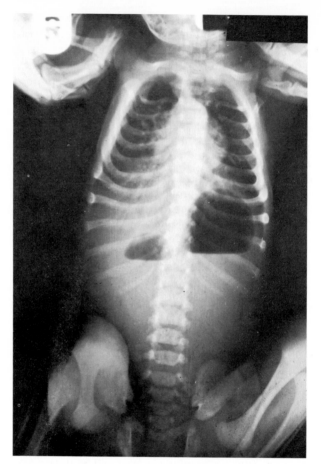

Fig. 11.43 Double air bubble in abdomen in duodenal atresia.

its positive reaction with specific tests such as the BM test or with Albustix. Rupture of the bowel may have occurred in utero resulting in meconium peritonitis. Areas of calcification may be seen on abdominal X-ray.

Hirschsprung's disease is due to absence of ganglion cells of Auer-bach's plexus in a segment of bowel in which peristalsis ceases, causing obstruction. There is delay in the passage of meconium but after the passage of a 'meconium plug' normal bowel movements may be present for a period of days, weeks or months before obstruction recurs. Diagnosis is by demonstration of the agan-glionic area on biopsy and treatment is surgical. A similar situation

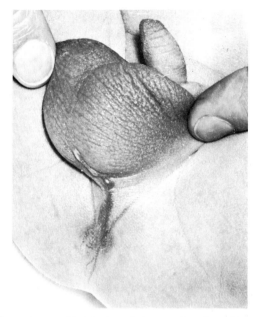

Fig. 11.44 Covered anus with intradermal sinus passing along the median raphe.

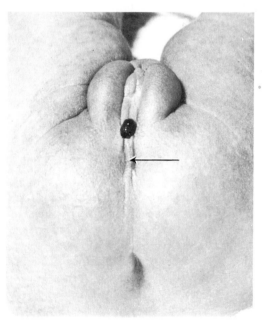

Fig. 11.45 Ectopic anus. The arrow indicates the normal site of the anus (Compare Fig. 11.10).

may be caused by a meconium plug which is not associated with Hirschsprung's disease. After a finger has been inserted into the rectum the plug is often passed and the obstruction relieved.

For more detailed discussion of the rare causes of intestinal obstruction in the newborn reference should be made to a textbook of neonatal surgery. In some cases of meconium ileus and meconium plug syndrome, a Gastrografin enema as well as giving diagnostic assistance may prove therapeutic. The Gastrografin acts by drawing water from the lower bowel mucosa into the bowel lumen and therefore, before this procedure is undertaken, care must be taken to ensure that the infant is adequately hydrated.

Vomiting later in the neonatal period may be due to hiatus hernia or pyloric stenosis.

The umbilicus

The umbilical cord normally contains two arteries and one vein.

A single umbilical artery is associated with an increased incidence of other congenital abnormalities.

Persistence of the allantois results in the discharge of urine from a patent urachus opening at the umbilical stump or the formation of a urachal cyst or sinus. These have to be distinguished from persistence of the omphalomesenteric duct from which faecal matter may be discharged at the umbilicus.

Exomphalos (Fig. 11.46) with protrusion of the bowel into a sac of peritoneum and amnion follows failure of the migration of the mesoderms (abdominal wall muscles) to close round the umbilical opening.

The sac, intact or partly ruptured, should be covered with sterile moistened swabs as initial management. Conservative treatment of the intact sac (with local application of 1% mercurochrome) has been recommended when there is no evidence of other abnormality in the bowel. There is now less enthusiasm for this form of therapy because of a risk of producing mercury poisoning. Corrective surgery or the insertion of a temporary silastic covering pouch is the more usual treatment. Hernia into the cord is a minor degree of exomphalos. The cord must be clamped distal to any bowel present to avoid intestinal obstruction and damage.

Gastroschisis in which the bowel protrudes without the protection of a covering sac requires early surgery (Fig. 11.47). Meanwhile the bowel should be covered with sterile moistened swabs.

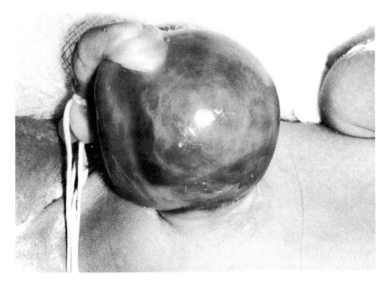

Fig. 11.46 Exomphalos.

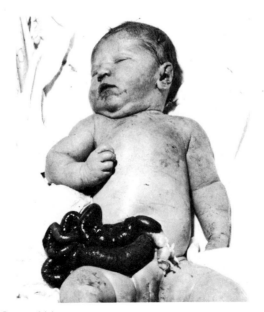

Fig. 11.47 Gastroschisis.

Urogenital system

Renal agenesis

Failure of the fetus in utero to pass urine results in oligohydramnios and a 'squashed baby' with large floppy ears and hands, deformities of the feet and characteristic facies (Potter's syndrome). The membranes of the placenta show fine nodules, amnion nodosum (Fig. 11.48). The commonest cause is failure of development of both kidneys — renal agenesis, but a similar picture follows complete obstruction to the flow of urine from, for example, urethral stricture (Fig. 11.49).

Obstructive uropathy. Infants with obstructive uropathy will have an enlarged bladder and kidneys. In either case there is insufficient functioning renal tissue to support life, no urine is passed and death occurs at or shortly after birth. Prenatal diagnosis of obstructive uropathies by ultrasound examination has resulted in fetal surgical procedures in an attempt to prevent renal damage, with somewhat disappointing results to date.

Prune belly syndrome. This is the association of absent abdominal wall musculature with cryptorchidism, hydronephrosis and hydroureter (Figs 19.6 and 19.7).

Cystic kidneys. Large renal masses at birth may also be due to multicystic disease which is generally unilateral and polycystic disease which is bilateral (Fig. 11.50). Survival is possible only if there is sufficient functioning renal tissue.

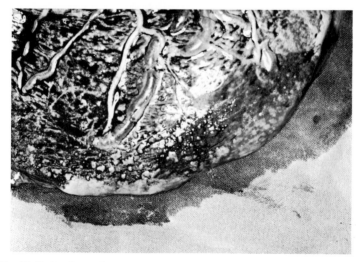

Fig. 11.48 Amnion nodosum.

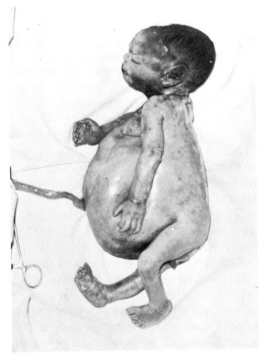

Fig. 11.49 Gross enlargement of kidneys, ureters and bladder secondary to complete obstruction of the urethra.

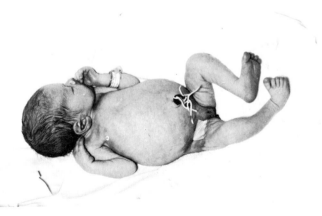

Fig. 11.50 Abdominal distension due to polycystic disease of the kidneys.

Exstrophy of the bladder. This condition is commoner in boys and is associated with epispadias, wide divarication of the recti abdominis muscles and the symphysis pubis (Fig. 11.11). Although unsightly it is not an immediate threat to life and surgical closure may be possible after a few years. Other abnormalities of the renal system may present at any age of infancy or childhood because they have predisposed to urinary tract infection.

Doubtful sex

The most urgent problems likely to arise in the genital system at birth are connected with the ascertainment of sex. In any infant where there is doubt about the external genitalia expert advice should be sought immediately so that a decision can be made as to which sex to announce to the parents.

Adrenogenital syndrome. Female infants suffering from the adrenogenital syndrome may have undergone virilization in utero and, as in the case of the girl shown in Figure 11.51, the urethra may pass through the clitoris and resemble a penis. Although the labia majora are fused and resemble a scrotum no gonads are palpable. Rapid help can be obtained from suitable staining of cells from the buccal mucosa. The presence of a chromatin body in the nucleus (Fig. 11.52) indicates that the infant has two X chromosomes and is probably female. Fluorescent staining can indicate the presence or absence of a Y chromosome (Fig. 11.68) but chromosome karyotype analysis, which takes two to three days is essential for a firm sex chromosome diagnosis. As some infants with

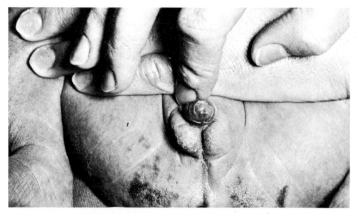

Fig. 11.51 Virilization of female infant in adrenogenital syndrome.

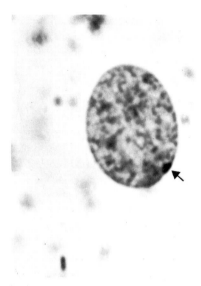

Fig. 11.52 Single chromatin (Barr) body in nucleus of buccal cell of a female infant. (Photograph by courtesy of the MRC Clinical and Population Cytogenetics Unit.)

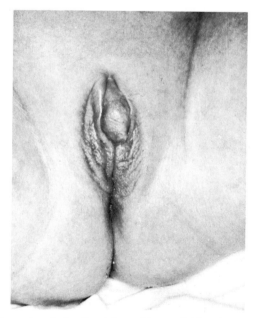

Fig. 11.53 External genitalia of an infant with a vestigial testis on one side and vestigial ovum on the other side.

adrenogenital syndrome also have adrenal failure, examination of plasma electrolytes is an essential early investigation. If there is a raised plasma potassium and lowered sodium and chloride the infant is at serious risk of early death unless given corticosteroids.

Intersex. Other forms of intersex (Fig. 11.53) will require detailed investigation, which often includes ultrasound and sometimes laparotomy, to examine the gonads. As such infants can often not function as either males or females and as the fetus is fundamentally female until acted upon by male hormones it is sensible when in doubt about the sex of a newborn infant to announce that it is female. When no sexual function exists it is easier for the patient and parents if the infant is brought up as female even though the chromosomoes are XY.

Less serious minor abnormalities of the external genitalia are more common and occur mainly in male infants.

Hypospadias. Failure of closure of the urogenital groove, leaving the meatal opening at the base of the glans penis or more proximally on the penis or scrotum (Fig. 11.54), results in hypospadias. No treatment is required in the neonatal period unless stricture of

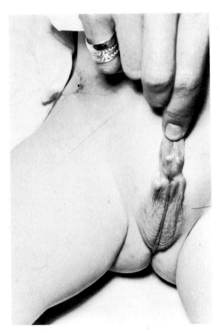

Fig. 11.54 Hypospadias.

the meatus prevents the normal passage of urine. Circumcision is contraindicated.

Epispadias. Less commonly the urethra may open on the dorsal surface of the penis. Treatment is surgical at a later stage of infancy.

Absence of testes. Failure of descent of one or both testes into the scrotum does not require treatment in the first month of life but is an indication for arranging regular follow-up examination. If neither testis is palpable buccal smear examination for sex chromatin and karyotyping should be undertaken.

Torsion of the testis. The presence of a hard reddish blue mass in the scrotum is suggestive of torsion of the testis and is an indication for immediate operation.

Hydrocele. A translucent swelling in the scrotum around the testis is indicative of a non-communicating hydrocele which will clear spontaneously (Fig. 11.55). A similar scrotal swelling extending towards the inguinal ring and which alters in size is suggestive of a communicating hydrocele which is often associated with an inguinal hernia. Surgical treatment is required.

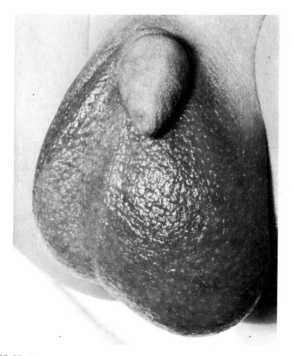

Fig. 11.55 Hydrocele.

Foreskin. The foreskin in the newborn is not normally retractable and no attempt should be made to extract the prepuce because attempts at retracting it may cause adhesion and the development of phimosis. Circumcision is only indicated medically if there is obstruction to urine flow by a narrow meatus, a rare occurrence.

Labial adhesions. In the female, labial adhesions can often be separated by simple traction.

Imperforate hymen. Bulging of the perineum in female infants occurs where there is obstruction by an imperforate hymen and an abnormal collection of vaginal fluid. Incision of the hymen relieves the situation.

Abnormalities of the sex chromosomes are considered later in this chapter.

Endocrine disorders

Hypothyroidism. The physical signs of athyrotic cretinism (hypothyroidism) are rarely evident at birth but may be suspected later in the first month of life because of sluggish movements and feeding difficulties including choking episodes. Prolongation of 'physiological' jaundice beyond the 10th to 14th day may be due to hypothyroidism and is often the first sign to suggest this possibility. The characteristic picture of the cretin is seldom evident until after one month of age. Routine screening of new-born infants by estimation of thyroid stimulating hormone (TSH) which is raised in congenital hypothyroidism is now being widely introduced and can be carried out on capillary blood spots collected on filter paper at five days after birth as for the Guthrie test which will be discussed later (see Fig. 11.75). Diagnosis can be confirmed by the demonstration of a low and falling level of T_3 or T_4 together with TSH concentrations greater than 50 $\mu U/ml$. Rarely there can be congenital hypothyroidism secondary to failure of TSH production which will not be detected by the TSH screening test. X-ray shows delayed epiphyseal development, and epiphyses present show stippling due to multiple centres of ossification. The ECG shows low voltage waves. Treatment is by a thyroid preparation such as sodium L-thyroxine, beginning with 20 μg daily (8–10 $\mu g/kg/day$). In some families with an inherited disorder of thyroid metabolism a goitre may be present at birth with evidence of hypothyroidism. Goitre may also appear in the infants of mothers treated with thiouracil during pregnancy.

Hyperthyroidism. Some mothers with present or past thyrotoxicosis have infants with transient hyperthyroidism who are flushed and overactive and who may develop heart failure secondary to tachycardia (200/min). Such infants should be treated with oral propranolol 2.0 mg/kg/day in divided doses six-hourly and/or with Lugol's iodine solution 0.1 ml three times daily. Antithyroid treatment with propyl-thiouracil 10 mg/kg/day should then be given for several weeks before cautiously weaning from therapy.

Adrenal failure. The frequency of haemorrhage into the adrenal glands is difficult to assess but it is seen at postmortem examination on infants who have collapsed suddenly. Occasionally a mass may be palpable in the flank. The differentiation from haemorrhage into the brain or lungs is difficult and all are liable to occur in infants with birth injury or a bleeding disorder (Chapters 12 and 18).

Congenital adrenal hyperplasia is most evident in female infants who have evidence of a virilizing effect in utero. Both male and female infants may present with vomiting and biochemical evidence of adrenocortical failure in that the plasma potassium is high and the sodium and chloride low. Treatment with sodium chloride by mouth or intravenously and fludrocortisone is life-saving. Urine collection for 17-ketosteroid, 17-OH steroid and pregnanetriol output measurement should be started. Increased values confirm the diagnosis and treatment with cortisone or prednisolone will be required. Such treatment is best controlled in a regional centre but the control of the electrolyte disorder is an urgent matter and should not be delayed.

Cushing's syndrome is rarely seen in the newborn period.

True diabetes mellitus is uncommon in the first month of life but must be remembered in an infant with polyuria and weight loss.

A transient form of diabetes mellitus with glycosuria and hyperglycaemia occurs in the newborn period. After a period when treatment with insulin may be required the infant appears to make a spontaneous recovery.

Persistent hypoglycaemia due to hyperinsulinaemia, caused by nesidioblastosis and other causes is dealt with in Chapter 17.

Skeletal system

Achondroplasia

The infant with classical achondroplasia (Fig. 11.56) presents little diagnostic problem at birth and can be recognized by X-ray examination in utero. The limbs are relatively short particularly in their

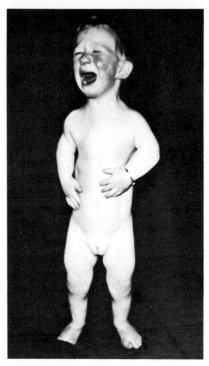

Fig. 11.56 Achondroplasia showing short proximal segments of the limbs.

proximal segments. Head size is a little larger than normal and although hydrocephalus is self-arresting in most infants with achondroplasia in others it is progressive and requires treatment. The bridge of the nose is flattened, the forehead prominent and the mandible may protrude. Lumbar lordosis makes the buttocks and abdomen prominent. Mentality is unaffected and parents often require firm reassurance on this point. Many cases arise from sporadic mutation but a dominant form of inheritance also occurs. No treatment is available for the skeletal abnormality in infancy.

Dyschondroplasias. There are several forms of abnormal growth of cartilage resulting in other forms of dyschondroplasia some of which, such as Conradi's disease (Fig. 11.57), are recognizable at birth. Morquio's disease and the other various forms of inherited mucopolysaccharide disorders do not become evident until later infancy or early childhood. Asphyxiating thoracic dystrophy (Jeune's syndrome) may present at birth with respiratory difficulty because of the small chest.

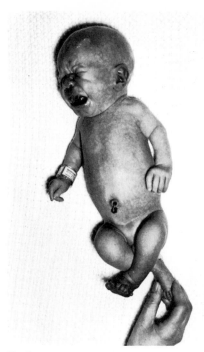

Fig. 11.57 Conradi's disease.

Osteogenesis imperfecta results in extremely fragile bones. In its severe form it affects the fetus in utero where fractures occur and the infant is born with shortened deformed limbs and X-ray shows multiple fractures. Many are stillborn. In those less severely affected survival may be possible but frequent fractures occur (Figs 11.58 and 11.59). No treatment other than protection and gentle handling is possible.

Cleidocranial dysostosis is inherited as a dominant character and causes abnormalities in the clavicles and skull. The cranial sutures are widely open and parts of the clavicles are missing. Treatment is not available and is not required as the condition causes no disability. The important of this condition lies in the differential diagnosis from other conditions. This is generally clear when the family history is known.

The lax hip

Laxity of the hip joint with partial or complete subluxation on suit-

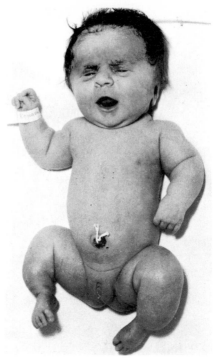

Fig. 11.58 Osteogenesis imperfecta.

able testing (Chapter 7) can be detected at birth relatively frequently. Subluxation or dislocatability is more common in females and in breech deliveries. A few infants whose hips later dislocate when weight-bearing is started may not show evidence of subluxation at birth, and in these the abnormality is in the structure of the acetabulum rather than in laxity of the joint. Lax hips can recover if diagnosed early and treated by being kept in a position of abduction using a rigid splint of the type shown in Figure 11.60. Regular follow-up of infants with lax hips is essential and in most centres this is arranged by the orthopaedic service. As there is an increased risk in the siblings of affected infants particular care must be taken in the initial examination and follow-up of infants in whose family there is a history of dislocation of the hip.

Talipes

The pressure of the uterine wall frequently produces positional

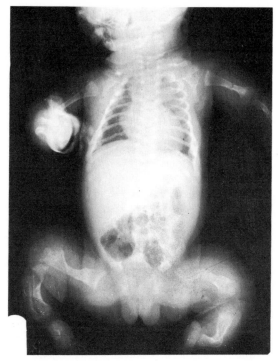

Fig. 11.59 Osteogenesis imperfecta with X-ray showing multiple fractures.

abnormality of the feet at birth which can be corrected by passive movements. As with the true club foot which cannot be corrected by passive movement the abnormality may be in equinovarus with the foot pointing downward and inward, calcaneovalgus with the foot pointing upward and outward, or metatarsus varus in which the forefoot only is angulated inwards. One or both feet may be affected.

Positional talipes is treated by frequent manipulation and stimulation of active movement.

Fixed club foot requires orthopaedic management with progressive splinting.

Scoliosis. Abnormalities of the vertebral bodies such as hemivertebrae produce scoliosis.

The skin

Abnormalities of the skin are readily discernible by parents and are frequently the cause of concern.

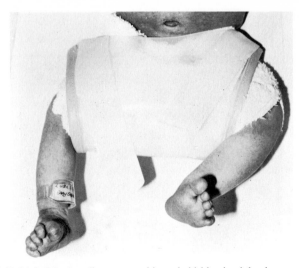

Fig. 11.60 Light plastic splint over napkin to hold hips in abduction.

Birthmarks

Minor abnormalities such as the smaller birthmarks, (mongolian) blue spots and urticaria neonatorum have been considered in Chapter 6. Larger naevi are most commonly of the port wine type (Fig. 11.61) or are pigmented (Fig. 11.62). Treatment is not required in the neonatal period.

Epidermolysis bullosa (Fig. 11.63) is a rare inherited condition in which pressure on the skin produces bullae which rupture leaving

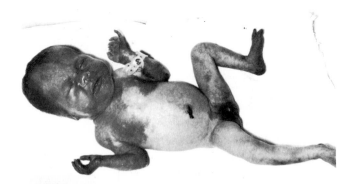

Fig. 11.61 Extensive port wine naevi.

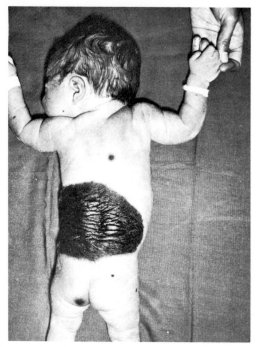

Fig. 11.62 Pigmented naevi.

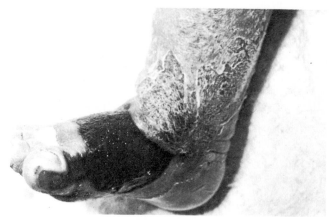

Fig. 11.63 Raw area over dorsum of foot following rupture of bulla in epidermolysis bullosa.

raw red areas which are readily infected. The mucous membranes are similarly affected in some infants, making feeding very difficult. Treatment is palliative by gentle handling and prevention of infection. The prognosis is poor in severe cases.

Collodion skin is evident at birth. The skin has a varnished appearance and cracks readily. As the abnormal skin is desquamated it is replaced either by normal skin or by skin showing signs of ichthyosis.

Ichthyosis, in which the skin is papery, dry and scaly, may also occur independently (Fig. 11.64).

Scalp defects. Defects of the skin, particularly over the scalp (Fig. 11.65), may be found at birth. These heal in a few weeks leaving a fibrous scar (Fig. 11.66).

Multiple congenital abnormalities

Congenital abnormalities do not always occur in single systems of the body but frequently several systems may be involved. Certain collections of abnormalities indicate a common aetiological cause as occurs in the rubella syndrome (Chapter 14), in the fetal alcohol syndrome and with chromosome abnormalities.

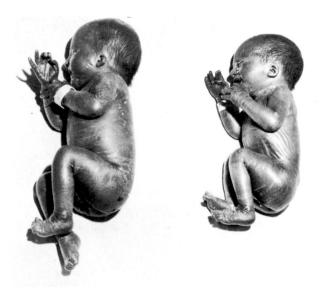

Fig. 11.64 Severe congenital ichthyosis in twins.

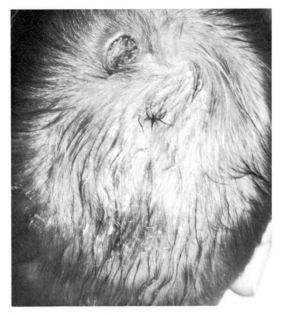

Fig. 11.65 Cutaneous defect of the scalp.

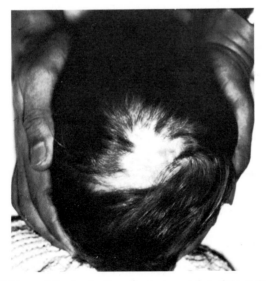

Fig. 11.66 Bald area following healing of cutaneous defect of the scalp.

The fetal alcohol syndrome, is being more frequently recognized. It is generally accepted that excessive consumption of alcohol during early pregnancy can harm the fetus. It is not clear at what level of alcohol intake the effect begins and whether or not there is a safe level of ingestion. The danger to the fetus is probably greatest in the first three months of pregnancy. In the fully established syndrome there is pre- and postnatal growth deficiency and delay in mental development. The head is small with narrow palpebral fissures and absent philtrum with a thin upper lip (Fig. 11.67). There may be deficiency development of the facial bones and a variety of abnormalities in the limbs, heart and elsewhere.

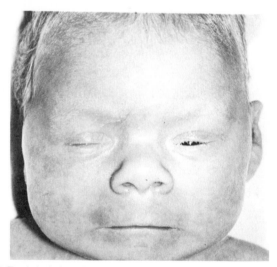

Fig. 11.67 Fetal alcohol syndrome.

Chromosome abnormalities

Buccal smears

Since 1959 it has been possible to examine cells for their sex chromatin content. The presence of a chromatin particle, made visible in the nucleus by suitable staining, indicates a 'resting' X chromosome. The number of X chromosomes present in a cell is one greater than the number of chromatin bodies. Normal females have one chromatin body and males have none. A female is said to be chromatin-positive and a male chromatin-negative. The relative

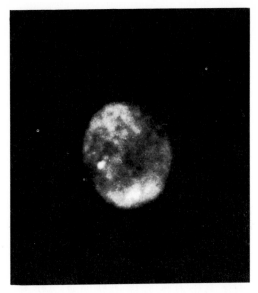

Fig. 11.68 Y chromosome demonstrated in buccal cell by fluorescent staining. (Photographs of Figures 11.68, 11.69 and 11.70 by courtesy of MRC Clinical and Population Cytogenetics Unit.)

simplicity and cheapness of the buccal cell examination for sex chromatin has allowed large-scale surveys of newborn populations to be carried out and the frequency of abnormalities of the X chromosome has been well established.

The Y chromosome. In 1971 it also became possible to recognize the Y chromosome in buccal smears using a fluorescein stain (Fig. 11.68). The incidence of abnormalities of the Y chromosome had by then been established by chromosome karyotype surveys of newborn male populations.

Chromosome karyotype analysis

Chromosome karyotype analysis is now carried out on capillary blood specimens (Fig. 11.69). Improvements in staining technique allow the 'banding' of individual chromosomes (Fig. 11.70). This increases the ease with which individual chromosomes can be recognized. Surveys of newborn populations using this technique are costly and at present routine chromosome karyotype analysis of all newborn infants cannot be justified other than for research purposes. Initially such surveys were limited to infants with a

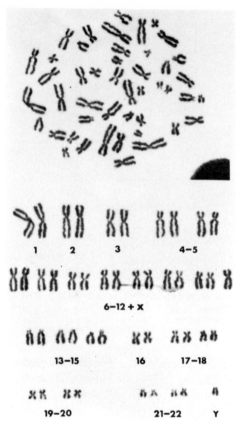

Fig. 11.69 Chromosome karyotype 46 XY of normal male infant.

congenital abnormality and it soon became evident that the great majority of abnormal infants had no recognizable chromosomal abnormality.

Most of the infants with a sex chromosome abnormality are apparently normal at birth but infants with the 45 X constitution can be diagnosed clinically. The presence of an additional autosome or deletion of part of an autosome results in physical abnormality. Screening of infant populations also reveals apparently normal infants in whom the chromosome pattern is rearranged without gain or loss of chromosome material (balanced translocations). Some infants show a mosaicism with a mixture of cells, some normal some abnormal. The incidence of the commoner chromo-

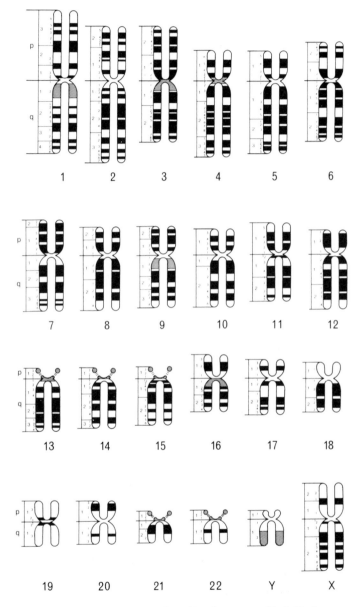

Fig. 11.70 Diagrammatic representation of band patterns of individual chromosomes.

Table 11.5 Incidence of abnormalities of chromosome karyotype occurring more frequently than 1 per 1000 livebirths in a survey of 11 129 infants in Endiburgh

Karyotype	Incidence (per 1000 livebirths)	
Sex chromosome abnormality		
47, XYY (extra Y)	1.58	1 in 664 males
47, XXY (Klinefelter's syndrome)	1.45	1 in 689 males
47, XXX (triple X)	1.41	1 in 709 females
Autosome abnormality		
47, 21 + (Down's syndrome)	1.53	1 in 654 both sexes

some abnormalities in infants in an Edinburgh hospital is shown in Table 11.5.

Sex chromosome abnormalities

Infant Turner's syndrome. Infants with a single X chromosome and no Y chromosome have 45 chromosome and female external genitalia but, because of gonadal dysgenesis, do not develop sexually.

At birth there is oedema of the extremities, abnormal nails, loose folds of skin in the neck and widely spaced nipples. Buccal cell testing shows them to be chromatin-negative. Associated abnormalities include coarctation of the aorta. The incidence of 45 X fetuses who are aborted is very much higher than the incidence of 45 X females at birth and this condition therefore occurs much more frequently than appears from the number diagnosed at birth. Although some girls have limited intellectual ability, the majority have IQs within the normal range and in some the associated growth restriction may be modified with hormone therapy.

Klinefelter's syndrome. Other sex chromosome abnormalities such as 47 XXY males (Klinefelter's syndrome) and 47 XXX females can only be recognized at birth by routine buccal cell examination or by chromosome karyotype testing.

Although the 47 XXY male can now be recognized by modifications of the buccal cell technique he has until recently been recognized only by routine chromosome karyotype screening. No physical abnormality is evident at birth.

Fragile X. Specialized techniques of chromosome examination have recently shown an abnormality of the X chromosome in males with mental handicap.

Down's syndrome

Down's syndrome had been diagnosed by the physical characteristics present for nearly 100 years before it was known to be associated with an extra chromosome number 21 giving a chromosome karyotype of 47 21 +. At meiosis when the gamete is formed the 21 chromosome pair fails to separate and two instead of one go to one gamete.

This is termed non-disjunction and after fertilization results in a trisomy, the presence of three chromosomes instead of the usual pair. Non-disjunction occurs more frequently the older the mother and Down's syndrome is more commonly found in children born to older mothers.

Rarely the extra chromosome results from the translocation of a 21 chromosome to another chromosome, e.g. number 15 of the parent who therefore has the genetic material from two 21 chromosomes and apparently has only 45 chromosomes. If the infant inherits a 15/21 translocation and a normal 21 chromosome from one parent and a normal 21 chromosome from the other parent he will apparently have 46 chromosomes but the genetic material from three 21 chromosomes and thus will have Down's syndrome. This type of inheritance is irrespective of parent's age. It accounts for less than 5% of cases of Down's syndrome.

Clinical features

The clinical features of Down's syndrome are recognizable at birth.

Birth weight is low for gestational age.

The head is round with a short anteroposterior diameter and the face is flat. The nose is small with forward-facing nostrils and a poorly formed bridge (Fig. 11.71).

Epicanthic folds may be present bilaterally and the palpebral fissures are slanting with the inner end below the outer.

The tongue tends to protrude and there may be a double alveolar margin resulting in a narrow palatal arch. Ear folds are poorly developed.

The hands may show a single transverse palmar crease (Fig. 11.72) and the little finger is often short and incurved (clinodactyly).

Feet. A gap may be evident between the big and second toes.

Muscular hypotonicity is a very characteristic finding.

It must be emphasized that each of the features mentioned may

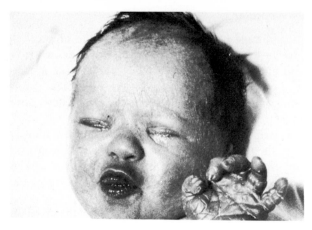

Fig. 11.71 Down's syndrome showing epicanthic folds, protruding tongue and short incurved fifth finger.

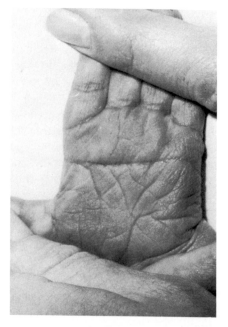

Fig. 11.72 Single transverse palmar crease in infant with Down's syndrome.

be present in a normal infant and not all the features are present in every infant with Down's syndrome. It is the number of these features present in one infant which arouses suspicion. In cases of doubt chromosome karyotype analysis should be carried out.

Mental retardation. The significance of the diagnosis is in the associated abnormalities likely to be present, principally mental retardation. This cannot be diagnosed at birth but it can be inferred from the physical features present. There is considerable variation in the ultimate level of intelligence and this is not related to the number of physical stigmata present at birth.

Other complications include congenital heart disease, particularly ventricular septal defect, duodenal atresia and leukaemia. Infants with Down's syndrome are particularly susceptible to upper respiratory infections.

The parents

As Down's syndrome is one of the few conditions in which mental retardation can be forecast from birth it is most important that great care is taken in informing the parents of the diagnosis and explaining its significance. This is discussed later in more detail but it is appropriate to mention it in this section as many mothers, particularly if elderly, are well aware of the increased risk of having a child with Down's syndrome. They are eager to have their own suspicions allayed if the infant is normal. If the infant has Down's syndrome, and mother suspects this, she may be afraid of voicing her suspicion. She may decide that she was wrong because she is certain that she would have been told but no one has said anything to her. Most mothers of affected children who have not been told feel let down by the staff whom they had previously trusted.

Risk of recurrence

The risk of recurrence after the birth of an infant with Down's syndrome to a mother with normal chromosomes is slightly greater than the risk to other women of the same age bearing in mind that the risk rises rapidly after 40 years of age. If mother has a balanced translocation involving a 21 chromosome the risk of further infants being affected is very high. Expert genetic advice is advisable to define the precise degree of risk which varies with the type of translocation. As translocations are not age-dependent it is important that the chromosomes of both infant and parents are examined when a young mother has an infant with Down's syndrome.

Other trisomies

Trisomy 18

Trisomy 18 may be suspected in infants with low-set abnormal ears, flexed and overlapping fingers, small jaw and mouth, rocker bottom feet, evidence of congenital heart disease and low birth weight (Fig. 11.73). No treatment is available and most die in infancy.

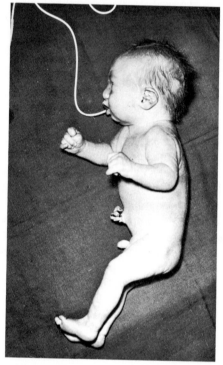

Fig. 11.73 Trisomy 18 showing low-set ears, micrognathia and flexion of middle digits with overlapping of fifth digit.

Trisomy 13

Trisomy 13 presents as multiple abnormalities including an abnormal facies with broad nares, cleft palate and microphthalmia, polydactyly, exomphalos, cerebral and cardiac defects (Fig. 11.74). The prognosis is poor.

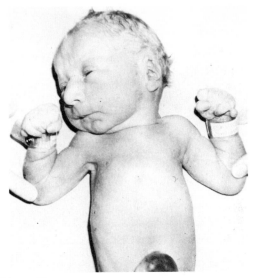

Fig. 11.74 Trisomy 13.

Cri du chat syndrome

This well-recognized syndrome in which there is deletion of part of an autosome is termed cri du chat syndrome after the mewing cry evident in such infants. They have oblique palpebral fissures with widely spaced eyes, low-set ears, a small jaw and may be mentally retarded.

METABOLIC DISORDERS

Recognition

Most metabolic disorders are present at birth and are therefore congenital abnormalities but they are not evident unless special investigations are carried out. Simplications in the techniques involved have now made it possible to screen whole new-born populations for a number of biochemical abnormalities.

Guthrie test. The Guthrie technique uses bacterial inhibition to detect such disorders as phenylketonuria, homocystinuria, tyrosinaemia, maple syrup urine disease and galactosaemia. Capillary blood is collected on prepared blotting paper and sent to a central laboratory which can carry out hundreds of examinations simultaneously. The test is normally carried out on the sixth day of life

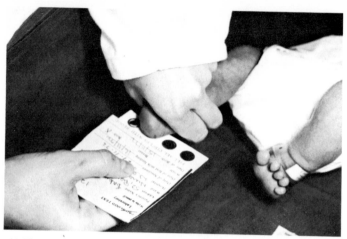

Fig. 11.75 Collecting blood for Guthrie test. This picture demonstrates a common error in collection of the capillary blood sample. The card should be held so that the site of bleeding is in contact with the unprinted side of the card. When the circle is 'filled' a satisfactory amount of blood has been obtained.

(Fig. 11.75). Estimation of TSH can also be carried out on blood collected by this method. Measurement of immunoreactive trypsin can be used to detect cystic fibrosis. There is obviously a limit to the number of conditions which can be tested for; hence only conditions where dietary or other treatments are available are included in routine screening programmes.

Chemical and chromatographic tests on urine are used in some conditions, e.g. organic acidurias, but are less easy to apply for routine screening.

Transient tyrosinaemia. Low birth weight infants may show a transient tyrosinaemia which is probably benign and which responds to treatment with ascorbic acid 25 mg daily.

Metabolic disorders are best managed in central units specializing in such conditions and referral is indicated.

Galactosaemia

Special mention must be made of the need for early diagnosis and management of the severe form of galactosaemia which presents as enlarged liver and jaundice shortly after either human or cow's milk feeding is introduced (Fig. 11.76). It is due to deficiency of an enzyme which converts galactose, one of the monosaccharides of lactose, to glucose. Treatment is the withdrawal of all feeds

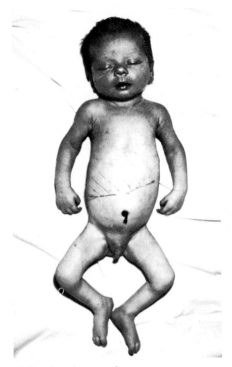

Fig. 11.76 Enlarged liver in galactosaemia.

containing lactose. With satisfactory dietary control the later severe complications of this condition can be prevented.

Telling the parents

It is no longer believed that abnormal infants should be separated from their families and nursed in special institutions. Home-care benefits the handicapped child. Some families have to be helped to accept affected children into their homes and be given support by the medical and social services. This support has to be given from birth if the abnormality is obvious and from the time when the diagnosis is confirmed if investigations have been indicated.

Trust. Parents are being asked to accept a considerable responsibility and it is essential that a trusting relationship is established with them from the beginning. This implies truthfulness and the willingness to answer direct questions. Absence of questions by parents about their infant does not necessarily indicate lack of concern or unawareness of the possibility of abnormality. Many parents expect doctors or midwives to take the initiative in explaining any abnormality present.

Early explanation rarely results in rejection but much depends upon the way in which the information is given. A terse announcement that a baby is abnormal will clearly distress and annoy parents. Similarly a false reassurance that all is well can be equally harmful. The procedure to be adopted in an individual situation has to suit the need of the moment.

A general policy for dealing with this problem should, however, be made in every nursery for the new-born. Whoever is to speak to the parents must have sufficient experience and authority to convince the parents that the doctor understands the situation and is capable of advising them. The significance of the abnormality, the likely prognosis, the facilities available for management and the probability of recurrence in further pregnancies must be known before the parents are approached.

Family doctor. It is often very helpful for the situation to have been discussed with the family doctor before the interview is arranged.

Father. Rarely father is best approached on his own before anything is said to his wife but in most circumstances they should be together during the early explanations.

Support for parents. Whichever approach is made it is essential that parents are given support during the hours and days after the original news has been given as initial reactions may not indicate the true state of their anxiety. Opportunity should be given for further interviews to answer questions and to confirm arrangements for home care and follow-up examinations.

Responsibility. Telling parents is clearly a matter of considerable responsibility and not one which should devolve on the most junior members of the team. Even the most junior student midwife, however, must appreciate that she may be asked crucial questions. If in doubt as to the answer always explain that you will arrange for a more senior person, whether nurse or doctor, who has the necessary information to answer the question as soon as possible.

Mourning the death of a baby. After a stillbirth medical and nursing staff may through pressure of work and other concerns ignore the mother's need to mourn the loss of her baby. Neonatal deaths may be treated similarly and the bereaved mother may be isolated and discharged from hospital in almost indecent haste. Other members of the family, especially the children, are frequently left in ignorance without one word of explanation.

Failure to mourn the loss of an infant stillbirth or neonatal death can severely affect the well-being of the family. Doctors and midwives should facilitate the process of mourning and so help the mother to adjust to her bereavement, by talking to her about the stillbirth or neonatal death and dispelling her inevitable feelings of shame and guilt. Most mothers welcome the opportunity to see and hold their dead baby and may like to have a photograph to take home. The mother may be encouraged to take an active part in the certification of a stillborn or died after birth. Finally mourning is facilitated by arranging and attending a funeral or cremation both for the infant who was stillborn and the infant who died shortly after birth. Many parents derive comfort from the fact that they know where their infant lies buried or where his ashes were strewn. By these means memories of the event are provided for the parents and so facilitate the process of mourning which normally continues in greater or lesser degree during the ensuing year and thereafter gradually diminishes.

FURTHER READING

Bowlby, J. (1980) *Attachment and Loss*, Vol. 3. *Loss. Sadness and Depression*. London: Hogarth Press.

Brent, R. L. & Beckman, D. A. (1986) Teratology. *Clinics in Perinatology*, **13**: 3. Philadelphia: Saunders.

British Medical Journal (1980) Screening for congenital hypothyroidism. **281**: 1.

Evans, D. R., Newcombe, R. G. & Campbell, H. (1979) Maternal smoking habits and congenital malformations: a population study. *British Medical Journal*, ii, 171.

Harris, R. (1980) Maternal serum alphafetoprotein in pregnancy and the prevention of birth defect. *British Medical Journal* i, 1199.

Jolly, H. R. (1980) Perinatal death and the family. In *Topics in Perinatal Medicine*, ed. Wharton, B. A. Tunbridge Wells: Pitman Medical.

Lancet (1980) Abnormal infants of diabetic mothers. i, 633.

Lewis, E. (1970) Mourning by the family after a stillbirth or neonatal death. *Archives of Disease in Childhood*, **54**, 303.

Ratcliffe, S. G., Axworthy, D. & Ginsborg, A. (1979) The Edinburgh Study of Growth and Development in Children with Sex Chromosome Abnormalities, *Birth Defects*: Original Article, **15**, 243.

Scrimgeour, J. B. (1978) *Towards the Prevention of Fetal Malformation*, Ediburgh: Edinburgh University Press.

Scrimgeour, J. B. & Cockburn, F. (1979) Congenital abnormalities. *Lancet*, ii: 1349–1352.

Smithells. R. W., Sheppard, S., Schorath, C. J., Seller, M. J., Nevin, N. C., Harris, R., Read, A. P. & Fielding, D. W. (1980) Possible prevention of neural-tube defects by periconceptional vitamin supplementation. *Lancet*, i, 339.

Turner, T. L. (1982) Fetal and neonatal complications of maternal drug therapy in pregnancy and labour. *Maternal and Child Health*, 7(11): 428–432.

12

Perinatal asphyxia

The introduction of fetal monitoring techniques has greatly reduced the problems of asphyxia in countries with well developed obstetric services. Early detection of fetal hypoxia, improved methods for induction, acceleration and safe delivery, together with improved paediatric resuscitation techniques (Chapter 4), have reduced not only mortality but also handicap. It was probably as a result of the 1958 British Perinatal Mortality Survey, published in 1963, that obstetricians and paediatricians became fully aware of the importance of differentiating between infants damaged by intrauterine hypoxia and those damaged by mechanical injury during the birth process. The subsequent introduction of fetal monitoring has improved our ability to make this important distinction. This has been important for our understanding of some of the causes of mental and physical handicap in later infancy and childhood and to stimulate the introduction of methods of management which prevent or reduce the incidence of such handicaps. It is very important that you should not confuse the terms perinatal asphyxia and perinatal injury particularly when talking to relatives of at risk infants where your words may contribute to later misunderstandings.

Asphyxia is a Greek word meaning without pulse which in modern usage has come to mean a state in which there is low blood oxygen (hypoxia).

Apnoea, which is also of Greek derivation, means without breathing movements. The terms asphyxia and apnoea are often loosely used interchangeably but we would urge you to use these words specifically. Hypoxia can result not only from asphyxia and apnoea but also from disorders of the cardiovascular system, the respiratory system, anaemia and poisonings.

Ischaemia, which literally translated means keeping back blood, is a condition of circulatory failure which can cause hypoxia or even be caused by hypoxia. Hypoxia can cause myocardial failure or peripheral vascular changes which produce the ischaemia.

Fetal hypoxia

Fetal hypoxia is likely to occur where there is interference with maternal oxygen uptake and distribution, interference with the normal function of the placenta or interference with fetal circulation and oxygenation.

Maternal hypoxia. Any condition which lowers the maternal blood oxygen will cause fetal hypoxia. Such conditions include environmental factors, such as high altitude or a smoke-filled atmosphere after a fire, pulmonary dysfunction, as during infection, cardiovascular failure, severe anaemia and some poisonings. Temporary apnoea, as may occur during a prolonged fit, may cause hypoxia.

Placental dysfunction. Poor development, premature separation, infarction and early degeneration of the placenta will reduce maternofetal blood gas exchange and cause fetal hypoxia. These conditions are more likely to occur when the mother suffers from preeclampsia or hypertension.

Obstruction to the cord. Interference to the fetal circulation through the cord can be caused by external pressure on the cord, by the cord being tightly stretched because it is too short or is looped round a part of the fetus, commonly the neck, trapped between fetal and maternal parts, or because there is a true knot in the cord.

Fetal anaemia. If the fetus is severely anaemic because of haemolysis or blood loss serious hypoxaemia of vital organs may occur.

Hypoxic tissue damage

Fetal tissues may be transiently compromised or permanently damaged through lack of adequate perfusion with oxygenated blood. Cerebral and brain-stem cells as well as the myocardium are to some extent protected by fetal vascular mechanisms which ensure that the circulation to the brain and heart are kept going at the expense of the supply of oxygen to other parts of the fetus such as muscles, kidneys, skin, gut and liver.

Brain cell death will occur if the nerve cells are deprived of oxygen, either because of hypoxaemia, or because of ischaemia, or as commonly occurs in perinatal asphyxia when there is a combination of these two.

Asphyxia results in a low PaO_2, a high $PaCO_2$ and concomitant acidaemia. When the PaO_2 falls to a critically low value, respiratory failure at cellular level takes place which is recognized on histology of the brain by swelling of the mitochondria and the accumulation of glycogen in the astrocytes. Asphyxia plays a part in 50% of stillbirths. Since intrapartum asphyxia predisposes to RDS then as many as a third of neonatal deaths are associated with asphyxia. The incidence of deaths from asphyxia due to placental and cord conditions has not fallen over the years to the same extent as deaths from mechanical trauma. With the improvements in perinatal care the total perinatal mortality has fallen but deaths from asphyxia and congenital abnormalities are rising as a percentage of the total perinatal mortality. The overall incidence of neonatal death from asphyxia has progressively fallen but in low birth weight infants asphyxia remains an important antecedent of mortality and morbidity. The longterm morbidity from perinatal asphyxia is in the region of 1.5 per 1000 deliveries for severe handicap and also 1.5 per 1000 deliveries for minimal brain damage. Although some degree of asphyxia at birth is common, asphyxial brain damage is fortunately rare.

Neonatal hypoxaemia

Hypoxaemia is a consequence of neonatal respiratory failure for which several causes can be recognized.

Central nervous system depression may involve depression of the respiratory centres. This may be caused by malformations of the brain or depression from trauma or infection, by intrauterine hypoxia due to dysfunction and premature separation of the placenta, by umbilical cord compression, by inadequate oxygenation of the maternal blood during eclamptic convulsions or during a general anaesthetic, and by the effects of drugs given to the mother.

Failure of aeration and alveolar ventilation may be caused by airways obstruction at any level. A common cause is failure to drain the respiratory passages of pulmonary fluid contaminated by mucus and meconium or more frequently in the condition known as 'wet-lung' syndrome (Chapter 16). Diaphragmatic hernia, pneumothorax or pneumomediastinum may lead to collapse of the lungs as a result of external pressure and may therefore limit gaseous exchanges. Pneumonia contracted after prolonged rupture of the membranes limits the passage of air into the alveoli and exchange of gases.

Failure of the pulmonary circulation except in such conditions as transposition of the great vessels and atresia of the pulmonary artery is a rare cause of respiratory failure. Persistence of fetal pulmonary vasoconstriction after birth (persistent fetal circulation) is the most common variety of this disorder.

Cerebral ischaemia

Failure of the systemic circulation for any reason is inevitably followed by ischaemic hypoxia. Occasionally, new-born infants are seen to be pale and collapsed and are found to be hypotensive with marked peripheral vasoconstriction. It can be difficult to determine whether this state of shock is due to disorder of the nervous, circulatory or respiratory systems.

Cerebral oedema. Some infants suffering from perinatal asphyxia develop cerebral oedema. This oedema may be the result of hypoxaemia and ischaemia but will also contribute to further hypoxaemia and ischaemia and is therefore an important factor in brain cell necrosis. It is critical for normal brain function to maintain adequate perfusion; where intracranial pressure rises above the blood pressure in the arteries supplying the brain, brain cell damage will result. If the increase in intracranial pressure is due to cerebral oedema, treatment for the oedema as well as maintenance of cerebral perfusion is necessary.

Interrelationship of systems

It is important to realize that successful adaptation at birth depends on the interrelationship of the central nervous system, the circulatory system and the respiratory system. Although only one of the systems may be under strain initially, depression of the remaining systems frequently follows and gives rise to a state of general depression and a vicious circle is established. Conversely, treatment of one system may break the cycle and lead to general improvement. If, for example, the depression is due to apnoea, IPPV will result in an improvement in the circulation and more oxygen will be supplied to the brain which in turn enables the establishment of spontaneous respiration and a lessening of the general depression. Similarly the successful treatment of cardiac failure will improve tissue oxygenation and correct depression of the central nervous system caused by previous hypoxia.

Oxygen-conserving adaptation

Faced with a gradual reduction in oxygen supply due to such conditions as preeclampsia and postmaturity the fetus reacts by means of oxygen-conserving adaptation of the fetal circulation, which is regulated by the autonomic nervous system. The blood flow and hence the oxygen supply to a number of less important parts of the body, such as the extremities, abdominal viscera and lungs, are reduced by vasoconstriction. The oxygen saved in this way then becomes available for use by the vitally important brain and heart.

Acidosis. Local tissue hypoxaemia leads to an increase in the formation of lactic acid with a rise in hydrogen ion concentration (lowering of pH) of the blood as a result of anaerobic glycolysis. Fetal blood sampling allows an estimate of the condition of the fetus before delivery. If acidosis is present it can be corrected at birth by the immediate intravenous injection of sodium bicarbonate/dextrose solution.

Effects of fetal hypoxia

Oxygen-conserving adaptation can be held responsible for many clinical conditions present at birth.

Light-for-dates infants. In conditions associated with prolonged fetal hypoxia there can be fetal growth failure. The affected fetus has poor energy (glycogen) reserves and responds poorly to subsequent acute perinatal asphyxia.

Skin. Generalized pallor of the skin represents an advanced stage of oxygen-conserving adaptation. Skin vasoconstriction may be so severe as to cause skin necrosis.

Meconium staining. Reduction of blood flow to the bowel is associated with hyperperistalsis and discharge of meconium, the time honoured sign of 'fetal distress'. In addition to discolouration of the amniotic fluid by the meconium and staining of the fetal nails, skin and umbilical cord, there can be major problems if the deep gasping movements associated with fetal hypoxia cause inhalation of the meconium-stained fluid. This may progress to meconium aspiration syndrome.

Adrenal haemorrhage may follow the delivery of a chronically hypoxic fetus and prove fatal. It is most likely to occur in term infants. If both glands are involved by massive haemorrhage, death follows rapidly. Unilateral or smaller bleeds are compatible with survival if the appropriate supportive therapy has been given. Ultrasonography is useful in the diagnosis of adrenal haemorrhage in the newly born infant and radiology some weeks later will often show confirmatory calcification.

Pulmonary vasoconstriction. The respiratory problems which frequently arise in postnatal life following intrauterine hypoxia may be a consequence of oxygen-conserving adaptation. As a result of pulmonary vasoconstriction there is reduced blood flow through the lungs. In some term and more frequently in preterm infants this may be associated with persistent patency of the ductus arteriosus and the condition of persistent fetal circulation.

Kidneys. Hypoxic kidney damage can result in anuria, haematuria and renal tubular damage. These problems are usually transient but can cause difficulties with water and electrolyte imbalance during the postnatal period.

Liver. Hypoxic liver damage can cause hepatic insufficiency which can cause jaundice, bleeding disorders and interfere with drug metabolism.

Gut. Bleeding can occur from acute gastric erosions, and gastric perforations can results from severe perinatal asphyxia. Ischaemic damage to the rest of the bowel can cause extensive damage with mucosal ulceration and perforation and predispose to necrotizing enterocolitis.

Clinical features of perinatal asphyxia

Clinical evidence of cerebral hypoxia manifests itself in many ways which alter during the first three days of life but may be modified by effective treatment. During the first 12 hours the infant is generally limp and unresponsive. The pupillary and oculomotor reflexes, however, may be normal. Breathing tends to be periodic with episodes of apnoea. Seizures may occur. During the next 12 hours baby may appear more responsive and may even appear normal; thereafter he may become over reactive with jitteriness and hypertonia. Usually by about the third or fourth day muscle tone relaxes so that the infant becomes progressively hypotonic. In some severely asphyxiated infants muscular hypotonia persists uninterrupted from birth. Surviving infants with severe brain injury generally become more stuporose and often have periods of respiratory arrest. Paralysis or incoordination of the muscles involved in swallowing, gagging and coughing which normally prevent milk from entering the trachea (bulbar palsy), abnormalities of eye movement and other features associated with brain-stem damage occur. There is depression of respiratory and other vital functions and death is common at this stage. The individual signs are described in more detail below.

Limpness. Muscular hypotonia and diminished muscle movement is characteristic during the first few hours, but may be followed by a period of jitteriness which in its turn is followed by a recurrence of muscular hypotonicity and progressive deterioration.

Respiratory pattern. Respirations can show almost any kind of abnormal variation and are often associated with bulbar palsy and an excess of mucus secretion. Initially there may be periodic breathing but later apnoea and more prolonged periods of respiratory arrest will occur during which the patient may die.

Cyanosis is common and is due both to diminished ventilation and to poor cardiac output and peripheral circulatory failure.

Irritability. Clinical signs of irritation may appear some 12 hours after birth. Their first appearance is rarely later than the second or third day of life. From being limp and quiet the infant becomes restless and may be heard to utter a high-pitched shrill cry. Twitching movements or jitteriness may occur in the extremities, the angles of the mouth or the eyes. In the most severe cases tonic convulsions develop. The limbs are frequently stiff with clenching of the fists.

The facial expression is that of an unnaturally wide-awake baby of many weeks and not of one a few days old, and seems to portray alertness and apprehension. The brow is wrinkled and shows an unnatural frown which increases with disturbance or movement. Responses to touch, light and sound are excessive to the point of being violent.

Eye and tongue movements may be normal initially but as progressive cell damage occurs and as the brain-stem becomes involved abnormal oculomotor and tongue movements become evident. Protrusive movements of the tongue are characteristic of intracranial irritation.

Head retraction occurs rarely but there is often some degree of stiffness of the neck in the absence of actual retraction.

The fontanelle if large may be bulging or feel tense or spongy on palpation. Sutures may widen in response to increased intracranial pressure, and regular measurement of head circumference must be made in any asphyxiated infant.

Feeding difficulty with the need to tube feed is common in the mature asphyxiated infant. The longer tube feeding is necessary the worse the prognosis. There is frequently associated vomiting and an increased risk of aspiration pneumonia.

Hypothermia with a temperature of 35 °C or less is common.

In summary the short-term effects of perinatal asphyxia include a combination of feeding difficulty, vomiting, limpness, hypothermia, apnoeic episodes, cyanotic attacks and convulsions especially when handled or disturbed. The Moro reflex may be absent and bulbar palsy and ophthalmoplegia may precede decerebrate rigidity. There may also be hypoglycaemia, hypocalcaemia hyponatraemia and disseminated intravascular coagulation caused by tissue damage and brain regulatory disturbances.

Prognostic signs

Convulsions, recurrent apnoea and hypothermia and prolonged tube feeding are indicative of a poor prognosis.

Early recognition

Any of the signs enumerated may appear in a baby with cerebral hypoxia. Diagnosis and treatment depend for success upon early recognition. The implied challenge is to anticipate and to observe the individual signs in the absence of the complete clinical picture and to realize their possible significance in relation to the antenatal and natal histories. The midwife has a special responsibility because more often than not she is the first individual to witness signs of intracranial disturbance, which in the early stages are liable to be stimulated by feeding and napkin changing.

Management of perinatal asphyxia

Antenatal

With careful antenatal supervision (Chapter 4) and obstetrical practice, damage from perinatal asphyxia can be reduced to very low levels. Avoiding circumstances favouring hypoxia, early recognition of situations which may call for episiotomy or instrumental delivery, and offsetting as far as possible the risks attendant upon preterm delivery, low birth weight and abnormal presentation all contribute to a reduced incidence of perinatal asphyxia.

After delivery

Quietness. The keynotes to care of the newly born infant with suspected intracranial disturbance are continuous, meticulous, careful clinical observation, the exclusion of all potentially disturbing stimuli, and the reduction to a minimum of handling of the baby. Weighing, measuring and bathing are dispensed with temporarily. Observation in an incubator allows for continuous observation without the need for excessive handling. Where not available the infant should be nursed in an open cot in a quiet, warm part of the nursery.

Monitoring. It is essential to monitor the respiratory rate and pattern and to detect periods of significant apnoea. In nurseries with full intensive care provision the severely asphyxiated infant might have heart rate, respiratory rate, central venous and arterial pressure, intracranial pressure and cerebral function (electroencephalogram) monitored continuously. Where such facilities are not available detection of apnoea using simple apnoea alarms (Chapter 10) is necessary.

The airway must be kept clear of mucus. Provided there is no excess of mucus, the head of the cot should be slightly raised.

Feeding. The decision as to whether feeding will be by breast, bottle or tube is determined by the condition of the individual baby. Fluid intake should be reduced in all but the mildest affected infant in order to reduce the risks of fluid overload due to impaired renal function and inappropriate antidiuretic hormone production. In the severest cases of asphyxial brain damage fluid intake should be reduced to 40–50 ml/kg/day until there is evidence of recovery. However, it is important to give adequate concentrations of glucose to prevent the development of hypoglycaemia and this will require frequent and regular estimation of blood glucose, attempting to keep the level at the upper end of the normal range. Urinary output should also be carefully recorded.

Anticonvulsants. For the infant who is extremely irritable or actually convulsing, anticonvulsant drugs should be used. It is most important, however, that their use to control signs should not be allowed to hide the necessity for establishing the cause of the convulsions. Hypoglycaemia, hypocalcaemia, hypomagnesaemia and other similar metabolic disturbances may occur in the infant with perinatal asphyxia and require specific treatment. Correction of these secondary disorders may be sufficient to abolish seizure activity. While awaiting the results of metabolic investigations, anticonvulsants should be given. Phenobarbitone 20 mg/kg stat intravenously or intramuscularly will usually control seizures and should be followed by maintenance doses of 5–10 mg/kg/day intramuscularly or orally given in two divided doses. Where phenobarbitone fails, phenytoin is often successful when given intravenously. This drug should never be given intramuscularly as it is poorly absorbed and causes local tissue damage. After an initial loading dose of 10 mg/kg, intravenous or oral treatment with 6–8 mg/kg/day in two divided doses is indicated. Oral suspensions of phenytoin require aggressive shaking before dispensing. Diazepam 0.5–1 mg/kg intravenously or rectally will also control seizures. Unfortunately repeated use may produce prolonged hypotonia and sedation and the preparation is usually only used in the emergency situation. Where these drugs fail thiopentone has been used with success, as has intravenous lignocaine. Access to laboratory estimation of blood concentrations of phenobarbitone and phenytoin is helpful in the management of seizures both in the acute and later stages. Anticonvulsants are often required for several weeks after the initial seizures have been controlled.

Dexamethasone given intramuscularly or intravenously in a tapering reducing dose from 4 mg daily has proved its value in the treatment of cerebral oedema in older children and adults but there is considerable doubt as to its efficacy in the newborn period. Mannitol 5 ml of 20% solution/kg, given intravenously, can effectively reduce cerebral oedema.

The treatment of bleeding disorders is considered in more detail in Chapter 17. However, all asphyxiated infants should be given prophylactic vitamin K intramuscularly at birth irrespective of their gestation. In severe cases it is wise to monitor the coagulation status by a clotting screen and to make appropriate corrections with screened blood products.

Prognosis

Experience gained as a result of following up infants asphyxiated at birth has taught that the Apgar score is unreliable as a screening test for cerebral damage. With good pre- and perinatal care an Apgar score of 3 or less in the infant at delivery is found in up to 5% of pregnancies. Only 0.15% of infants, however, will eventually be found to have a permanent neurological handicap associated with perinatal asphyxia. The paediatric neurologist has learned that an infant who is neurologically completely normal on recovery from his initial disturbance has an excellent prognosis irrespective of the birth history or subsequent events. Increasing knowledge of the normal pattern of neurological behaviour in the new-born period and the first few weeks of life is making it easier for paediatric neurologists to make a more accurate prognosis at an early stage.

Expert knowledge and skill is essential for this type of forecasting. Even with that knowledge it is still necessary to follow any infant in whom hypoxia has been suspected at a suitable centre over several years.

Minimal brain damage

Such long-term follow-up into school age has revealed some children with learning and coordination problems which are not readily demonstrable on routine neurological examination but which cause sufficient difficulty to the child to result in a sense of frustration. Because of difficulty in fine movements such children may not be able to function in the school setting at the level expected for their degree of intelligence. This may lead to emotional problems and add to their schooling difficulties.

Minor impairment of sensory function particularly of the special senses may similarly cause educational problems.

Assessment centres

Assessment of minor as well as major handicap requires the coordinated investigation of a number of specialists. This can best be organized in the form of assessment centres which are now well established. Further development of such centres and a review of their findings will in the future give us a more accurate assessment of the significance of perinatal asphyxia in the production of long-term handicap.

FURTHER READING

Brown, J. K. (1976) Infants damaged during birth — perinatal asphyxia. In: *Recent Advances in Paediatrics*, Ed. Hull, D., vol. 5, 57–88. Edinburgh: Churchill Livingstone.

Dear, P. R. F (1986) Hypoxia and the neonatal brain. In: *Recent Advances in Paediatrics*, Ed. Meadow, R., vol. 8, 139–156. Edinburgh: Churchill Livingstone.

de Crespigny, L. Ch. (1984) Intraventricular haemorrhage. In: *Perinatal Practice*, Ed. Bennett, M. J., vol. 1, 157–181. Chichester: John Wiley.

Lancet (1980) Towards the prevention of intraventricular haemorrhage. i, 236.

Pape, K. E., Blackwell, R. J., Cusick, G., Sherwood, A., Howang, M. T. W., Thornburn, R. J. & Reynolds, E. O. R. (1979) Ultrasound detection of brain damage in preterm infants. *Lancet*, i, 1261.

Pape, K. E. & Wigglesworth, J. S. (1979) Haemorrhage, Ischaemia and the Perinatal Brain. *Clinics in Developmental Medicine 69/70*. London: Heinemann for Spastics International Medical Publications.

Philip, A. G. S. & Allan, W. C. (1985) Neonatal intracranial haemorrhage and cerebral oedema. In: *Perinatal Practice*, Ed. Crawford, J. W., vol. 2, 95–117. Chichester: John Wiley.

Volpe, J. J. (1980) Evaluation of neonatal periventricular — intraventricular haemorrhage. *American Journal of Diseases of Children*, **134**, 1023.

13

Perinatal injuries

There has been a progressive and gratifying decline in the incidence of 'mechanical' birth injuries within the last two or three decades. Although intracranial injury in the newborn presents a dramatic clinical picture, minor injuries such as bruises, abrasions, lacerations, haematomata and fractures must not be neglected. Damage to tissues increases the risk of infection.

Prevention

Trauma widely interpreted is an inevitable accompaniment of the mechanics of birth even when delivery is spontaneous and uncomplicated. The nature of the injury varies greatly and, depending upon the site and severity, may be of minor or major significance. A doctor or midwife must therefore always be on the alert to reduce to the minimum the risk of an infant being seriously injured and to recognize damage to tissues without delay. This can be done by exercising the maximum care when undertaking antenatal supervision, when conducting a delivery and when carrying out subsequent nursing procedures.

Antenatal injury

Induction of labour. Antenatally superficial trauma, generally of minor degree, can occur following the use of a catheter for the rupture of membranes, the application of a scalp electrode and obtaining blood by buttock and scalp sampling (Fig. 13.1).

Caesarean section. Occasionally the incision during Caesarean section will include some part of the fetus.

Injury during delivery

Mechanical birth injury during delivery is most likely to be severe in the presence of one or more of the following situations:

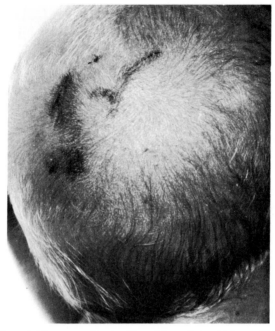

Fig. 13.1 Superficial trauma of scalp. Caused by catheter during artificial rupture of membranes.

Disproportion of the size of the fetal head for the maternal pelvis
Excessive uterine contractions (augmented labour)
Abnormal presentations
Low birth weight
Instrumental delivery
The following situations further contribute to the risk of injury:
Firstborn infant
Elderly mother
High parity mother

Postnatal injury

Successful delivery is not an assurance that the newly born infant is no longer exposed to the risks of trauma. As the factors causing postnatal injury differ from those causing ante- and intrapartum injury they will be considered separately at the end of this chapter.

TYPES OF BIRTH INJURY

It is important to consider trauma according to the structures involved and according to whether it is of temporary or long-term significance.

Injury to the superficial tissues

Damage to the superficial tissues of presenting parts may take the form of simple bruising or the skin may be abraded.

A caput succedaneum consists of oedematous swelling and bruising in the superficial tissues of the presenting part of the fetus. In vertex presentations the caput is not sharply defined and it may extend across the lines of the sutures (Fig. 13.2). If the presentation is abnormal the 'caput' will be formed elsewhere (Figs. 13.3 and 13.4). It 'pits' on pressure, is present at birth and disappears in the course of a day or two. The tissues involved are those encircled by the 'girdle of contact' formed by the maternal soft passages, and the oedema is the result of interference with local venous return.

Abrasions are sometimes present in the skin over a caput succedaneum and unless particular care is taken may allow the entry of organisms leading to infection and suppuration.

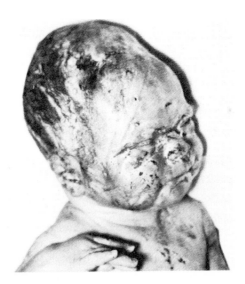

Fig. 13.2 Caput succedaneum over vertex.

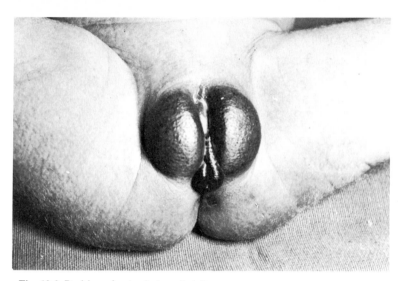

Fig. 13.3 Bruising of vulva in breech delivery.

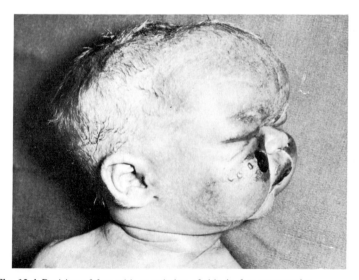

Fig. 13.4 Bruising of face with excoriation of skin in face presentation.

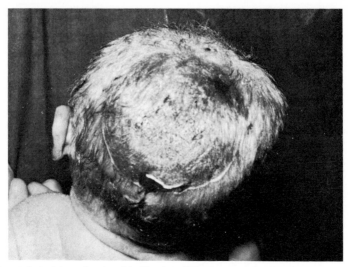

Fig. 13.5 Bruising of scalp with abrasions following use of vacuum extractor.

Bruising and minor abrasions of the scalp not infrequently result from applications of a vacuum extractor (Fig. 13.5). Tissues within the encircling site of application tend to be oedematous.

Cephalhaematoma (subperiosteal haematoma) is a swelling consisting of blood situated more deeply between the periosteum and the underlying skull bone. A cephalhaematoma is evidence of the escape of blood from capillaries damaged as a result of the separation of periosteum from the bone. The swelling may cover a part or the whole of one or other of the parietal bones (Fig. 13.6) or the occiput (Fig. 13.7) but does not extend across sutures. It is not usually present at birth but becomes evident on the second or third day. Thereafter it may increase in bulk and in extent for a few days. It is well defined, may persist for a number of weeks or even months, but invariably disappears completely. At first fluctuant, the swelling becomes firmer as absorption of fluid due to osmosis takes place. In the course of a few days a firm ring may be felt surrounding the swelling. This is evidence of commencing calcification which sometimes extends to form a localized hard elevation around the site of the original swelling. A cephalhaematoma may be unilateral or bilateral (Fig. 13.8).

In general neither a caput succedaneum nor a cephalhaematoma need cause concern. They do not distress the infant. There is no need to place the baby in any special position, and it is sufficient

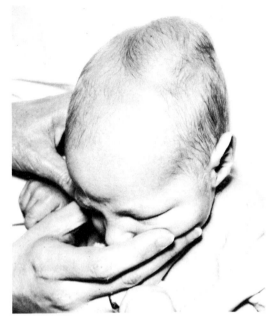

Fig. 13.6 Left parietal cephalhaematoma.

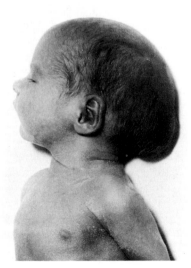

Fig. 13.7 Occipital cephalhaematoma.

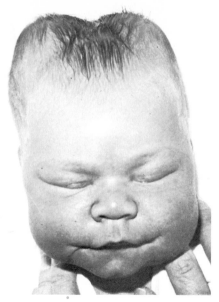

Fig. 13.8 Bilateral parietal cephalhaematomas.

to keep the scalp clean. Localized swelling of the scalp, especially if large and unsightly, may distress the mother. She can be confidently assured that the swelling will disappear completely and (should she raise the question) that it will certainly not interfere with the baby's normal development. Active treatment is seldom required and the need for a blood transfusion is exceptional. Aspiration may introduce infection and is contraindicated. Jaundice may follow lysis of the contained blood. Infants with cephalhaematoma should be given vitamin K_1 prophylaxis, by either the oral or intramuscular route, in a dose of 1 mg for term or 0.5 mg for preterm infants.

Subaponeurotic haemorrhage (subgaleal haemorrhage) occasionally results from application of a vacuum extractor. This may be confused with a caput succedaneum as the swelling extends across the lines of the sutures. This is potentially a more dangerous complication and the infant must be observed carefully as deaths have been reported as a result of excessive blood loss. Vitamin K_1 prophylaxis is indicated.

Forceps marks. Inevitably superficial trauma of some degree accompanies the application of forceps (Fig. 13.9). The injury may

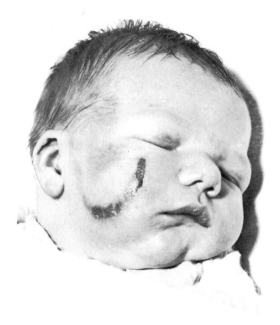

Fig. 13.9 Bruising and abrasions due to the application of forceps.

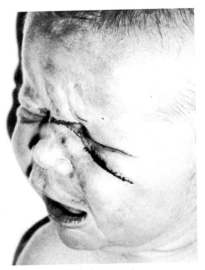

Fig. 13.10 Accidental incision of left cheek during emergency Caesarean section.

be scarcely perceptible and consists only of indentation, hyper-aemia or minimal abrasions. On the other hand there may be a comparatively deep laceration which requires suturing.

Accidental incision (Fig. 13.10) of the face or buttocks occasionally occurs during Caesarean delivery. Such injuries are easily overlooked in a hurried initial examination following delivery only to be discovered later as the cause of severe blood loss. Suturing may be required and particular care must be taken in the repair of lesions affecting the face.

Subcutaneous fat necrosis takes place in areas subjected to undue pressure or along the line of forceps pressure, appearing a week or two after delivery as small areas of reddened induration. Typically it occurs over the upper arm, lower jaw or back. No treatment is required but resolution may take several months.

Injury to the eyes

Subconjunctival and retinal haemorrhages occur most frequently after a difficult delivery and almost always disappear spontaneously within a month. Temporary blockage of the nasolacrimal duct by a small haematoma can occur after abnormal local pressure by forceps blades; no treatment is necessary. Injury accounts for a small proportion of cases of glaucoma.

Injury to muscle

Sternomastoid tumour. This tumour sometimes appears in the body of a sternomastoid muscle when delivery has involved excessive rotation or gross lateral extension of the neck. The tumour appears a number of days after birth, and among babies born in hospital is frequently first discovered after and not before discharge home. It is usually situated in the lower half of the muscle, and may be relatively small or visibly imperceptible (Fig. 13.11). Extending the neck by gently pulling into the sitting position makes the swelling more obvious. Hard and painless, the tumour does not fluctuate, occurs most commonly after a breech delivery and eventually disappears spontaneously. There are doubts concerning the exact nature of the pathology. Some authorities regard the swelling as a haemorrhage into torn muscle, whilst others believe that it is a desmoid or fibrous tumour completely unrelated to injury. A reduced incidence of the disorder during the past decade supports the trauma theory.

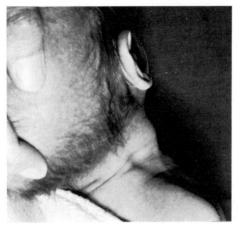

Fig. 13.11 Sternomastoid tumour.

Treatment commonly consists of parental reassurance and daily passive movements of the infant's head and neck to maintain a full range of movement. A rare complication is shortening of the muscle leading to torticollis.

Injury to peripheral nerves

Paralysis

Paralysis as a result of damage to a peripheral nerve may be temporary or permanent.

Temporary loss of function occurs following damage by local pressure effects, particularly where the nerve is superficial and lying over bone. In most cases such injury is the equivalent of bruising. Normal function is restored within a few days as the bruising subsides.

More prolonged loss of function occurs if the axon is torn but the neurolemmal sheath remains intact, as may happen in the lesser traction injuries. Function will be restored as the axon regrows inside the sheath and nerves reach the motor end-plates.

Permanent paralysis follows complete division of axon and sheath as may occur with accidental incision or after a severe traction injury.

Injury leading to temporary paralysis

Facial paralysis follows pronounced pressure on the facial nerve beyond the point where it leaves the skull at the stylomastoid foramen. Most commonly the damage is due to pressure by the blade of forceps but it can occur during normal delivery, possibly due to excessive pressure on the ramus of the mandible by maternal parts. Evidence of facial paresis consists in diminished movement of the affected side of the face. The mouth is drawn over to the uninjured side when the infant cries. Although milk may 'dribble' out of the dependent angle of the mouth there is no interference with sucking. On the injured side the eye frequently, but by no means always, remains partly open (Fig. 13.12). Restoration of normal function and disappearance of the paresis may be complete in a few days, and in any event are usually complete within two or three weeks of birth.

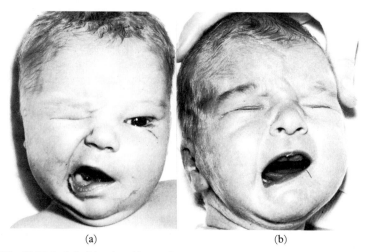

(a)   (b)

Fig. 13.12 Left facial palsy: (a) complete; (b) partial.

In the mild case no treatment is required. Where the eye of the affected side remains open it should be kept clean and drops of sterile normal saline or methylcellulose instilled to prevent corneal ulceration.

Radial palsy (Fig. 13.13) is characterized by wrist drop, ability to grip with the fingers and voluntary extension of the fingers with the wrist in the dropped position. Palsy is usually detected within a few hours of birth. Spontaneous recovery in the course of days, weeks or several months takes place. The condition is probably due to interference with blood supply to the nerve as a result of

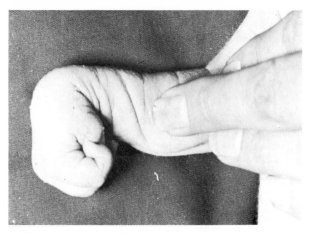

Fig. 13.13 Wrist drop due to radial nerve palsy.

abnormal compression or traction. Bruising or later fat necrosis over the anterolateral aspect of the upper arm is sometimes present. Difficult labour accounts for the majority of cases. Exceptionally the palsy may be bilateral as when pressure on both arms has been exerted by a uterine contraction ring.

Obturator and external popliteal palsies (Fig. 13.14) are uncommon findings and are examples of nerve damage caused by sustained traction on the nerve involved consequent upon the intrauterine position of the limb. The palsies are detectable at birth and according to their severity disappear spontaneously within days or a few weeks.

Sciatic palsy is usually the result of unskilled intramuscular injections into the buttocks but can follow the injection of drugs into the umbilical artery. To prevent the former it is wise to limit intramuscular injections to sites overlying the vastus lateralis muscles of the thigh.

Injury leading to prolonged or permanent paralysis

Brachial palsy. The nerves forming the brachial plexus pass from the spinal cord to supply the upper extremities. Damage to the plexus may follow excessive rotation, stretching or lateral flexion of the neck during delivery of the shoulders in a vertex presentation, or of the aftercoming head in a breech presentation. The clinical picture of brachial palsy varies according to the nerves of the plexus which have been damaged.

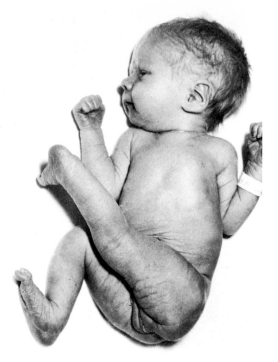

Fig. 13.14 Left obturator palsy.

Erb's palsy. In Erb's palsy (Fig. 13.15), which results from damage to cervical nerve roots 5 and 6, the arm is rotated internally and hangs limply from the shoulder, the elbow is extended, and the hand is partially closed with the palm directed outwards and posteriorly. Although movements of the hand and fingers are possible, the infant cannot raise the arm. Flexing a deflexed head to allow delivery may damage the spinal cord resulting in a bilateral palsy. The majority of cases recover completely, some in a matter of weeks and others after a number of months. Where damage has been particularly severe, paralysis may persist permanently and be accompanied by wasting of muscles.

Methods of management differ. Most paediatricians favour encouragement of free movement of the limb rather than strapping or splinting. Passive movements are commenced two or three weeks after birth to prevent contractures. In severe cases, specialist orthopaedic advice should be sought.

Klumpke's paralysis is a rare condition involving nerve roots

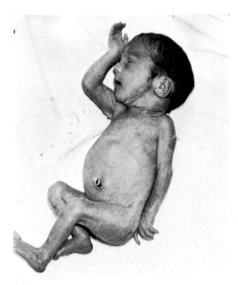

Fig. 13.15 Left Erb's palsy.

cervical 8 and thoracic 1. The clinical features are wrist drop, flaccid paralysis of the hand with absence of the grasp reflex and sometimes local swelling and redness. A splint is applied which extends the wrist at the same time as keeping the hand flat. Complete recovery is rare.

Horner's syndrome (Fig. 13.16) with ptosis, enophthalmos, constriction of the pupil and absence of sweating on the affected side of the head and face is caused by damage to the cervical sympathetic nerves. As the cervical sympathetic nerves run with the nerve root of thoracic 1 Klumpke's paralysis and Horner's syndrome may coexist.

The entire brachial plexus may be ruptured following excessive traction and results in a permanent flaccid paralysis of the arm with wasting of all muscles.

Phrenic nerve paralysis causes paralysis of half of the diaphragm on the side concerned. As the phrenic nerve arises from the same cervical nerve roots as are affected in Erb's palsy the two conditions may coexist (Fig. 13.17).

Other causes of paralysis

Although not due to injury it is important to recognize that

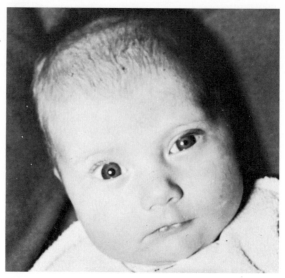

Fig. 13.16 Horner's syndrome on left side showing ptosis, enophthalmos and constricted pupil.

permanent paralysis of the angle of the mouth may be due to congenital absence of the labial branch of the seventh cranial nerve, which has been associated with congenital heart disease. Mobius' syndrome is permanent bilateral paralysis of the facial and swallowing muscles due to agenesis of cranial nerve nuclei.

Injuries to internal organs

Recognition. Injuries to internal organs are much less common than superficial injuries. Because they are, in general, less obvious on external inspection and as their diagnosis relies on the correct interpretation of a number of clinical signs which may also arise from other causes, the recognition of internal injuries requires constant awareness of the possibility of their occurrence and alertness and good observation to recognize the presenting signs.

Abdominal organs

The organs most likely to be involved are those least well protected by a covering of bone. Abdominal organs are therefore particularly prone to injury not only during and after birth, but antenatally as

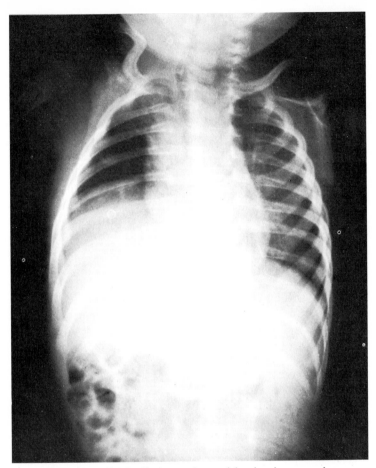

Fig. 13.17 Elevation of right diaphragm due to right phrenic nerve palsy.

well. The needle used at amniocentesis may rarely penetrate the fetal abdomen and damage any of the enclosed organs.

The liver

Occasionally difficulty in delivery results in bleeding from veins on the surface of the liver with the subsequent formation of a subcapsular haematoma. If bleeding persists the capsule ruptures and haemorrhage into the peritoneal cavity takes place. The liver may be ruptured in the course of a breech delivery if the infant's trunk is grasped too firmly. Similar injury can take place during mismanaged artificial respiration using techniques of manipulating the infant which have now been abandoned.

The spleen

The spleen may be injured at the same time as the liver for the same reasons. Occasionally the spleen only will be ruptured.

Subcapsular haematoma. Injury to the liver or spleen or both may result in haemorrhage below the capsule without rupture of the capsule. Suspicion should be aroused if, in the absence of external haemorrhage, there are increasing pallor, restlessness and dyspnoea, a low body temperature and slight fullness of the abdomen. Local swelling in the neighbourhood of the liver or spleen with local tenderness may be detectable. Ultrasound examination of the abdomen may be helpful. Examination of the infant must be reduced to a minimum. Immediate blood transfusion and operative intervention may be required.

Rupture of liver or spleen may occur immediately during trauma or follow development of a subcapsular haematoma and will then not occur until several hours after birth. The infant shows signs of collapse and unless given a blood transfusion and operative repair of the tear within a short period death will ensue.

The skeleton

Almost any bone in the body may be the site of a fracture, but the incidence of fractures in relation to the number of difficult deliveries is small.

The clavicles

The clavicles (Fig. 13.18) are fractured with greater frequency than is generally supposed. Such fractures are sometimes found unexpectedly after a normal delivery, cause no trouble and require no treatment other than protection of the infant's arm from excessive painful movement. This can be achieved by nursing the arm on the affected side alongside the trunk within the infant's clothing. Occasionally the fractured clavicle may only be detected days or weeks after delivery when callus formation becomes apparent.

The long bones

Long bones (Fig. 13.19) are liable to fracture when difficulty is

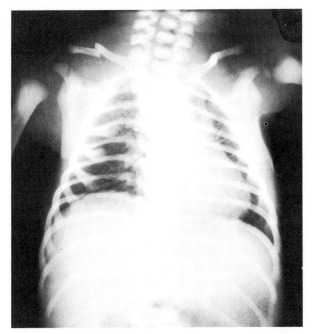

Fig. 13.18 Fracture of right clavicle.

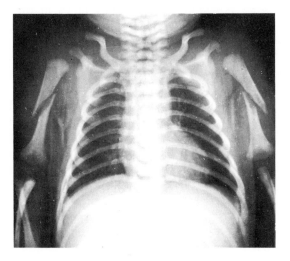

Fig. 13.19 Fracture of both humeri.

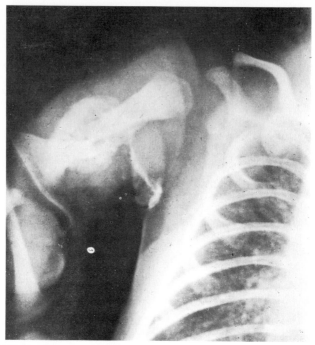

Fig. 13.20 Fractured humerus showing massive callus formation three weeks after birth.

experienced in bringing down extended limbs in the course of delivery. Healing is invariably rapid because of the speed with which callus formation takes place (Fig. 13.20), and there is rarely permanent deformity. The occurrence of a fracture is sometimes suspected by the obstetrician during delivery and can result from inexpert handling of babies.

The presence of apparent paralysis, more especially if associated with deformity of a limb in a newly born baby, should always raise the question of fracture. Handling should be minimal, and instead of being dressed the infant should be covered with a warm blanket. Movement of the trunk and limbs must be avoided as far as possible. If the infant is in obvious distress, the affected limb may be lightly bandaged to the trunk or the other leg.

Epiphyseal injuries (Fig. 13.21) are uncommon, usually occur in the course of breech delivery, and on clinical examination may be indistinguishable from fracture. The upper epiphyses of the femur and humerus are the most commonly affected. Separation of the

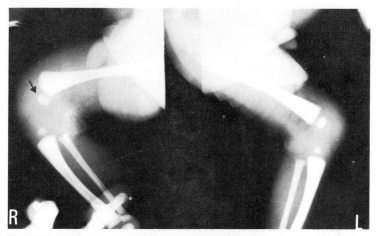

Fig. 13.21 Displaced epiphysis. Lateral views of knee joint showing displaced lower right femoral epiphysis. Delivery was by the breech. Clinical signs consisted of swelling of the thigh and immobility of the limb. (By courtesy of Mr J. M. Fitton, FRCS.)

epiphyses may be accompanied by dislocation in which event application of a splint is necessary.

The skull

Fractures of the skull are not uncommon.

Linear fractures without displacement are the most common and are the result of difficult deliveries where there is fetopelvic disproportion. No treatment is indicated.

A depressed fracture (Fig. 13.22) may occur where labour has been allowed to proceed despite a maternal pelvic deformity and where excessive pressure has been exerted by the sacral promontory. The depression usually disappears spontaneously and operative elevation is seldom required. Where delivery has been precipitate the cranium should be examined for any obvious damage (Fig. 13.23). Should injury to the head be suspected, the baby must be observed for clinical evidence of cerebral irritation. Circumstances such as delivery into a lavatory pan and falls onto the floor make this especially necessary. Traumatic separation of the squamous and lateral parts of the occipital bone (occipital osteodiastasis) is due to suboccipital pressure when the infant is forcibly hyperextended with the head trapped beneath the symphysis pubis during the process of breech delivery. The

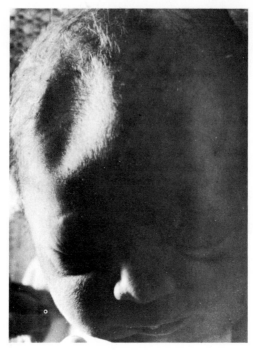

Fig. 13.22 Depressed fracture of the skull which disappeared spontaneously in six months.

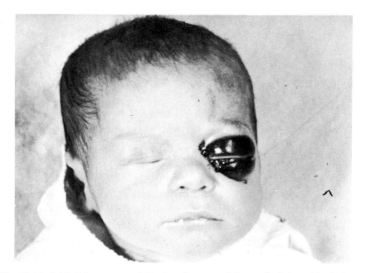

Fig. 13.23 Orbital haematoma following fracture of the roof of the orbit during forceps delivery.

squamous occipital bone is displaced forward damaging underlying structures including the occipital sinuses and cerebellum. Such an injury is usually fatal. Vertebral artery damage can also result from cervical hyperextension.

The spine

Fractures of the spine are rare, result from excessive traction during breech delivery and are usually fatal, although fractures and dislocations of the cervical vertebrae may produce paraplegia.

Mechanical brain injury

Moulding

Moulding of the fetal head is a necessary accompaniment of vaginal delivery, but the structural adaptability of the skull to varying pressures and tensions protects the skull and its contents from damage. This adaptability depends upon the normal elasticity and partial mobility of the fetal skull bones, the fact that the cranial sutures are not closed, and upon the detailed structure and attachments of the supporting falx cerebri and tentorium cerebelli. Damage occurs when the moulding is of unusual degree, is excessively rapid or is applied in an abnormal direction, or when the infant is grossly post mature.

Compression head injury (excessive moulding) occurs in a variety of circumstances, including disproportion between the fetal head and the maternal pelvis or birth passages, rigidity of the pelvic floor and prolonged or violent uterine contractions. Instrumental delivery and certain obstetrical manipulations entail the application of abnormal forces. Moulding may be excessive in an occipitoposterior position, and may develop rapidly in precipitate deliveries and in a proportion of breech deliveries. It must be emphasized, however, that the severest degree of moulding can occur without there being any clinical evidence of intracranial damage.

Venous obstruction

Successful delivery depends upon a balance between the stresses involved and the ability of the fetus to withstand those stresses. Venous obstruction consequent upon breech delivery may lead to cerebral bleeding — as the trunk is subjected to pressure during its passage through the maternal canal, the contents of the aftercoming skull become congested and the combination of congestion and cranial distortion increases the possibility of damage.

The cord may become coiled round the infant's neck. Descent of the fetus into the pelvis may then tighten the cord and compress structures in the neck of the fetus. At the same time cord circulation is impaired. Both venous obstruction and hypoxia will contribute to the ensuing haemorrhage (Fig. 13.24).

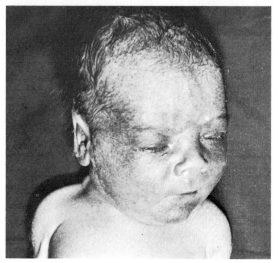

Fig. 13.24 Petechiae over the face and scalp secondary to venous congestion caused by the cord coiled round the neck.

Falx cerebri. Gross moulding of the fetal head may result in tearing of the dura and massive intracranial haemorrhage. The falx cerebri and tentorium cerebelli are the structures most liable to tearing, and when this occurs there is always a serious risk of fatal haemorrhage from involvement of one of the large veins or sinuses. If copious and not arrested, the bleeding may spread over the surface of the cerebrum giving rise to clinical signs, or it may spread down and around the brain-stem, threatening death from the pressure exerted on vital centres. The prevention of post-term delivery and prolonged labour has resulted in a reduction in this type of birth injury from 5 per 1000 to less than 1 per 1000 live births over recent years.

Subdural haematoma

Bleeding into the subdural space is the consequence of tears in the vessels in the falx cerebri and tentorium cerebelli, most commonly at the site where the straight cerebral vein (vein of Calen) drains from the brain into the dural venous sinuses. This venous blood loss does not usually cause any immediate increase in intracranial pressure. Signs of increased pressure rarely develop in the first week of life and may not appear until after the neonatal period. Findings suggestive of a subdural haematoma include failure to thrive, disinclination to feed and inactivity. There is no constant time in relation to delivery when clinical signs first appear. Subsequently vomiting and convulsions may occur. The fontanelle may be moderately full and the occipito-frontal circumference may have increased excessively. Percussion of the skull may produce a 'cracked-pot' sound. Retinal haemorrhages are frequently present. In present-day practice one would expect to have made the diagnosis using transillumination of the skull, computerized axial tomography (CAT) scanning or magnetic resonance imaging (MRI) before signs of increasing intracranial pressure become evident. Ultrasonography can sometimes detect larger subdural collections but is not generally as effective as CAT or MRI. If the subdural collection extends over the cerebral cortex it may be detected by inserting a short bevelled needle into the subdural space at the lateral angles of the anterior fontanelle. Occasionally aspirations from these sites can reduce intracranial pressure. If the subdural haematoma becomes encysted and is not accessible to needle drainage it may be necessary to treat surgically.

Intraventricular and intracerebral haemorrhage

Intraventricular haemorrhage rarely occurs from trauma. It most commonly occurs in extremely low birth weight, preterm infants (Chapter 9) where it remains the commonest cause of death. It can, however, occur in term infants who have experienced perinatal asphyxia. Haemorrhage occurs in the poorly supported capillary vessels in the subependymal layer overlying the lateral ventricles of the brain with subsequent rupture into the ventricular spaces.

Intracerebral haemorrhage is fortunately rare but can follow severe trauma. It is usually associated with severe hypoxia.

Haemorrhagic diseases. Primary haemorrhagic disease, due to vitamin K deficiency, may aggravate the severity of bleeding from injured tissues in the newborn infant but it is now rare following the routine use of prophylactic vitamin K. The likelihood of haemorrhage is particularly great in the case of low birth weight

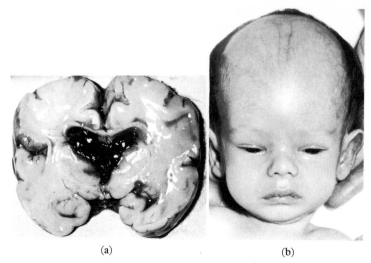

(a)   (b)

Fig. 13.25 (a) Intraventricular haemorrhage. (b) Enlargement of head three days before death.

infants in whom impaired clotting is frequently associated with intrapartum hypoxia and secondary haemorrhagic disease (Chapter 17).

Differential diagnosis. Clinically it is difficult to differentiate signs of intracranial injury from hypoxia but a full history, especially if it contains intrapartum monitoring information, is of value. Occasionally clinical signs may be localized to one half of the body and this will help distinguish focal lesions in the brain such as subdural haematoma.

Diagnosis. Diagnosis by non-invasive mobile real-time echo-encephalography is employed in most centres. This will reliably detect most periventricular and intraventricular haemorrhages and many intracerebral haemorrhages. Computerized axial tomography can be similarly employed but requires moving the infant to the equipment and exposure to radiation. The diagnosis of subdural haematoma can be suggested by the above methods but often requires tapping for confirmation. Lumbar puncture will confirm subarachnoid haemorrhage but there are serious risks if there is evidence of increased intracranial pressure.

Management of intracranial injury

The principles of management are identical to those of the infant suffering perinatal asphyxia as the two conditions frequently coexist. Careful observation, monitoring and nursing in a quiet environment are necessary. The method of feeding and feed volumes must be carefully considered. In severely injured infants anticonvulsants may well be necessary and treatment to reduce cerebral oedema may become an emergency. Vitamin K prophylaxis is necessary and severe coagulation defects require replacement therapy. The treatment of an encysted subdural haemorrhage is by repeated aspiration or continuous drainage. Open operation is sometimes required. Neither intracerebral nor intraventricular haemorrhage are treated surgically although occasionally they may produce hydrocephalus which may require surgical drainage.

Prognosis. The majority of minor and moderate degrees of mechanical brain injury fortunately cause little long-term sequelae. Trauma is less likely to produce severe handicap than asphyxia and the handicap is more likely to take the form of cerebral palsy.

Postnatal injury

After delivery the infant continues to be exposed to risk of injury either from his own actions or from those of his attendants.

He may scratch his own face (Fig. 13.26) or cause local abrasions

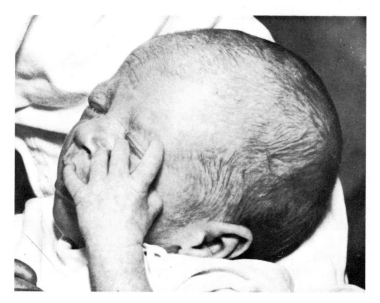

Fig. 13.26 Scratching — a possible cause of minor superficial injury.

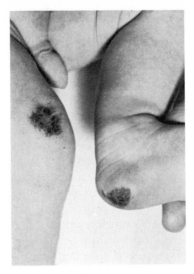

Fig. 13.27 Abrasions caused by rubbing.

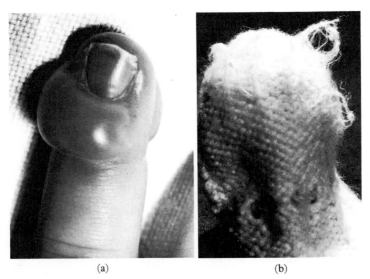

(a)   (b)

Fig. 13.28 The results of constriction of a digit (a) by loops of nylon thread. The fingerless glove in use is shown turned inside out (b).

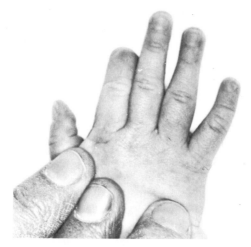

Fig. 13.29 Loss of distal phalanx of index finger following constriction by a loose thread in a mitten.

by rubbing a knee with the heel of the opposite leg (Fig. 13.27). Burns may occur due to lapses in nursing technique in the use of electric blankets. The use of unsuitable napkins or careless attention to napkin changing can give rise to local irritation. Loose threads inside a mitten may occlude the circulation in a finger and lead to gangrene with possible loss of part of a finger (Figs. 13.28 and 13.29). Overzealous attention to the hygiene of the mouth, too vigorous extraction of mucus from the pharynx (especially during resuscitation), and impatient use of the feeding bottle can all injure the buccopharyngeal mucous membrane. Mismanagement of physiological engorgement of the breasts may lead to tissue destruction and suppurative mastitis. These are instances of avoidable trauma which, if they occur, are a reflection on the standards of nursing care.

FURTHER READING

Braun, J. K. (1976) Infants damaged during birth. In: *Recent Advances in Paediatrics*, Ed. Hull, D., vol. 5, 35–56. Edinburgh: Churchill Livingstone.

Casaer, P., Eggermont, E. & Volpe, J. J. (1986) Neurological problems in the newborn. In: *Textbook of Neonatology*, Ed. Roberton, N. R. C., 527–604. Edinburgh: Churchill Livingstone.

Haas, R. & Davies, P. (1980) Iatrogenic hazards in the newborn intensive care unit. In: *Topics in Perinatal Medicine*, Ed. Wharton, B. A. Tunbridge Wells: Pitman Medical.

Walker, C. H. M. (1985) Birth trauma. In: *Perinatal Practice*, Ed. Crawford, J. W., vol. 2, 71–94. Chichester: John Wiley.

14

Infection

The fetus in utero is protected from infection by his isolation from the external environment. This protection is not absolute but the fetus is in a very much safer situation than the newborn infant who is exposed to invasion by the organisms of whatever environment he may enter. Under favourable circumstances this invasion is accomplished without harm to the infant and some benefit may accrue. This is termed colonization, as opposed to clinical infection which occurs when the number or virulence of the organisms encountered overwhelms the defence mechanisms of the infant. As many of the factors involved in the colonization of infants are under the control of those caring for the newborn, most infections are preventable. Adequate preventive measures depend upon a knowledge of the source and spread of organisms and of the infant's capacity to resist invasion. With this knowledge a logical policy of management can be prepared and kept under review. This chapter will therefore deal with the general principles involved in preventing infection as well as discussing the diagnosis and management of particular infections. As the effect of infection alters as pregnancy progresses, the fetus as well as the newborn infant will be considered.

INTRAUTERINE INFECTION

Transplacental infection

While the uterine membranes are intact the most probable route by which infection can reach the fetus is via the maternal bloodstream across the placenta into the fetal circulation.

Rubella

From extensive studies of non-immune pregnant women exposed

366

to the virus of rubella it is clear that this virus readily crosses the placenta and affects the fetus.

Incidence. When the mother has been infected in the first four months of pregnancy, 20–25% of the infants will show evidence of intrauterine infection.

Abortion. In the very early stages of pregnancy the infected embryo may die and be aborted. During the first eight weeks, when the organs are developing (organogenesis), transplacental rubella infection may cause abnormal development of one or more organs but allow life to continue.

The heart, eyes and ears are the commonest sites of abnormality (Chapter 11). Infection acquired at later stages in pregnancy produces more disseminated evidence of infection in those infants who survive to delivery.

Purpura occurs because of thrombocytopenia due to bone marrow damage; the liver and spleen are enlarged because of hepatitis and there may be jaundice.

The long bones on radiological examination often show evidence of areas of translucency and increased density due to infection.

Retinal pigmentation is evident on ophthalmoscopy.

Microcephaly may be present at birth or be noted on later examination and is caused by cerebral damage leading to brain atrophy and frequently mental retardation. It is important to remember that the infant may continue to excrete live virus from throat and urine for some weeks to months after birth and be a potential risk to pregnant women.

Prevention

There is no treatment for rubella virus infection. Following exposure a degree of passive protection can be given by the injection of specific antirubella IgG where this is available.

Immunization. Knowledge of the harmful effect of rubella infection in pregnancy is widespread and causes great anxiety to many mothers. In pregnant women with no natural immunity who have been exposed to infection the question of a therapeutic termination of pregnancy has to be considered seriously. The development of an effective rubella vaccine of the attenuated 'live' variety provides a more efficient means of eliminating this problem. Schoolgirls who have not acquired immunity from the natural infection should be offered immunization before childbearing age. It is also important that women health workers and teachers should be offered protection and that pregnancy should be avoided by appropriate contraceptive advice for three months after immunization as it has been reported that the vaccine can cause a degree of fetal damage. Pregnant women who are found to be non-immune during pregnancy should be immunized afterwards prior to further pregnancies. Since the incidence of rubella in a community rises and falls in a cyclical fashion it is important to maintain levels of protection. It is hoped that this will provide complete protection during later pregnancies. With wider application of prophylactic immunization it should be possible to eliminate rubella as a problem during pregnancy. In many countries, a policy of immunizing boys and girls is followed in order to reduce and eventually eliminate the 'wild' rubella virus from the population. A combined mumps, measles and rubella (MMR) vaccine is usually employed.

Other virus infections

Rubella has been selected from the virus diseases because it is a common condition and readily recognized. It has therefore been relatively easy to establish a connection between rubella infection in the mother and abnormality in the fetus. Other virus infections cross the placenta and several are known to be associated with an increased incidence of abortion. In infections such as measles, chickenpox, smallpox, vaccinia and herpes simplex the fetus may be infected and if the infection occurs late in pregnancy the infant may be born with the characteristic rash of the infection. This can produce severe systemic illness in the infant. Figure 14.1 shows an infant of 2 days with chickenpox. Mother developed her rash one day after the infant. It is possible to reduce the severity of the illness by the use of hyperimmune gamma globulin if given to the mother in the incubation period.

Other intrauterine infections

Other intrauterine infections may become evident only after the infant has been delivered as the mothers have shown no evidence of illness during pregnancy. Typical of these is cytomegalovirus (CMV) infection.

Cytomegalovirus infection. As the mother will rarely have symptoms it is often not possible to fix the time of infection. Infection is probably transplacental during the period of maternal viraemia. The infant may be stillborn or alive but ill. In those severely

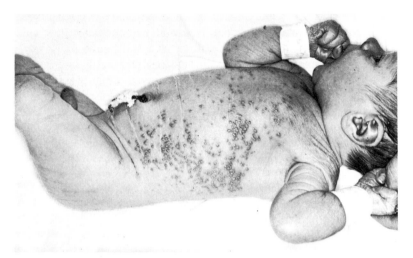

Fig. 14.1 Chickenpox on second day of life. Mother developed her rash the following day.

infected there is enlargement of the liver and spleen, jaundice, haemorrhage, purpura, choroidoretinitis and often a severe pneumonitis. There may be evidence of encephalitis with cerebral calcification on X-ray examination. Treatment with antiviral agents and hyperimmune specific immunoglobulin may modify the illness but in the severest cases many infants still succumb or are severely damaged.

In other infants culture of virus from the urine and throat and the presence of cytomegalovirus specific IgM will confirm that the virus has crossed the placenta prenatally. Long-term follow-up of such infants into childhood may, however, demonstrate evidence of cerebral dysfunction or deafness.

Herpes simplex. Neonatal manifestations of systemic herpes simplex infection reflect the fact that the organism invades liver, lungs, adrenal, brain, skin and mucous membranes. The infection is rarely acquired transplacentally but from the mother during vaginal delivery or subsequently. Mother may or may not show evidence of oral or vulval herpetic lesions. Where lesions of the vulva are present Caesarean section should be advised to diminish the risk to the infant.

Hepatosplenomegaly, jaundice, dyspnoea, purpura, thrombocytopenia, signs of encephalitis and circulatory collapse may be present. Occasionally there may be localized infection affecting only the skin, eyes and mouth or an encephalitis without other evidence of systemic infection. Neonatal herpetic infections are frequently severe and have a high mortality and morbidity.

Herpes simplex virus can be cultured relatively easily and direct fluorescent antibody testing of vesicle scrapings when present will allow a rapid diagnosis. The virus may also be isolated from the mouth or nasopharynx, the eyes, urine, blood and cerebrospinal fluid. Cultures from the mother's cervix or from labial lesions will also prove positive. Treatment is extremely difficult and combines the use of specific immunoglobulin and drugs such as Acyclovir and Vidaribine.

Hepatitis B (HB). Neonatal infections with this virus are almost always acquired during birth from maternal secretions and/or blood when the mother is an active carrier. The carrier rate is greater in some populations than in others and worldwide HB infections are a major health problem. High risk groups include drug addicts and women of Chinese, Asian, sub-Saharan African and Haitian origin. Neonatal manifestations are variable and include fulminant hepatic necrosis, chronic persistent hepatitis, mild focal necrosis or may even be asymptomatic. Later complications include portal hypertension and primary liver cancers. The infant is most at risk when mother has acute HB hepatitis during the third trimester and at delivery, or is e antigen positive. Protective immunization of susceptible women of child-bearing age and of infants in endemic areas and in susceptible women and children in non-endemic areas will reduce the risks to the individuals and also to the community. This is because infected infants act as carriers and excretors of the virus and a continuing reservoir of infection.

Infants at risk should be given specific immunoglobulin as soon as possible after birth (within 4 hours) followed by immunization with HB vaccine within the first day and repeated at one month and six months.

Acquired immune deficiency syndrome (AIDS). AIDS is a disorder which is increasingly recognized in mothers and infants. The presence of the infection is confirmed by measurement of antibody against the human immunodeficiency virus (HIV) previously known as human T-lymphotrophic virus type III (HTLV-III) and lymphadenopathy associated virus (LAV). Manifestations of AIDS may not become evident for some months after birth and include failure to thrive, chronic diarrhoea, hepatosplenomegaly, lymphadenopathy and interstitial pneumonia. Thrombocytopenia may be an early feature. The mother may be asymptomatic or show features of the disease which, in addition to the features found in the infant, may include Kaposi's sarcoma and *Pneumocystis carinii* pneumonia. The virus may also be shed in breast milk of affected mothers. Infected blood and blood products are also a risk to recipient infants. At the present time there is no treatment or immunization available and mortality is very high. Mothers who abuse intravenous drugs, have multiple partners, particularly homo/heterosexual partners, or are from Central Africa or Haiti are in the high risk category and should probably have their HIV status checked in pregnancy.

Toxoplasmosis. Similar clinical features are found in infants with congenital toxoplasmosis due to transplacental infection with a protozoon, *Toxoplasma gondii*, which frequently causes intracerebral calcification, microcephaly, choroidoretinitis and severe mental retardation. Diagnosis is usually made using the toxoplasma dye-test.

Syphilis. Some non-viral maternal infections such as syphilis can be recognized by antenatal serological testing. Where infection is present, appropriate treatment in early pregnancy will prevent infection of the fetus, which does not occur before the fourth month and is more likely to occur later in pregnancy. Affected infants may be stillborn. Those born alive have an enlarged liver and spleen and develop snuffles, a watery and later purulent nasal discharge. A skin rash appears from the second week onward. X-ray of the long bones shows osteochondritis and periostitis in about 90% of affected infants. Treatment with penicillin is highly effective.

Ascending infection

Prolonged rupture of membranes (PROM)

Prolonged rupture of membranes allows organisms present in the maternal vagina to spread to the amniotic cavity and to infect the fetus. Most paediatricians now accept that a period of rupture greater than 24 hours constitutes prolongation.

Intrauterine pneumonia. The resulting infections are generally in the form of a bronchopneumonia, and the organisms isolated include non-haemolytic streptococci, *Escherichia coli* and other Gram-negative bacteria, *Listeria monocytogenes* and *Candida*. Death may occur before delivery but in those born alive prompt and appropriate antibiotic and antifungal therapy may prevent death.

Bacterial swabs taken from high in the mother's vagina (HVS) and from the ear of the infant, in which infected liquor may have been trapped, can give early indication of the organisms involved as will gastric aspirate.

Treatment. Opinions differ as to the advisability of giving antibiotic treatment to the mother when membranes have ruptured prematurely or to the infant following delivery. Our policy is to swab any mother who has PROM and her infant and to give prophylactic antibiotics to those infants who have been exposed to PROM for longer than 36 hours. Mothers who are pyrexial or have pathogenic organisms in the HVS are given appropriate antibiotics. An alternative policy is that of *careful* bacteriological screening and observation of infants suspected of having suffered intrauterine infection so that the appropriate antibiotic therapy can be started at the first clinical sign of infection.

Intrapartum infection

The differentiation between infection acquired in utero following rupture of the membranes and infection acquired during passage of the fetus down the birth canal is mainly one of timing.

The organisms acquired are similar but the infant infected during delivery may not show clinical evidence of infection for a day or more after birth.

Listeria monocytogenes

Listeria monocytogenes infection acquired before delivery generally presents at birth as aspiration pneumonia, but meningitis has been observed. Other infants present later in the first week of life with signs of septicaemia and meningitis. In these infants infection was probably acquired during delivery. Treatment with intravenous ampicillin alone or in combination with penicillin or gentamicin has proved effective if given sufficiently early.

Group B streptococci

Experience, has shown that infection with group B haemolytic streptococci is an increasing danger to newborn infants. Some infants infected in utero or during delivery become seriously ill shortly after birth with bacteraemia and generalized signs including dyspnoea and cyanosis which may lead to a mistaken diagnosis of idiopathic respiratory distress syndrome or congenital heart disease. Treatment at this stage must be intensive and will include intravenous Penicillin and correction of hypotension and shock. Resuscitation with plasma, blood or exchange transfusions may be required. Despite these measures the death rate is high. Other infants do not develop signs of infection for several days and often have meningitis. In such cases with later onset, treatment with Penicillin or other appropriate antibiotic is more successful.

In some centres where the incidence of group B streptococcal infection is high, routine screening of high vaginal swabs taken from mothers in late pregnancy or when they are first admitted in labour is advocated and prophylactic Penicillin given to mother and infant.

Chlamydia trachomatis

Infants delivered through a birth canal infected by *Chlamydia trachomatis*, which is a sexually transmitted pathogen, are liable to develop conjunctivitis (inclusion conjunctivitis of the newborn) and may develop pneumonia later. This form of ophthalmia has been observed in up to 10% of cases in some nurseries and should be suspected when the conjunctivitis is resistant to traditional treatment. One per cent tetracycline drops or ointment locally to the eye and systemic erythromycin are indicated.

Gonorrhoea

Infants of mothers suffering from gonorrhoea are liable to a severe form of conjunctivitis due to contamination of the conjunctival sac during delivery. With the present increase in the incidence of gonorrhoea, gonococcal ophthalmia neonatorum is once again appearing. Diagnosis may be delayed by the use of chloramphenicol eye drops which suppress clinical signs without eradicating the infection in many cases.

Prophylaxis. The use of prophylactic antiseptic eye drops (e.g. 1% silver nitrate) is associated with a chemical conjunctivitis in some infants and is not fully effective in preventing infection.

Prenatal screening of mothers, particularly of those with a vaginal discharge, and appropriate treatment of those shown to be infected is the most effective prophylaxis for the infant. Unfortunately gonococcal infection may be atypical and not suspected clinically. The affected infant should be treated with penicillin given locally and systemically.

Other organisms

Other organisms including Gram-negative bacilli and *Candida* may be acquired in sufficient numbers during delivery to cause subsequent clinical infection of the skin or deeper tissues, particularly where there has been a break in the skin surfaces.

Postnatal infection

The great majority of infants are free of organisms when labour begins and pick up only small numbers during delivery. Swabs taken from skin surfaces after birth produce growths of organisms of the type found in the maternal vagina and rectum.

Environment

During the first few days of life these are generally replaced by other organisms acquired from the infant's immediate environment. It is important that wherever possible the infant should be colonized by the mother's own commensal organisms and these will include *Staphylococcus epidermidis* from the skin and *Bacillus bifidiis* from the nipple if the infant is breast-fed. In the 1950s the predominant organism in most hospital nurseries was the *Staphylococcus aureus* and many studies were made of the pattern of spread of this organism in the progressive colonization of individual infants.

These studies showed that the infant's nose, throat, umbilicus, axillae and perineum which are normally sterile at birth became colonized within the first few days of life. The umbilicus is the first site to be colonized. Of the skin sites the perineum and axillae tend to become heavily colonized. The spread of organisms from one infant to another may take place by contact with attendants' hands, common surfaces with which more than one infant comes into contact or from the dust suspended in the air. New organisms are introduced by infected attendants or by symptomless carriers.

Although much of our knowledge of the spread of organisms in nurseries came from studies of staphylococci these organisms are no longer the dominant organisms in most nurseries and their place has been taken by a variety of Gram-negative organisms including *E. coli*, *Bacillus proteus* and *Pseudomonas pyocyanea*. Less is known about the method of spread of these organisms. As they flourish in a moist environment they are often called the 'water bugs'. They are particularly likely to contaminate incubators, suction apparatus and ventilators, the very environment and equipment used in nursing preterm and low birth weight infants. In the UK and Europe the group A β-haemolytic streptococcus was a major cause of maternal and infant mortality and morbidity before *Staphylococcus aureus* became predominant, and now the group B β-haemolytic streptococcus is a major cause of concern. Different countries have had slightly different experiences but it is critically important that each maternity and neonatal unit should be vigilant as to the types of microorganisms present and their sensitivities to antimicrobial therapy.

Viruses

Our knowledge of viral colonization of the newborn infant is relatively scanty. As has been shown, clinical viral infections occur in the newborn and it is reasonable to suppose that infants can be colonized by viruses without clinical infection when the defence mechanisms are sufficient to contain the number of viruses encountered.

Resistance to infection

Clinical infection will appear in the infant only where the number or virulence of the organisms present is greater than the infant's ability to resist infection.

The balance may be upset by an overwhelming number of invading organisms or by lack of resistance on the part of the host.

Defence mechanisms

At all ages the body provides a number of defence mechanisms against infection.

The skin and mucous membranes remain our first and principal line of defence. During delivery the skin may be abraded and any break offers a route of access for organisms. Resuscitative measures are liable to damage the mucous membranes of the nose, mouth, pharynx and larynx.

The inflammatory response is well established before birth but the newborn infant has poor ability to concentrate the response at the site of infection.

Immunoglobulins

Maternal immunuglobulins do not cross the placenta with the exception of IgG, which crosses to the fetus in significant amounts. This transfer occurs mainly during the last trimester of pregnancy and maternal IgG gradually disappears from the infant during the first few weeks of life.

Fetal immunoglobulins IgG, IgM and probably IgE are produced from about midterm onwards but in the absence of an antigenic stimulus during pregnancy there is little no IgA or IgM in the cord blood. Where intrauterine infection has occurred IgM specific for the infecting agent will be present in the cord blood.

Newborn immunoglobulins. IgA appears in secretions after birth before it appears in the serum. Synthesis of IgM is increased from shortly after birth but the process is slower in immature infants. IgG synthesis is slower to develop. As antibodies against Gram-negative bacteria belong mainly to the IgM group the relative lack of IgM in the newborn may explain their susceptibility to Gram-negative infection. Maternal IgG, on the other hand, grants temporary protection to many virus diseases.

Human breast milk

As explained in Chapter 8 human breast milk contains several factors such as IgA, lactoferrin, lysozymes and cells which contribute to the reduction of infection within the gastrointestinal tract. Specific antibodies to infections to which mother has recently been exposed appear in breast milk within a few days.

Immunological competence

Contrary to earlier belief it is now clear that the newborn infant is immunologically competent to deal with infection. It would appear, however, that the male is less efficient than the female in resisting infection as is shown by the male preponderance in morbidity and mortality from infective causes. There is evidence to suggest that immunoglobulin synthesis is related to a gene locus on the X chromosomes thus favouring females, who have a greater genetic diversity having inherited one X chromosome from each parent.

Spread of organisms in nurseries

Organisms spread in nurseries by both direct and indirect pathways

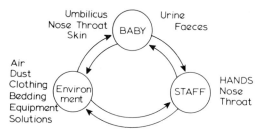

Fig. 14.2 Circle of contact whereby infection is transferred.

through movement of air and dust, on the hands or clothing of attendants and by contact with shared surfaces. Figure 14.2 illustrates the chief sources of infection and the circles of contact whereby infection is spread. Recognition of such pathways of spread is essential to the planning of prophylactic measures to prevent infection in the newborn.

Superficial infections such as conjunctivitis may be a slight risk to an individual baby but a major source of infective material to other babies. Deep infections such as septicaemia are a major risk to the infant concerned but not necessarily to other infants.

Prevention of infection

Many of the factors involved in the spread of infection are controllable, and with good policy planning and effective application of these policies some prenatal and almost all postnatal infections are preventable. In units where careful attention is paid to preventive measures neonatal infection is a rare cause of death or morbidity. There is, however, a risk that the success achieved in preventing infection leads to relaxation of precaution and a return of infection.

The preventive measures necessary involve the design of hospitals, wards and equipment, the planning of nursery and domestic procedures, the encouragement of breast feeding, knowledge of the environmental flora and policy decisions with regard to the use of antiseptics and antibiotics.

Design of hospitals and wards is generally outside the control of hospital, medical, nursing and domestic staff, but the other measures are more readily controllable. In each case several branches of the profession are involved and decisions are best made by those involved meeting for discussion and agreement. Much as the authors dislike the proliferation of committees this is one situation where a committee appears to be the best solution. The following factors have to be kept in mind.

Good architectural design of nurseries avoiding dust traps and allowing easy cleaning together with planning which prevents excessive movement of personnel, help to reduce the number of airborne organisms.

Design of equipment should bear in mind the possibility of organisms becoming trapped in inaccessible areas and allow for the effective disinfection of all equipment used. This helps to reduce sources of organisms previously often not suspected.

Disposable equipment should be used in all situations where it is financially justifiable.

Space between cots in nurseries where these have to be used reduces the risk of infection but increases nurse's work. A compromise has to be reached.

Ventilation. A flow of air from a clean source is essential. Discharged air is likely to be contaminated and care has to be taken to avoid passing infection to some other area of the hospital. If air conditioning is considered necessary, precautions must be taken to ensure absolute cleanliness of the air source, ducting and machinery involved.

Hand washing. Adequate facilities for hand washing for staff, parents and visitors is essential. These facilities should include hot water, appropriate soaps or antibacterial cleaning fluids and disposable hand towels.

Control of Infection Committee

The planning and supervision of these preventive measures involves several branches of the health professions. Coordination is best arranged through a Control of Infection Committee on which the interested parties should be represented.

Nursing procedures

Rooming-in with baby nursed alongside his mother has many advantages apart from reducing the amount of contact with other infants and thus reducing the risk of infection. Adequate space must be allowed in the postnatal wards for this purpose.

Breast feeding. Measures to encourage and promote breast feeding have already been discussed in Chapter 8.

Cot nursing the infant reduces periods of common contact in changing or bathing rooms.

Cohort nursing, whereby batches of infants born about the same time are nursed together in small nurseries, is aimed at reducing the number of infants with whom an individual infant comes in contact. The small nurseries are emptied as each cohort leaves and thoroughly cleaned before the next cohort is admitted. Such a system is costly in space and equipment and is not always justifiable. It is, however, an important means of management when infections such as gastroenteritis have occurred in a nursery.

Hand washing after contact with any infant or its excreta is the most important personal factor in preventing the spread of infection and cannot be over-stressed. The senior members of each profession involved must set the example for their juniors and be prepared to be considered obsessional. All visitors to the units must comply with the hand washing regulations.

Antiseptic and antibiotic policies should be discussed and decided by the Control of Infection Committee. Any change in the environmental flora should lead to a reassessment of the antiseptics and antibiotics being used.

By careful application of the factors mentioned above the amount of antibiotic used in a nursery can be reduced and it should be the aim to use antibiotics as sparingly as is consistent with the safety of the infants. The use of antibiotics prophylactically has not been shown to be useful and may be harmful if used excessively. Similarly the unnecessary use of gowns, masks and overshoes can lead to their abuse. Hence they are usually only employed for specific indications such as blood culture or lumbar puncture procedures.

CLINICAL INFECTION

Clinical infection will occur where there has been a failure of preventive measures and the degree of colonization overwhelms that infant's resistance to infection. This may occur because of the number of organisms or the virulence of the organisms involved or because of the failure of the resistance of the infant.

Gram-positive organisms

When staphylococci and other Gram-positive organisms such as pyogenic streptococci are the causative organisms the first clinical signs of infection are often superficial and therefore visible with clinical signs of inflammation in the form of redness, swelling and production of pus. Blood spread to the deeper organs such as the lungs and bones may follow.

Gram-negative organisms

With Gram-negative organisms the reverse is frequently the case and infection presents in a widespread form with bacteraemia, urinary tract infection and meningitis. In such a situation the infant is systemically ill with a variety of clinical signs which are not specific to infection. It is unusual for a local site of inflammation to be obvious.

In this chapter infection will be divided into superficial visible infection and the less obvious deep systemic infection. This division is artificial and there is a considerable overlap between the two types. The distinction is, however, useful clinically and therapeutically. Superficial infections are more likely to contaminate the environment, and whereas they may be less of a risk to the individual affected they may create a greater risk to other infants. Deep infections are a more immediate threat to the infant concerned but, with the exception of gastroenteritis, are less likely to be a risk to other infants. Antibiotic therapy is essential for the management of deep infection but may not be called for in superficial infection.

Superficial infection

Although the nose, throat, umbilicus and groins are the first sites to be colonized by organisms the commonest sites of superficial infection are the conjunctiva and the skin.

Sticky eye

Sticky eye occurring in the first day of life is only rarely associated with bacterial infection and cleansing with saline is the only treatment required provided that swabs have been taken for culture.

Conjunctivitis

Conjunctivitis occurring after the first day or two of life may be due to a variety of organisms including chlamydia and viruses (Fig. 14.3). Treatment should not be started until adequate specimens have been taken for bacteriological examination. The infant should be isolated and all swabs used for wiping the eyes kept in a disposable bag and burned. The mother should be asked about any vaginal discharge before delivery: bacteriological reports may be a available to help in the choice of treatment. Chloramphenicol

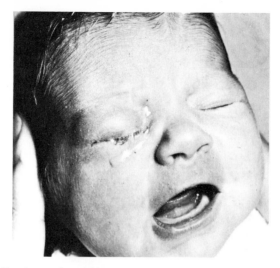

Fig. 14.3 Purulent conjunctivitis.

eye drops (1%) or neomycin ointment (1%) are a suitable initial therapy remembering that the irrigant effect may be as important as the antibiotic effect. If the response is not satisfactory, increase in frequency of treatment is more important than increase in number of drops per instillation. The risk of masking gonococcal infection has already been noted earlier. Should the initial smear or culture suggest the presence of gonococci, treatment should be changed to a combination of local and systemic penicillin. Chlamydia infection may be treated with erythromycin systemically and tetracycline ointment (1%) locally.

Skin infection

Skin infection with staphylococci has been markedly reduced since the introduction of skin washing preparations containing suitable antiseptics.

Pustules are the commonest presentation and present (Fig. 14.4) as small 1 to 2 mm vesicular projections containing pus and surrounded by an area of erythema. The yellow colour of the pustule distinguishes it from papular urticaria (Chapter 6). Rupture of the pustule leaves an ulcerated area and discharges highly infective material.

Pemphigus. Larger vesicles, particularly over the buttocks and

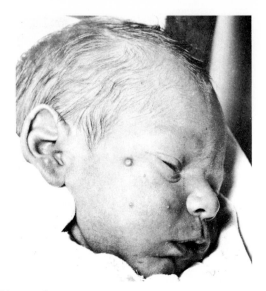

Fig. 14.4 Skin pustules.

trunk, may occur with staphylococcal or streptococcal infection and are termed *impetigo* or, in their most severe forms, *pemphigus*.

Ritter's disease. A more severe but fortunately rare form of skin infection produces exfoliation of large areas of skin (Fig. 14.5) and is called *Ritter's disease or exfoliative dermatitis*.

Prevention. The most important aspect of treatment is prevention of contamination of the skin by the methods described above.

Isolation and barrier nursing are necessary for the child with skin infection.

Antiseptics, antibiotics. In the milder cases with skin pustules local antiseptic washes containing chlorhexidine, povidone iodine, hexachlorophane (3%) or a similar preparation are often sufficient to control infection but in more severe cases of pemphigus and exfoliative dermatitis a systemic antibiotic is necessary. Penicillinase resistant penicillins such as flucloxacillin are generally the most suitable choice.

The demonstration that hexachlorophane under particular circumstances could enter the body and be found in the brain of very small infants led to the withdrawal of this preparation in many hospitals. In some of these, staphylococcal infection recurred. With specified limitation of use it is generally accepted that infants can be safely washed with solutions containing hexachlorophane (3%)

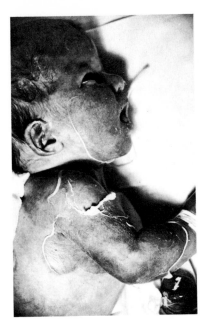

Fig. 14.5 Exfoliative dermatitis (Ritter's disease).

and benefit by protection against staphylococcal infection. Hexachlorophone should be rinsed off after use and should not be used for more than seven days consecutively.

Flexures. Skin infection particularly in the flexures such as the axillae and groins may be due to Gram-positive and Gram-negative organisms. Between the buttocks and occasionally around the neck and behind the ears *Candida* may be responsible. These sites are normally moist and poorly ventilated. Exposure and drying aid in treatment. Local antiseptic preparations such as surgical spirit, 4% povidone iodine or 1% gentian violet in spirit may also be used.

Paronychia

Paronychia is infection occurring in the nail folds of the skin. It is an added risk to the infant because of the ease with which he can infect other parts of his body by scratching. Because of the tightness of the skin around the nails the oedema of inflammation produces a rapid rise in pressure and infection may spread to proximal and deeper tissues (Fig. 14.6). In addition to the general treatment of skin infection the infant's limb should be immobilized

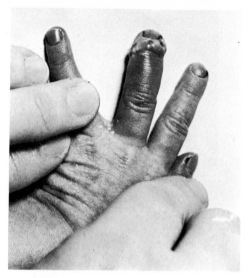

Fig. 14.6 Paronychia.

and mitts applied so that he cannot scratch himself or his mother's breast with the infected finger.

Abscesses

The scalp, ears and face may be injured during delivery and local infection follow. Infection of the subcutaneous tissue gives rise to abscess formation. This may be seen in the infant's breast particularly if it is engorged (Fig. 14.7). Laceration of the skin also allows access for organisms to deeper tissues and abscesses may be formed. A subcutaneous haemangioma is an ideal culture site for invading organisms.

Omphalitis

The umbilical stump is colonized early and occasionally clinical infection, omphalitis, occurs with spread to the surrounding skin. Further spread of infection may occur along the umbilical vein to the liver where abscess formation may occur. Thrombophlebitis may also occur and lead to portal vein thrombosis and resulting portal hypertension.

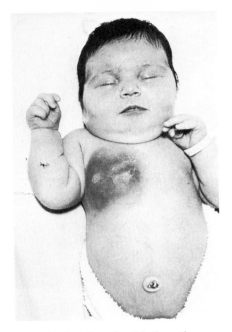

Fig. 14.7 Untreated mastitis in infant of a diabetic mother.

Stuffy nose

Stuffy nose is the commonest manifestation of infection of mucous membranes and varies from a slight mucoid nasal discharge to a profuse mucopurulent discharge which seriously hampers breathing during feeding and therefore causes the infant distress. Viruses or a combination of virus and bacteria are generally responsible. Decongestant nose drops such as 0.5% ephedrine in saline relieve symptoms and the condition generally clears without further treatment. Should the infection pass down the respiratory tract a more serious situation develops.

Thrush (oral candidiasis)

The mouth is a relatively common site of infection particularly with *Candida albicans* producing thrush. This generally presents as a white coating of the tongue (Fig. 14.8) which cannot be removed with a spatula as can milk curds. Spread to the mucous membranes of the gums, cheeks and soft palate produces a deeper form of

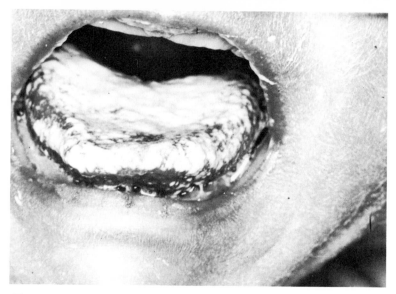

Fig. 14.8 Extensive thrush on the tongue.

infection which is more difficult to eradicate. It is important therefore to recognize monilial infection as early as possible. Treatment with local application of 1% aqueous gentian violet or by drops of nystatin or miconazole is indicated. Spread of thrush downwards into the gastrointestinal tract can produce a severe form of infection which in debilitated infants may prove fatal. This is a particular risk where wide-spectrum antibiotic therapy has been given for other forms of infection. Systemic candidiasis can also occur in debilitated infants.

Deep infections

As has been mentioned earlier, the signs of infection in the organs and deeper tissues are non-specific and this applies particularly to infection with Gram-negative organisms (Fig. 14.9) when there is rarely any superficial sign of inflammation as often occurs with Gram-positive infections.

Bacteraemia

Many deep infections are accompanied by bacteraemia and infection may occur simultaneously in several parts of the body. Low

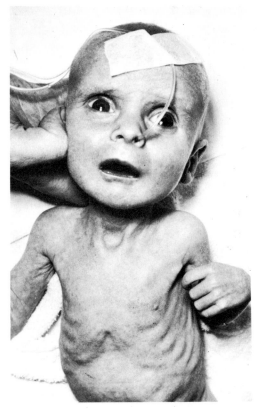

Fig. 14.9 Seriouslly ill infant with Gram-negative bacteraemia and meningitis.

birth weight infants are particularly prone to such infection. Infants dying of such infection may show at postmortem examination that there has been pyelonephritis, meningitis, pneumonia, osteomyelitis, arthritis or pericarditis (Fig. 14.10). The liver and spleen are frequently enlarged and abnormal as the result of circulating toxins. Widespread haemorrhage often occurs and death follows bleeding into the adrenal glands, lungs or brain. Microscopical examination in such cases often shows evidence of disseminated intravascular coagulation (Chapter 17).

Clinical presentation

Clinically such infants present with inactivity, feeding difficulty, weight loss, and these progress to circulatory collapse with a

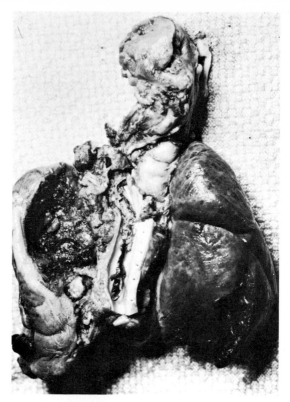

Fig. 14.10 Postmortem specimen of infants who had widespread staphylococcal infection with pyopneumothorax, mycotic aneurysm of the aorta and thrombosis.

greyish pallor, episodes of cyanosis and rapid, shallow breathing and poor pulse. The abdomen becomes distended, the liver and spleen are large, jaundice and haemorrhages may develop. There may be hypothermia or hyperthermia.

Pyelonephritis should be suspected as a source of bacteraemia where there is enlargement of one or both kidneys and pyuria.

Meningitis is not always diagnosable clinically in the ill infant (Fig. 14.9) who may show little in the way of neck stiffness. The fontanelle may be tense or bulging and the infant irritable. Lumbar puncture is an essential part of the investigation of all seriously ill infants.

Pneumonia as part of a generalized infection acquired before or at birth is termed congenital pneumonia. Postnatally acquired pneumonia may result from aspiration from airborne infection or as a complication of other conditions such as respiratory distress syndrome or cerebral haemorrhage. In addition to the general signs of severe illness there is disturbance of respiration ranging from tachypnoea to gasping with apnoeic spells. Cough may occur initially but becomes less frequent as the general condition deteriorates.

Osteomyelitis generally affects the metaphyses of the long bones and may spread to the adjacent joint. In addition to the general signs of bacteraemia there is localized tenderness and swelling with pseudoparalysis.

Septic arthritis is a common complication of osteomyelitis. More than one joint may be affected.

Peritonitis may occur as a result of bacteraemia or secondary to perforation of the bowel.

Gastroenteritis may present with generalized symptoms of collapse and dehydration before there has been much in the way of vomiting or diarrhoea, and differentiation from parenteral infection is difficult. Deterioration may occur rapidly and early recognition and treatment of fluid and electrolyte disturbance is essential.

Investigations of deep infections

Although physical examination may indicate the main site of infection it is essential that adequate specimens be obtained to check the possibility of infection at other sites before treatment is started. The bacteriological investigations suggested are shown in Table 14.1. Our experience shows that urine culture is the investigation most likely to be omitted unless its importance is appreciated. Techniques for obtaining urine including suprapubic aspiration of the bladder are described in Chapter 19. In addition to bacterial

Table 14.1 Specimens to be taken for bacteriological examination in suspected deep infections

Swabs from
    Nose
    Throat
    Ear
    Umbilicus
    Groin
Blood cultures
Urine (preferably by suprapubic aspiration)
Stool
Cerebrospinal fluid

and viral cultures, blood should be collected for white cell count and immunoglobulins and virus antibody titre.

Antibiotics

Once the bacteriological specimens have been obtained antibiotic treatment should be started. The choice of individual antibiotic depends on knowledge of the antibiotic sensitivity of the likely invading organism or of the environmental flora (see below).

Intravenous fluids are generally required both to restore the circulation and to correct coexistent metabolic disorders. Where bleeding is occurring the cause must be defined and appropriate treatment given (Chapter 17).

Intensive therapy. Severely infected infants require intensive therapy and where suitable facilities do not exist early transfer to a suitably equipped centre is advisable before the infant deteriorates to a state which would make a journey unjustifiable. This implies close observation and recognition of the earliest signs of infection.

Prognosis of deep infections

In spite of advances in antibiotic therapy the mortality from serious deep infections, particularly in low birth weight infants, remains high. Even with adequate therapy and survival the infant may be left with a handicapping disorder such as hydrocephalus. The importance of preventing the spread of infection in nurseries for the newborn cannot be over stressed.

Source of infection

Outbreaks of infection in nurseries indicate a break in the preventive measures employed. With low birth weight infants nursed in incubators the problem is often a local one involving one infant only. When several large well babies become infected, however, a source of infection with access to many infants has to be sought. This may be a member of staff or a mother who has a clinical infection or who is a carrier.

Spread may occur by direct contact or indirectly by common objects handled. The maximum risk occurs if an infected person is involved in preparing feeds. The common types of organisms to be introduced into nurseries by adults are streptococci, staphylococci, shigellae and salmonellae.

Epidemics

Epidemics of skin and umbilical infection have been virtually eliminated by skin antisepsis. Gastroenteritis remains the main
epidemic infection in nurseries. A wide range of organisms
including salmonellae, typeable *E. coli* and viruses may be
involved.

Epidemic diarrhoea of the newborn is a serious threat to nurseries
and, should an outbreak occur, treatment of the individual infant
must be accompanied by control of the epidemic. This involves
barrier nursing of affected infants and cohort nursing of clean
babies for whom separate clean accommodation and staff must be
available. Should such measures fail the unit may have to be closed
to further admissions until the outbreak has been controlled.
Consultation between all members of the nursing, medical, laboratory and administrative staff is essential to make sure that each
understands the other's position. Rapid planning will frequently
curtail an outbreak before it is established.

Transferable drug resistance. The ability of organisms to transfer
drug resistance to previously sensitive organisms can cause major
problems in treatment if antibiotics are used unnecessarily. Co-
ordination and planning are again essential.

Antibiotic policies

Antibiotic policies are frequently talked about, less frequently put
into effect. Nurseries for the newborn are suitable situations in
which to formulate and test antibiotic policies. Our own experience
has convinced us of the advantage of a firm policy for the use of
antibiotics which limits the primary choice to a single antibiotic or
antibiotic combination, the choice of which is based on knowledge
of the environmental flora.

Prophylactic antibiotics

Opinions differ as to the advisability of using antibiotics prophylactically. We have progressively reduced the use of antibiotics in
the absence of suspected clinical infection without evidence of
increase in infection. An antibiotic policy must be based on local
information and no single policy is universally applicable.

Education of unit staff

Throughout this chapter stress has been laid on the importance of policy decisions in the prevention and control of infection in hospital nurseries. Advances in the understanding of sources and spread of organisms have provided a basis on which sound policies can be based. The responsibility for carrying out such policies rests with the staff of the unit concerned. Education of new members of staff is essential, and regular reviews of results and reassessment of policy decision are necessary to maintain a high standard of vigilance and efficiency. Without these, infection continues to be a potential hazard to all infants in newborn nurseries.

FURTHER READING

Alder, V. G., Burman, D., Simpson, R. A., Fysh, J. & Gillespie, W. A. (1980) Comparison of hexachlorophane and chlorhexidine powders in prevention of neonatal infection. *Archives of Disease in Childhood*, 55, 277.

Committee on Infectious Diseases Report (1986) 20th edn., Red Book. Illinois: American Academy of Pediatrics.

Davies, P. A., (1980) Pathogen or commensal? *Archives of Disease in Childhood*, 55, 169.

Hanshaw, J. B. (1979) A New cytomegalovirus syndrome *American Journal of Diseases of Children*, **133**, 475.

Peevy, K. J. & Chalhub, E. G. (1983) Occult group B streptococcal infections: an important cause of intrauterine asphyxia. *American Journal of Obstetrics and Gynecology*, **146**, 989–990.

Remington, J. S. & Klein, J. O. (Eds) (1983) *Infectious Disease of the Fetus and Newborn Infant*. Philadelphia: Saunders.

Rudd, P. J. & Carrington, D. (1984) A prospective study of chlamydial, mycoplasmal and viral infections in a neonatal intensive care unit. *Archives of Disease in Childhood*, **59**, 120–125.

Speck, W. T., Fanaroff, A. A. & Klaus, M. H. (1979) *Neonatal Infections in Care of the High Risk neonate*, 2nd edn, ed. Klaus, M. H. & Fanaroff, A. A. Philadelphia: Saunders.

15

Jaundice

Jaundice is the commonest abnormal physical sign in the newborn period, so much so that jaundice is described as being 'physiological' in the majority of affected infants. As jaundice may be associated with cerebral dysfunction and death it is clearly not always physiological and must be considered as a potentially serious condition. To understand the investigation and management of a jaundiced infant it is useful to have some knowledge of the metabolism of the pigment bilirubin which is the cause of the yellow discoloration of the tissues known clinically as jaundice.

Physiology

Bilirubin is a breakdown product of haemoglobin which is released when red blood cells die and their membranes rupture. Two main forms of metabolism of bilirubin occur in the body, conjugation which takes place in the liver and photodecomposition which takes place in the skin under the influence of light. Bilirubin is not soluble in water but is taken up by fatty tissues and is soluble in fat solvents. It is carried in the plasma bound to albumin.

Hepatic conjugation

On arrival at the liver two transport globulins Y and Z carry bilirubin from its albumin carrier across the liver cell membrane into the liver cell where conjugation with glucuronic acid takes place. This changes fat-soluble bilirubin to water-soluble bilirubin diglucuronide which can then be excreted in the bile. The laboratory will report fat soluble bilirubin as unconjugated or indirect-acting bilirubin, and water-soluble bilirubin diglucuronide as conjugated or direct-acting bilirubin. This process is catalysed by the enzyme glucuronyl transferase which is not present in sufficient quantity in the first few days of life to deal with all the bilirubin presented to the liver. The level of bilirubin in the blood rises causing jaundice. In term babies enzyme activity is generally sufficient to deal with the bilirubin load by the third or fourth day of life, but in preterm babies it may not be present in the quantities required until the sixth or seventh day. Jaundice is therefore likely to be more marked in preterm infants. Jaundice from this cause is due to immaturity of liver function. It is also important to realize that the lifespan of neonatal red cells is shortened to 90 days (cf. 120 days in adults), leading to an increased breakdown load, and that other globins (e.g. myoglobin) share the same breakdown pathway. In addition, the enterohepatic circulation in the upper intestine is capable of reconverting conjugated (water-soluble) bilirubin into unconjugated (fat-soluble) bilirubin, which is absorbed and thus requires reprocessing.

Hepatic excretion

Excretion of conjugated bilirubin into the bile canaliculi is an active process.

Obstructive jaundice occurs when the liver is unable to excrete conjugated bilirubin into the gastrointestinal tract by the bile duct system. The problem may occur in the liver cell, the intrahepatic biliary system or in the extrahepatic bile ducts. Particularly when the liver cell is involved both conjugated and unconjugated bilirubin may be abnormally raised in the blood and tissues.

Photodecomposition

Photodecomposition of bilirubin to water-soluble isomers takes place in the skin under the stimulus of blue light and is not dependent on enzyme action. The isomers are excreted in the urine. How much bilirubin is decomposed depends on the area of skin exposed to light, the wave length and intensity of the light and the length of exposure. In a clothed infant under normal lighting conditions the amount is probably small and special conditions have to be created to make this method of disposal of bilirubin of clinical importance. This is described later in this chapter as phototherapy.

Pathology

Bilirubin encephalopathy

If neither of these pathways is sufficient to dispose of the bilirubin

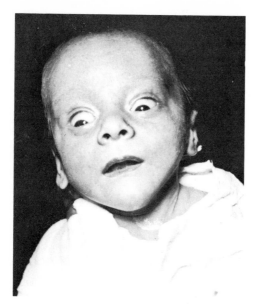

Fig. 15.1 Sunsetting appearance of eyes in infant with kernicterus.

formed the level of bilirubin in the serum rises progressively and
the infant becomes increasingly jaundiced as bilirubin passes from
blood into the skin and other tissues such as the brain. This latter
occurs when the ability of plasma albumin to bind unconjugated
bilirubin is exceeded and will occur early if there is acidosis or
other competitors (e.g. drugs) for albumin sites. Brain cells do
not tolerate the presence of bilirubin, and cell death may occur.
The effect of this is called bilirubin encephalopathy, which is
evident clinically as lethargy, disinclination to feed, drowsiness
and eventually coma. A sunsetting appearance of the eyes may be
seen (Fig. 15.1). As brain damage increases, twitching, convulsions
and episodes of cyanosis occur. Recovery is possible in all but the
most severely affected infants but there are frequently permanent
residual signs in the form of high tone nerve deafness and cerebral
palsy of the athetoid type.

Kernicterus

Where death results from bilirubin encephalopathy, examination
of the brain shows areas of yellow discoloration in the basal nuclei
and other parts of the brain and spinal cord (Fig. 15.2). These are
due to deposition of bilirubin and cell death. The condition is

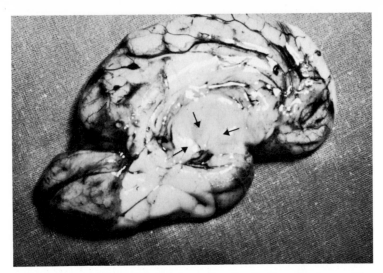

Fig. 15.2 Brain of infant of 28 weeks' gestation who died from kernicterus. The arrows indicate where yellow staining was evident.

termed kernicterus. Treatment of kernicterus is impossible and management must aim at forestalling the passage of bilirubin into brain cells. This can best be done by recognizing those infants in whom bilirubin encephalopathy is liable to occur, watching their progress carefully and applying treatment at a stage when the risk of brain damage exceeds the risk of the treatment proposed. It is therefore necessary to be able to assess the chances of brain damage occurring in any jaundiced infant and to know the relative dangers of possible therapeutic regimens.

Contributory factors

Hyperbilirubinaemia. The risk to the infant increases with progressive rise of serum unconjugated bilirubin but the level of bilirubin at which encephalopathy occurs varies from infant to infant.

Acidosis, hypoglycaemia, hypoxia and the presence in the blood of substances such as free fatty acids which compete with bilirubin for albumin-binding sites are other factors involved. We have seen kernicterus in severely acidotic immature infants in whom the serum unconjugated bilirubin did not exceed 220 μmol per litre (13 mg per 100 ml). Healthy mature infants have had unconjugated bilirubin levels of 427 μmol per litre (25 mg per 100 ml) or more and shown no evidence of bilirubin encephalopathy. The serum unconjugated bilirubin level remains, however, the best means available at present of assessing the risk of brain damage in jaundiced infants.

Albumin-binding capacity. When the molar concentration bilirubin/albumin exceeds 1/1 the albumin-binding capacity is likely to be exceeded and the infant is in danger. This ratio corresponds to a serum unconjugated bilirubin level of 350 μmol per litre (20 mg per 100 ml) at an albumin concentration of approximately 3 g per dl (3 g per 100 ml). It must be stressed, however, that immature acidotic infants are at risk at unconjugated bilirubin levels well below 350 μmol per litre (20 mg per 100 ml).

CLINICAL CAUSES

Our chief concern in the management of the jaundiced infant is the prevention of bilirubin encephalopathy. As bilirubin is no longer toxic once it has been made water-soluble it is important to differentiate those causes of non-obstructive jaundice which are associated with high levels of unconjugated bilirubin from those causing obstructive jaundice in which conjugated, water-soluble, bilirubin is a major cause of jaundice. As the risk of bilirubin encephalopathy is highest in non-obstructive jaundice, and as this is much more common than the obstructive type, it will be dealt with first and at greater length.

Non-obstructive jaundice

The commoner factors likely to increase the serum unconjugated bilirubin and to produce a non-obstructive jaundice are shown in Table 15.1.

Immaturity of liver function

Adequate liver function is essential for the conjugation of bilirubin and its excretion into the biliary tract. In some term infants and in the majority of preterm infants liver function is temporarily inadequate. The more mature the infant the more rapidly does liver function mature to cope with the load of bilirubin presented. The longer the delay until such maturity of function occurs the greater the risk of bilirubin rising in the serum to levels which may produce bilirubin encephalopathy.

Table 15.1 Causes of non-obstructive jaundice

IMMATURITY OF LIVER FUNCTION
    Jaundice of immaturity
    Physiological jaundice
INHIBITION OF LIVER FUNCTION
    Breast milk jaundice
HAEMOLYTIC ANAEMIAS
    ABO incompatibility
    Rh incompatibility
    Glucose-6-phosphate-dehydrogenase
      (G6PDH) deficiency
    Spherocytosis
    Haemoglobinopathies
    Severe infections
    Drug sensitivity
    Extravasated blood
Other rare causes
    Hypothyroidism
    Crigler-Najjar syndrome
    Congenital pyloric stenosis
    Malrotation of the intestine
    Cystic fibrosis

Time scale

Time is therefore of great importance in the assessment of jaundice. The earlier the jaundice appears and the longer it persists the greater is the risk to the infant. In healthy term infants physiological jaundice, which is due to a relatively minor degree of hepatic immaturity, appears on the second or third day of life and clears in two or three days as liver function improves. In preterm infants the onset is also on the second or third day but persists for longer and may not reach its maximum until the end of the first week of life.

Jaundice in the first 24 hours. Jaundice appearing on the first day of life must never be accepted as physiological and is highly suggestive of a haemolytic anaemia or of severe liver dysfunction as may occur in infection.

Persistence of jaundice. Similarly, any jaundice which persists for more than 10 to 14 days after birth must always be investigated thoroughly with particular reference to signs of obstructive jaundice. If there is no evidence of biliary obstruction the possibility of hypothyroidism has to be considered, as persistent jaundice in the neonatal period may be the first clinical evidence of this condition.

Haemolytic anaemias

The incidence of haemolytic anaemia varies according to the racial background of the infant. In European countries Rh incompatability was until recently the most frequent cause of severe haemolytic anaemia. As shown below, preventive treatment may soon make this problem a rarity. Throughout the world incompatibility of the fetus and mother for the ABO blood groups is the most frequent potential cause of haemolytic anaemia but fortunately it seldom results in severe degrees of jaundice. In some Mediterranean races, in Negroes and Far Eastern races deficiency of the enzyme glucose-6-phosphate dehydrogenase (G6PDH) is a much commoner cause of haemolytic anaemia than Rh incompatibility. Abnormalities of red cell membrane in such conditions as thalassaemia and elliptocytosis are associated with unusual haemoglobins and are a cause of haemolysis in certain races.

Antenatal detection of such haemolytic anaemias is now possible in some centres by the examination of fetal blood taken from cord vessels in utero by fetoscopy.

Blood group incompatibility

Blood group incompatibility occurs when the fetus has inherited from its father a blood group such as the Rh factor which is not present in the mother. Should fetal red blood cells pass across the placenta into the mother in sufficient numbers she may become sensitized to these foreign red cells and produce an antibody (immunoglobulin) which promotes the destruction of the foreign cells. Should such an immunoglobulin pass back to the fetus across the placenta it will cause haemolysis of the fetal cells, haemoglobin will be released and break down, with resulting anaemia and the production of bilirubin. In utero this bilirubin is excreted via the placenta into the maternal circulation and dealt with by the mother. If the placenta has not been able to excrete all the bilirubin presented the infant at birth may be slightly jaundiced and jaundice is likely to increase rapidly. The infant may also be anaemic and have a large liver and spleen due to increased intrauterine haemopoiesis. Where haemolysis has been very marked in utero the degree of anaemia can be sufficient to cause cardiac failure with the accumulation of oedema which, when severe, is called *hydrops fetalis* (Fig. 15.3). In severe cases haemorrhage may occur into the skin or deeper tissues. The infant may be stillborn.

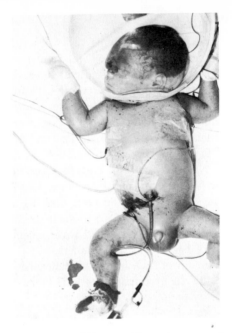

Fig. 15.3 Hydrops fetalis successfully treated by exchange transfusions.

ABO incompatibility

Incompatibility of the ABO blood groups leading to jaundice can occur in the situations shown in Table 15.2. Ninety per cent of group O, A and B mothers produce natural blood group antibodies of the IgM type. These are of large molecular size and cannot cross the placenta to attack the fetus. In the remainder of the natural blood group antibody is of the IgG small molecular size variety and is able to cross the placenta with the potential for haemolysis of fetal red cells. This is particularly likely when the mother is group

Table 15.2 ABO incompatibility

Mother's group	Fetus, group	
	Compatible	Incompatible
O	O	A, B, AB
A	O, A	B, AB
B	O, B	A, AB
AB	O, A, B, AB	

O and the fetus group A. The antibody is present before pregnancy so all pregnancies have an equal chance of being affected. Fortunately the haemolytic anaemia produced is usually mild and the jaundice can usually be controlled with phototherapy. Where both ABO and Rh incompatibility occur in the same pregnancy the ABO incompatibility frequently protects mother from being sensitized by Rh-positive fetal cells.

Rh incompatibility

Prevention

Rhesus (Rh) incompatibility occurs where mother is Rh-negative and father and fetus Rh-positive. Among European races approximately 15% of the population is Rh-negative. It is now possible to prevent almost all Rh-negative women from being sensitized by Rh-positive cells from the fetus. The passage of cells from the fetus to mother is likely to occur late in pregnancy most frequently during labour, particularly where there are such complications as toxaemia of pregnancy, Caesarean section and breech delivery. It can also occur in such situations as threatened abortion, external version and amniocentesis. Fetal red cells can be recognized in mother's blood by the acid elution technique (Kleihauer test). Injection of an immune anti-D (Rh) globulin into mother destroys the fetal red cells before sensitization takes place. Where Rh-negative mothers are adequately supervised throughout all pregnancies it should therefore be possible to eliminate almost completely Rh incompatibility as a cause of jaundice in infants.

Sensitization

Women may be sensitized to the Rh and other factors which they do not themselves possess by means other than pregnancy. These generally involve the injection of blood or blood products containing the antigen. This is now fortunately an unusual occurrence but in spite of the widespread use of preventive measures the possibility of blood group sensitization must always be kept in mind as a cause of jaundice in the newborn.

Antenatal recognition

Some blood group incompatibilities can be recognized antenatally by examination of maternal serum and liquor amnii as discussed in Chapter 4. Such examination may indicate that a fetus is severely affected and in danger of dying within a few days. In such situations the obstetrician and paediatrician have to consult together to decide whether it is safer to induce labour and accept the risk of delivering the infant prematurely, or to transfuse the infant in utero in an attempt to prolong fetal life until the risk of the haemolytic anaemia outweighs the risk associated with that period of gestation.

Intrauterine transfusion. In general transabdominal intrauterine transfusion is preferable to induction of labour before 32 weeks gestation but the advantage lies with delivery after 32 weeks. It is now possibly by use of fetoscopy to transfuse directly via the umbilical vein in early pregnancy in severe Rh incompatibility. Other techniques in antenatal treatment involve reduction in maternal antibody level by plasmaphoresis. Decisions of this nature should only be made at centres used to dealing with such problems. With the decreasing incidence of Rh incompatibility it is important that sensitized mothers be referred for advice as to management to a limited number of regional centres who can maintain the high standard of judgment based on experience necessary to produce a successful outcome.

Other causes of haemolytic anaemias

In spite of the likely continuing decline in the incidence of Rh incompatibility, jaundice in infants will remain a major problem for those managing nurseries for the newborn because of the other factors involved in the production of jaundice. With the increase in movement of families between countries there is need for awareness of causes of jaundice which were previously rare in this country. These include deficiency of the enzyme G6PDH, which results in increased liability to haemolysis, the presence of abnormally shaped red blood cells (e.g. spherocytosis) and the presence of an abnormal haemoglobin within the cell. Infections, particularly with Gram-negative organisms, must always be looked for where jaundice is otherwise not satisfactorily explained. Drugs such as Synkavit, the synthetic analogue of vitamin K, in doses of 15 mg or more per day are associated with an increase in haemolysis. Extravasated blood as in a large bruise or cephalhaematoma increases the load of bilirubin and may be a significant contributing cause of jaundice.

Inhibition of liver function

Breast milk jaundice. Substances which may impair liver function include some steroids. The increased incidence of jaundice in breast fed infants may be related to a steroid contained in the milk of some mothers giving rise to 'breast milk jaundice'. Infants of mothers who have been taking the 'pill' shortly before conception occurred are reported to have higher levels of bilirubin than infants of mothers who were not on the 'pill'. Novobiocin is believed to inhibit the activity of glucuronyl transferase.

Breast feeding jaundice. The majority of breast-fed infants who develop jaundice do so because of the increased enterohepatic circulation of bilirubin. This is aggravated by the sluggish upper bowel transit time caused by the lower fluid intake of these infants in the first few days of life.

Rarer causes of jaundice

The persisting jaundice associated with hypothyroidism is due to depression of enzyme activity whereas in families with the Crigler-Najjar syndrome there is inherited deficiency of glucuronyl transferase. In infants with obstruction of the pylorus or small intestine, jaundice may, at least in part, be non-obstructive and due to the active enterohepatic circulation and clears with correction of the obstruction to the bowel.

Obstructive jaundice

Obstructive jaundice has a greenish tinge which may be distinguishable clinically from the purer yellow of jaundice associated with raised levels of unconjugated bilirubin. Observation of the stool and urine is important in any infant with jaundice. Where the jaundice is of obstructive type the urine will be dark brown in colour due to the excess of bile pigments (but not of urobilinogen) and the stools are very pale in colour and will be white in the early stage of complete obstructive jaundice. Blood examination will show raised levels of conjugated bilirubin which will fall if the obstruction is relieved.

Obstructive jaundice can be due to hepatitis or to abnormality of the bile duct system.

Hepatitis

Hepatitis may be due to infection, to the toxic effect of certain chemical substances or to inherited abnormality.

Infective hepatitis evident at or shortly after birth would have been acquired antenatally by the passage of organisms across the placenta. Syphilis, cytomegalic inclusion body disease and toxoplasmosis are acquired by this method. During delivery viruses such as *Herpes simplex* or bacteria such as *Listeria monocytogenes* may be acquired and cause hepatitis within a few days of birth. Infection may be introduced into the umbilical vein following umbilical sepsis, particularly if a catheter has been introduced through the infected area. Further spread of infection to the liver occurs by the portal venous system, and multiple liver abscesses or a more generalized hepatitis follows. All of these conditions will be associated with jaundice and enlargement of the liver. In addition there are often enlargement of the spleen and signs of more generalized infection (Chapter 14).

Chemical hepatitis. More rarely hepatitis may also occur in the first week of life because of the deposition of toxic chemical substances in liver cells. Jaundice due to such hepatitis may be the presenting sign of galactosaemia (Chapter 11).

Alpha-1-antitrypsin deficiency. Some infants with hepatitis have a deficiency of the enzyme alpha-1-antitrypsin. This deficiency is inherited as an autosomal recessive and there is a 1 in 4 risk of other children in the family being similarly affected. The severity of hepatitis varies in different families but in some may lead to early death from liver failure or later death from cirrhosis. No treatment is available.

Abnormalities of the bile ducts

Obstructive jaundice occurs shortly after birth where there is mechanical obstruction or where the bile ducts fail to develop or are destroyed by intrauterine hepatitis caused by organisms such as the cytomegalovirus. A cyst of the bile duct (choledochal cyst) may result in intermittent or permanent obstruction of the biliary system. The differential diagnosis between hepatitis and mechanical obstruction of the bile ducts can be difficult during the first month of life. If galactosaemia and alpha-1-antitrypsin deficiency have been excluded by the appropriate blood tests and there has been no evidence of bile in the stools for one month, liver biopsy may be necessary to establish the diagnosis.

Assessment of the jaundiced infant

Clinical assessment must bear in mind significant information obtained from the mother's antenatal history which may clearly suggest Rh incompatibility or other cause of haemolytic anaemia such as congenital spherocytosis which has an autosomal dominant inheritance.

Time of onset

Infants who are active and feeding well and in whom the onset of jaundice occurred after 24 hours of age require less urgent investigation than the sick infant who has become jaundiced on the first day of life. In such an infant urgent investigation is necessary to establish the cause of jaundice and to apply appropriate treatment in the hope of preventing the onset of bilirubin encephalopathy and kernicterus.

Rate of increase in depth of jaundice

Jaundice which deepens rapidly and which is accompanied by a rise in serum bilirubin at a rate greater than 10 μmol/litre an hour requires urgent investigation as to possible causes such as haemolysis or infection.

Associated features. The jaundiced infant who remains well and active and who continues to feed well is a less urgent problem than the infant who demonstrates other features such as pallor and lethargy or in whom there is enlargement of the liver, or spleen, purpura or other evidence of bleeding.

Investigation. Such infants require urgent investigation and treatment including maternal and infant blood grouping, direct Coomb's test, full blood count, reticulocyte count, blood and urine culture, examination of the urine for reducing substances other than glucose. Other investigations such as red cell fragility, red cell enzymes, and haemoglobin electrophoresis may be necessary.

When preliminary investigations do not establish the diagnosis and if the infant's condition is deteriorating, referral to a regional centre for more detailed investigation will be indicated.

TREATMENT

The treatment of the jaundiced infant must include both the correction of the underlying condition causing the jaundice where this is possible and the protection of the infant from the potentially harmful effects of bilirubin. Investigation to establish the cause of the jaundice is therefore an essential part of the management of the jaundiced infant. Similarly it is necessary to assess the urgency of the need for treatment. The majority of jaundiced infants suffer no ill effect from their short period of mild jaundice and require no treatment other than that of close observation.

Prophylaxis

Reduction of the incidence of preterm delivery and the early institution of feeding have already been discussed in Chapters 4, 8 and 9.

Phototherapy

Phototherapy, which changes bilirubin into non-toxic, water-soluble isomers can be achieved by exposing the infant to a potent source of blue light. This is most readily carried out in an incubator with the infant fully exposed apart from the eyes which should be covered by a mask made from non-irritant material (Fig. 15.4). It is, however, perfectly possible to provide phototherapy in a cot,

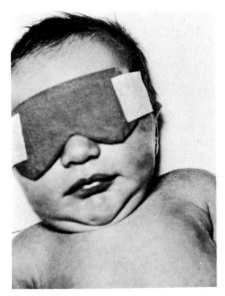

Fig. 15.4 Mask for protecting eyes during phototherapy.

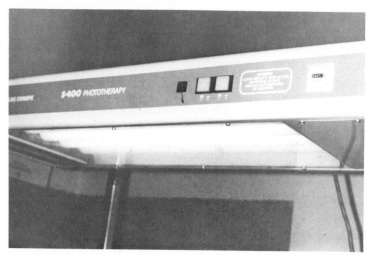

Fig. 15.5 Phototherapy unit with both blue and white tubes.

provided the naked infant is kept in a sufficiently heated environment which should preferably be shared by mother. In Britain natural day-light varies so considerably in intensity that it cannot be relied upon to provide an adequate source of blue light for a long enough period each day.

Phototherapy units provide an artificial source of light the characteristics of which will depend largely on the type of fluorescent tube used (Fig. 15.5). Experimental evidence has shown that blue light in the wavelength range 425 to 475 nanometres is the most effective in causing a fall in serum bilirubin. At this wavelength the minimum effective radiance is 15 μW/cm^2 and saturation is reached at 585 μW/cm^2. Accurate measurement of radiance within the appropriate wave band requires sophisticated spectroradiometers which are expensive and not readily available. Most commercially available phototherapy units will, however, produce a satisfactory radiance if correctly operated and maintained.

Indications. As phototherapy is more effective in preventing a rise in serum bilirubin than in reducing a high level of bilirubin, treatment should be given to jaundiced infants as soon as their serum bilirubin reaches 250 μmol per litre (15 mg per 100 ml) in term infants and 170 μmol per litre (10 mg per 100 ml) in preterm infants. Some paediatricians prefer to expose the infant to phototherapy intermittently for limited periods of say four hours with an interval of four hours. This appears to be almost as effective as continuous exposure, allows other infants to share the use of the light source and may interfere less with mother-infant interactions.

Length of treatment. As skin colour is no longer a useful indication of depth of jaundice in infants under treatment with phototherapy it is necessary to take blood for serum bilirubin estimations to decide on the length of treatment required. This is likely to vary with the gestational age of the infant being longest in the most immature infants. Phototherapy is most suitable for the treatment of jaundice due to immaturity of liver function but may also be used prophylactically in infants with haemolytic anaemias. In such cases a particularly careful watch must be kept on the serum bilirubin as photo-decomposition may not be sufficient to deal with the bilirubin being released. It has, of course, no effect on the associated anaemia.

Side effects of phototherapy initially caused concern particularly with regard to the possibility that brain growth might be disturbed. This has been disproved and is no longer a cause for concern. Infants being treated by phototherapy lose an increased amount of water, both through the skin and in the stools. The fluid intake, therefore, has to be increased during phototherapy to compensate for this.

Enzyme induction

It is possible to induce enzyme activity in the fetus by giving phenobarbitone to the mother antenatally. At birth the infant is therefore better prepared to deal with the load of bilirubin presented to the liver. Giving phenobarbitone to the infant from birth has a similar but delayed effect and is therefore less valuable. As it is not possible to recognize antenatally all mothers who will deliver their infants before term or to recognize at birth all infants who will become jaundiced, treatment with phenobarbitone would have to be given unnecessarily to large numbers of mothers and infants to make sure that all infants who were due to become jaundiced had been treated in time. This raises ethical problems. As there is no evidence that treatment with phenobarbitone has any advantage over phototherapy the authors prefer the latter.

Early feeding

Early feeding helps to reduce the danger of high bilirubin levels by reducing the risk of acidosis and preventing the rise of free fatty acids which compete with bilirubin for albumin binding sites.

Correction of acidosis

Correction of acidosis by intravenous alkali will restore the capacity of albumin to bind bilirubin.

Albumin infusion

The place of infusions of salt-free albumin to boost albumin binding capacity has not been settled. Given intravenously in a maximum dose of 1 g per kg body weight as a replacement for an equal volume of blood this method has proved safe in very small infants (below 1 kg) and may prevent the need for exchange trans-fusion in infants seriously ill for other reasons. The authors, however, have not used this method of therapy except along with exchange transfusion in an attempt to manage severe Rh isoim-munization.

Exchange transfusion

The object of an exchange transfusion is to remove blood containing harmful substances such as bilirubin from a patient and to replace it by healthy donor blood. Similarly, blood of low packed cell volume (PCV) can be replaced by blood of normal PCV so that severe anaemia can be corrected without overloading the circu-lation. In the same ways, polycythaemia (high PCV) can be treated to lower the PCV. In Rh incompatibility Rh-positive cells can be replaced by Rh-negative cells. The procedure is generally carried out through a catheter in the umbilical vein. In immature infants it is common practice to perform exchange transfusion through both umbilical arterial and venous catheters simultaneously to reduce swings in the infant's blood volume. Various techniques can be employed and some of these are discussed in Chapter 20.

Risks

In all procedures there is a risk to the infant which depends upon a number of factors such as the skill and experience of the oper-ators, the type of donor blood used and the technique involved. 'Unexplained death' during exchange transfusion is in well ordered centres now very much rarer than previously but the complex physical and chemical changes which take place during exchange transfusion still constitute a risk for infants. The decision as to when this method of treatment should be employed depends upon knowledge of the risk to the infant of the condition being treated, the availability of other safer methods of treatment and the risk of exchange transfusion in the unit concerned. Only when the risk of exchange transfusion is less than the risk of the infant developing bilirubin encephalopathy should exchange transfusion be the treatment of choice.

Expertise. As a result of the falling incidence of Rh incompatibility, fewer exchanges are carried out, and the subsequent loss of expertise may lead to greater risk to the infant. Because of reduced number there may be long periods without serious mishap and it becomes difficult to assess the risk involved.

Complications. Even with experienced staff, however, the risk of exchange transfusion itself is probably not lower than a mortality rate of 1 in 100 transfusions. Non-fatal complications such as portal vein thrombosis, hepatitis, and cytomegalovirus infection from donor blood also have to be borne in mind. There is also an increased risk of necrotizing enterocolitis and septicaemia.

Indications

It therefore follows that knowledge of the risk to the infant of the degree of anaemia or jaundice present is equally important when considering the indications for exchange transfusion. In each infant more than one factor is likely to be involved and the ultimate decision is therefore a clinical one and should not be made entirely on laboratory evidence. As clinical impressions are difficult to quantify some laboratory guide-lines are useful.

Laboratory criteria. We recommend that exchange transfusion be carried out in patients with proven blood group incompatibility for the following indications: at birth and in the first 72 hours of life, a cord or venous haemoglobin of 10 g per dl (10 g per 100 ml) or less; at any age jaundice with early signs of bilirubin encephalopathy or a serum unconjugated bilirubin exceeding the guidelines in Fig. 15.6.

In older, well term infants with no cause other than hepatic immaturity for jaundice the indications for exchange transfusion are early signs of bilirubin encephalopathy or a serum unconjugated bilirubin of 425 μmol per litre (25 mg per 100 ml).

In infants with Rh or other causes for haemolytic anaemia we have not found that the bilirubin level in cord blood is a useful

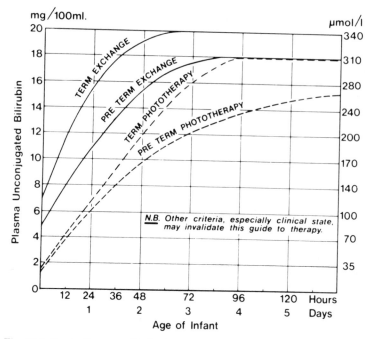

Fig. 15.6 Graph of suggested indications for exchange transfusion and phototherapy.

indication of the need for immediate exchange transfusion. Early exchange transfusion in such infants does little to prevent the need for subsequent exchange transfusion and may increase the total number of transfusions required.

The urgency of treatment must always be assessed. Where the prenatal findings in a Rh-sensitized mother suggest a severely affected infant arrangements must be made in good time before delivery so that an immediate exchange transfusion can be carried out at birth. This will be required in severely anaemic and oedematous infants (hydrops fetalis) — (Fig. 15.3) — from whom peritoneal and pleural fluid may have to be aspirated to allow respiration to continue. Jaundiced infants are not such urgent problems provided that frequent assessment of their clinical state has been made and that the rate of rise of serum bilirubin is known. Estimations at four hourly intervals of serum-bilirubin allow a useful graph to be plotted, and the pattern of further development can be estimated with a surprising degree of accuracy. A rapid rise to 250 μmol per litre (15 mg per 100 ml) followed by a slower rise may indicate that dangerous levels of bilirubin will not be reached. If an exchange transfusion is carried out in such an infant who is well at a level of say 300 μmol per litre (17 mg per 100 ml) serum bilirubin, the bilirubin may fall but rise again with the entry of bilirubin from the tissues into the blood stream. A second transfusion may then be required. If the first transfusion had been delayed the second transfusion might not have proved necessary.

Donor blood

Blood for exchange transfusions must be fresh (less than 48 hours old) accurately tested for compatibility and restored to the infant's true packed cell volume (approximately 60%) by withdrawal of plasma (e.g. 100 ml). Rh negative blood of appropriate ABO group is used for Rh-sensitized infants. It should if possible be collected from known hepatitis B, HIV, cytomegalovirus negative donors. The preferred anticoagulant is citrate phosphate dextrose rather than acid citrate dextrose. Heparinized blood is seldom used for the management of jaundiced infants. The blood must be slowly warmed to body temperature. Where citrated donor blood is used injections of calcium gluconate are commonly given at regular intervals because of the production of hypocalcaemia by the citrate. These are not indicated in all infants and others prefer to give 1 ml of 10% calcium gluconate slowly intravenously only when the infant shows electrocardiographic evidence of hypocalcaemia.

Procedure

Monitoring. Observation of the infant during exchange transfusion is of first importance to detect the earliest changes in general condition, body temperature, pulse rate and volume and irritability. Many centres use monitors to record heart rate, respiration temperature etc, but where such monitors are not available, good clinical observation can be as effective, provided that there is no relaxation of concentration.

Temperature control. Maintenance of a stable body temperature may require special arrangements for heat control. This may be an incubator, overhead heating panel or heating pad below the infant (Fig. 15.7). Continuous recording of the infant's skin and core temperature is extremely useful but if not available can be replaced by frequent recording of the infant's skin and rectal temperature.

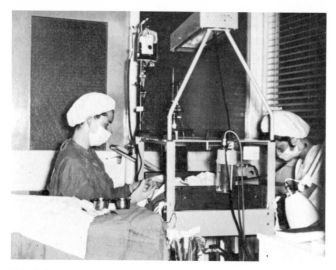

Fig. 15.7 Exchange transfusion being carried out in a controlled environment.

Volume control. Careful control of the volumes of blood removed and transfused is essential to prevent changes in the infant's blood volume. Where mechanical control is not available the importance of careful recordings of the volumes used in each cycle cannot be over-stressed. Each cycle of removal and replacement should not exceed 10% of the infant's blood volume. It is customary to perform a twice blood volume exchange (160 ml/kg) which removes 85% of the infant's blood.

Access of resuscitation. Particularly where several leads from recording instruments are involved it is important to ensure that free access to the infant's head is always available in case of vomiting or the need for resuscitative procedures. To reduce the risks of vomiting and inhalation the stomach should be kept empty throughout the procedure.

Prevention of infection. As the umbilical vein is a ready source of entry for pathogenic organisms antiseptic and aseptic precautions must be rigidly enforced. It is useful to take a bacteriological swab from the umbilicus before cannulation and after the transfusion to send the distal end of the catheter for bacteriological examination. Most centres prefer to give prophylactic antibiotic cover following an exchange transfusion.

Effectiveness

Exchange of red cells. A mathematical study of the effectiveness of exchange transfusion in removing an infant's red cells shows a decrease in efficiency, as the exchange proceeds, as more and more of the blood being removed is donor blood.

Removal of bilirubin. When the indication for the exchange transfusion is jaundice a different pattern emerges. As the serum level of bilirubin falls a gradient is established and bilirubin passes from the tissues into the blood. This movement is encouraged by the provision of 'clean' albumin in the donor blood. Thus more bilirubin can be removed from the body than was in the blood at the beginning of the transfusion. This advantage can be further improved by priming the infant with albumin 1 g per kg body weight at least 30 minutes before the exchange, and the priming can be repeated during the procedure. Whether the advantage gained is justified is debatable. Even without priming with albumin the mass of bilirubin removed may be as much as 150% of the bilirubin in the infant's plasma before exchange transfusion. The speed of transfusion is of some importance and there are advantages from increased safety and increased bilirubin output in not exceeding a rate of exchange of 2 ml per kg body weight per minute.

Cord stump. Following withdrawal of the umbilical vein catheter bleeding should be controlled by pressure and the umbilical cord stump dusted with antibacterial powder. If bleeding persists a ligature should be inserted to control the bleeding but this is not often required. It is advisable to leave the stump exposed so that any secondary bleeding can be observed quickly.

Prevention

The prevention of maternal Rh sensitization, the recognition and early treatment of affected infants together with contraceptive advice or sterilization of mothers liable to have further seriously affected infants should progressively reduce the problem of Rh imcompatibility. It is less easy to forecast further development in relation to jaundice of immaturity which is now the most frequent cause of possible bilirubin encephalopathy. Better understanding of the metabolic processes involved has already reduced the frequency of the most severe forms of this condition, and as safer forms of therapy are introduced it can be hoped that this cause of jaundice will be less of a problem in the future.

Treatment of obstructive jaundice

Urgency. The treatment of obstructive jaundice is less urgent unless the cause in infective, in which case rapid identification of the causative organisms and appropriate antibiotic or other treatment is indicated.

Infective

It is unfortunately only in the case of bacillary infections and syphilis that satisfactory therapy exists. Toxoplasmosis may respond to pyrimethamine (Daraprim) plus sulphadiazine or spiramycin but in infants infected before birth and showing evidence of hepatitis at delivery the outlook is poor. In other forms of hepatitis due to virus infection no treatment other than supportive is available but the prognosis is not necessarily poor. Evidence of spontaneous recovery may not be seen for several weeks.

Galactosaemia

The treatment of galactosaemia is withdrawal of lactose containing food from the diet.

Surgical treatment

Surgical treatment of obstructive jaundice should not be undertaken until conditions such as alpha-1-antitrypsin deficiency and galactosaemia have been excluded.

In case of obstructive jaundice where there is no evidence of viral infection and other causes have been excluded, ultrasound and radiological examination of the biliary system and possible surgical exploration have to be considered from about one month of age so that the rare cases of operable extrahepatic biliary obstruction shall not be allowed to progress to cirrhosis.

FURTHER READING

Bowman, J. M. (1986) Haemolytic disease of the newborn. In: *Textbook of Neonatology*, Ed. Roberton, N. R. C., 469–483. Edinburgh: Churchill Livingstone.
Cashore, W. J. (1980) Free bilirubin concentrations and bilirubin-binding affinity in term and pre-term infants. *Journal of Pediatrics*, **96**, 521.
Chandra, R. K. (Ed.) (1979) *The Liver and Biliary System in Infants and Children*. Edinburgh: Churchill Livingstone.

Cockington, R. A. (1979) A guide to the use of phototherapy in the management of neonatal hyperbilirubinaemia. *Journal of Pediatrics*, **95**, 281.

Cohen, A. N. & Ostrow, J. D. (1980) New conceptsin phototherapy: photoisomerization of Bilirubin IX potential toxic effects of light. *Pediatrics* **65**, 740.

Harper, R. G., Sia, C. G. & Kierney, C. M. P. (1980) Kernicterus 1980 *Clinics in Perinatology*, **7**, 75.

Poland, R. L. & Ostrea, E. M. (1979) In *Neonatal Hyperbilirubinaemia in Care of the High Risk Neonate*, 2nd. edn, ed. Klaus, M. H. & Fanaroff, A A. Philadelphia: Saunders.

Roberton, N. R. C. (1986) Neonatal jaundice. In: *Recent Advances in Paediatrics*, Ed. Meadow, R., 157–183. Edinburgh: Churchill Livingstone.

Tan, K. L. (1977) The nature of the dose response relationship of phototherapy for neonatal hyperbilirubinaemia. Journal of Pediatrics **90**, 448.

16

Dyspnoea and cyanosis

The healthy baby generally breathes within a few seconds of birth. Once established, respirations assume a rhythmic, although not precisely regular, pattern. Inspiration and expiration through the nose follow each other in uninterrupted succession with preterm babies breathing at a rate of about 55 per minute and mature babies 45 per minute. Normally breathing is diaphragmatic, rather than thoracic, with indrawing of the lower ribs and intercostal spaces on inspiration.

DYSPNOEA

The terms dyspnoea and respiratory distress are applied to breathing which is difficult, distressed, laboured or rapid. Dyspnoea usually assumes the form of rapid shallow breathing which is often accompanied by more pronounced costal recession (Fig. 16.1). In any condition in which there is obstruction of the upper airways or decreased lung compliance (lack of elastic recoil) as in some forms of congenital heart disease with a left to right shunt, costal recession becomes very much greater. With increasing dyspnoea breathing takes place through the mouth. Inspiration is accompanied by backward movement of the head and expiration by a characteristic grunt.

Silverman score

In an effort to evaluate the degree of severity of dyspnoea Silverman introduced a scoring system based on five objective signs (Table 16.1). Each sign is given a score and the total score can range from 0 to 10. Silverman scoring is of particular value in assessing improvement or deterioration rather than as an indication for treatment. Some clinicians use a score of 6 or more on two occasions, or over 6 on one occasion, as an indication for arranging

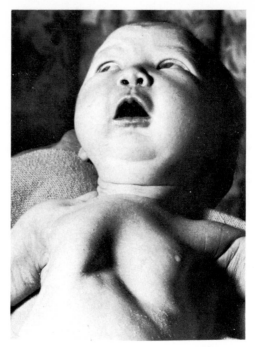

Fig. 16.1 Costal recession in dyspnoeic infant.

Table 16.1 Silverman assessment of dyspnoea

Sign	Score 1	Score 2
Respiratory rate	Over 60	Over 80
Chest recession	Slight	Marked
Grunt	Heard with stethoscope	Heard without stethoscope
Nostril dilation	Slight	Marked
Cyanosis	Slight	Marked

for blood gas analysis but, as in all clinical situations, assessment of the infant may indicate blood gas analysis at lower scores.

Causes of dyspnoea

A great variety of disorders cause dyspnoea (Table 16.2). In preterm babies the commonest causes of dyspnoea are the respiratory distress syndrome and pulmonary haemorrhage, whilst in term infants aspiration and pneumonia head the list.

Table 16.2 Causes of dyspnoea

OBSTRUCTION OF THE UPPER AIRWAY
  Nasal obstruction
  Choanal atresia
  Laryngeal obstruction
  Tracheal compression
LUNG PARENCHYMAL DISEASE
  Primary atelectasis
  Secondary atelectasis
  Respiratory distress syndrome
  Pulmonary haemorrhage
  Pneumonia
  Emphysema
  Pneumothorax
  Wilson-Mikity syndrome
  Transient neonatal tachypnoea
INTRATHORACIC DISORDERS
  Developmental defects of the lung
    Pulmonary agenesis
    Pulmonary cysts
    Pulmonary sequestration
  Disorders of the diaphragm
    Hernia
    Paralysis
  Oesophageal atresia
  Intrathoracic tumours and cysts
  Pleural effusion
MISCELLANEOUS DISORDERS
  Heart failure
  Intracranial lesions
  Severe anaemia
  Febrile conditions
  Metabolic acidosis

Obstruction of the upper airway

Nasal obstruction. Obstruction of the nasal passages in the newborn is a frequent finding. It varies considerably in degree. Complete obstruction may result from bilateral choanal atresia (Chapter 11). Obstruction by nasal secretions is recognized by the noise (snuffles) in the nose accompanying inspiration and expiration. A discharge from the nose is rarely seen in the newborn, although on occasion dried particles of mucus can be detected adherent to the nostrils. Discharge, when present, tends to drain posteriorly into the nasopharynx.

Stuffy nose syndrome. Not all nasal secretion is due to infection. The nasal mucous membranes of the newborn infant are notably susceptible to changes in temperature and humidity of the atmosphere. Nasal swabs taken from babies born in hospital often give growths of staphylococci on culture but these organisms may not belong to pathogenic strains. A combination of staphylococci and an adenovirus appear to be the cause of what is called the stuffy nose syndrome, which is descriptive. Neither organism on its own produces the same effect. Even when it is the result of infection, nasal catarrh is not accompanied by symptoms of general systemic disturbance unless spread to the pharynx, trachea or bronchi takes place. Signs and symptoms if present are essentially local and take the form of mild to moderate dyspnoea and of difficulty in feeding. Unable to breathe effectively through the nose, the infant has periodically to release his grasp of the areola or teat in order to breathe through his mouth.

Snuffles, an early sign of congenital syphilis, is now rarely seen in this country.

Treatment of nasal catarrh is only necessary where feeding difficulties arise.

Decongestant nasal drops such as 0.5% ephedrine in saline serve to relieve the vascular congestion of the mucous membranes. One drop is instilled into each nostril before feeds as required. If the discharge is purulent a close watch should be kept for early signs of descent of infection as bronchitis in the newborn can rapidly assume serious proportions.

Pierre-Robin syndrome (Fig. 11.21). In this congenital malformation complex there is usually a central cleft palate and extreme micrognathia, so the poorly supported tongue falls backwards into the cleft, thus occluding the pharynx and nasal passages. Management is difficult and depends on careful postural management of the infant in the prone position, or occasionally on the need for suturing the tip of the tongue to the gum margin. With time, as the lower jaw grows, the problems of respiration resolve.

Laryngeal obstruction

Laryngeal obstruction giving rise to congenital laryngeal stridor may be first noticed at birth or at any time during the first two weeks of life. If the obstruction is severe it gives rise to marked inspiratory stridor which becomes worse in the presence of a respiratory infection.

Laryngomalacia. The condition has been variously ascribed to an unusually soft larynx which collapses on inspiration (laryngomalacia), an epiglottis of abnormal shape and size, and redundant aryepiglottic folds. Phonation is unimpaired but stridor is present and is usually more severe when the infant is agitated, reducing in intensity during quiet respiration — no treatment is usually indicated.

Laryngeal web. Stridor is present and phonation may be abnormal in the presence of a laryngeal web. This requires surgical correction.

Laryngeal stenosis. Stridor present in both inspiration and expiration can result from laryngeal stenosis. This can also follow prolonged endotracheal intubation.

Oedema of the larynx and epiglottis may follow tracheal intubation at birth when stridor will also be present both in inspiration and expiration. Placing the baby in the prone position improves the airway and relieves the stridor.

Tracheal compression

Tracheal compression from a vascular ring (Fig. 16.2) or from a mediastinal tumour is rare.

A *vascular ring* is in effect a double aortic arch which encircles and compresses both the trachea and oesophagus. The condition should be suspected in the presence of dyspnoea and swallowing difficulty. In order to improve the airway the baby holds his head in extension. Forcible flexion of the head may completely occlude the airway. The diagnosis is confirmed by barium swallow examination and surgical removal of the accessory arch relieves all symptoms.

Lung parenchymal disease

Primary atelectasis

During fetal life the lungs are not required for ventilation and are filled with fluid. With the first breaths after delivery air fills the bronchial tree and the alveoli are progressively expanded and fill with air. Areas of the lung, however, may not expand and in these areas there is primary atelectasis. If the total area of primary atelectasis is small the clinical effect is minimal, but if larger areas fail to expand, there is dyspnoea and cyanosis.

If a major bronchus remains filled with fluid a whole lung or lobe of a lung may fail to expand. In severe circumstances laryngoscopy and aspiration of the trachea and major bronchi by a suction catheter passed through the larynx may be required. When the obstruction is relieved expansion of the alveoli follows.

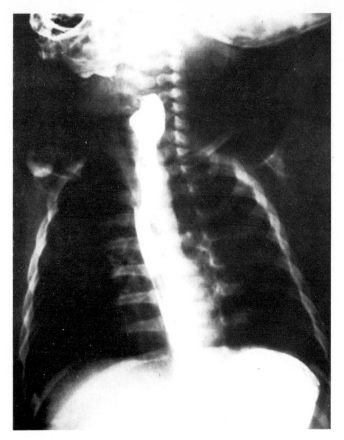

Fig. 16.2 Vascular ring compressing the oesophagus and trachea.

Secondary atelectasis

Aspiration syndromes. A baby may aspirate fluid into the lungs before, during or after birth, the mortality being high in those who aspirate meconium.

Meconium aspiration is most frequently seen where there has been prenatal hypoxia with intrauterine gasping before delivery. Efforts must be made to reduce further intrusion of meconium into the lung at delivery. If possible the infant should have its airways cleared of meconium before spontaneous respiration commences. Respiration may be delayed by compressing the thorax between the hands of a helper whilst the pharynx is cleared, the infant intubated and trachea sucked clear. The consequence of meconium aspiration is a severe pneumonitis which may prove lethal to even robust term infants who have been further compromized by their perinatal hypoxia. Meconium-stained liquor which is much more common is a less sinister problem and seldom causes significant respiratory problems.

If inspiration takes place after premature separation of the placenta the lungs may be filled with maternal blood. This also leads to a severe form of pneumonitis.

Aspiration pneumonia. Aspiration of infected amniotic fluid or vaginal secretions is a common cause of postnatal penumonia. It is generally agreed that conditions tending to produce fetal hypoxia cause the fetus to gasp in the uterus or birth canal. When aspiration has occurred in utero it often follows fetal distress marked by the presence of heavy meconium staining of the amniotic fluid.

Postnatal aspiration of gastric contents may be found in infants who have vomited or have neuromuscular disease leading to a poor gag reflex.

The aspiration of foreign material leads to severe irritation of the lungs with congestion, oedema and haemorrhage resulting in patchy emphysema, atelectasis and secondary collapse.

Physical signs. The baby may be severely hypoxic at birth requiring immediate intubation and intermittent positive pressure ventilation. On examination of the chest there will be tachypnoea, costal recession, dullness on percussion and crepitations on auscultation. The baby continuously produces mucus which is stained with meconium or blood.

X-ray examination of the chest shows coarse, irregular densities together with focal areas of emphysema and collapse. The domes of the diaphragm are usually flattened.

Treatment. Thorough clearing of the airway at birth should be followed by aspiration of the stomach aimed at preventing further vomiting and aspiration. The baby is nursed in an incubator with extra oxygen as necessary. Some infants may require ventilatory assistance. Antibiotics are given to prevent *E. coli* pneumonia, which commonly complicates meconium aspiration. It may be necessary to correct metabolic acidosis (Chapter 12).

Prognosis. Babies who aspirate small amounts of amniotic or vaginal contents generally do well and recover within two or three days. Deaths are common following massive aspiration associated with intrauterine hypoxia. Some develop pneumomediastinum and/or pneumothorax as a result of progressive emphysema. This may absorb spontaneously in mild cases but may require the insertion of intercostal drains in more severely affected infants. Others develop pneumonia as a result of aspirating infected liquor, maternal secretions or meconium.

RESPIRATORY DISTRESS SYNDROME

The respiratory distress syndrome (RDS) occurs most commonly in preterm babies. Other predisposing factors include perinatal asphyxia, maternal diabetes and severe antepartum haemorrhage.

Aetiology

Pulmonary immaturity. RDS is more common in preterm infants but may occur in some term infants. The immaturity of such infants' lungs is related to inability to produce sufficient amounts of surfactant which acts as a surface tension reducing agent.

Surfactant

Surfactant is a phospholipid secreted into the alveoli by type II pneumocytes. The most active components are dipalmitoylphosphatidylcholine (DPC) and phosphatidylglycerol (PG). It has a half life of about 14 hours. Formation begins quite early in gestation and surfactant can be found in the fetal lung at 24 weeks. There is an increase in production at about the 34th week coincident with a rise in fetal cortisol levels. This rise in surfactant level is mirrored in the amniotic fluid by an increased lecithin:sphingomyelin ratio indicating accelerated lung maturation and a reduced risk of RDS. Intrauterine infection, exposure to certain drugs in utero, maternal toxaemia, premature rupture of the membranes and even normal labour advance pulmonary maturation whereas uncontrolled maternal diabetes and severe asphyxia retard maturation. Surfactant production is sometimes enhanced when the mother is treated with corticosteroids such as betamethasone and dexamethasone provided she has been in labour, is between 30 and 32 weeks' gestation and has treatment for 48 hours. Surfactant reduces the surface tension within the alveoli and allows the lungs to expand normally at birth. In the absence of surfactant the alveoli collapse on expiration thereby increasing the work of breathing and leading ultimately to death as a result of exhaustion and respiratory failure.

Diminished lung compliance resulting from lack of surfactant makes it more difficult to expand the lungs and as a consequence there are atelectatic portions of the lungs.

There is also increased pulmonary vascular resistance because of hypoxia and right to left shunting of blood through the foramen ovale and ductus arteriosus. Vasodilatory prostaglandins are neutralized in the lungs of adults. In the fetal circulation prostaglandins bypass the lungs by way of the shunts already mentioned and dilate large arterial vessels including the ductus arteriosus.

It is clear that lack of surfactant is of major importance in the aetiology of RDS. This deficiency is mainly a failure of adequate production. The antenatal assessment of fetal lung maturity by measurement of amniotic fluid lecithin:sphingomyelin ratio was discussed in Chapter 4.

Persisting pulmonary vasoconstriction. It will be recalled that one of the consequences of oxygen-conserving adaptation accompanying intrauterine hypoxia (Chapter 5) was persisting pulmonary vasoconstriction after birth with marked increase in the right to left shunting of blood through the ductus arteriosus. Many authors believe that the resulting reduction in pulmonary blood flow contributes significantly to deficiency or absence of surfactant.

The ductus arteriosus. Patency of the ductus arteriosus may in RDS lead to a worsening of the condition particularly in the most immature infants. Cardiac failure may follow and should be treated with diuretics and careful attention to fluid balance. Surgical closure may be necessary.

Pathology

The overall mortality rate for RDS in preterm deliveries is under 10% in those of 1000 g and more at birth and less than 5% in those who established spontaneous respiration at birth but as high as 30% in infants requiring assisted ventilation from birth. In infants weighing less than 1000 g the mortality from RDS is closer to 50%

At postmortem examination the lungs are found to be atelectatic with a typical eosinophilic hyaline membrane (Fig. 16.3) lining the alveoli and terminal bronchioles. The origin of the membrane is doubtful but it is probably formed as a result of exudation of fibrin from pulmonary capillaries.

Pulmonary hyaline membrane disease is to be regarded as a pathological and not a clinical diagnosis.

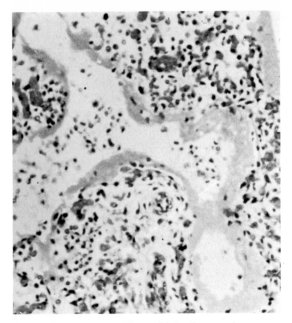

Fig. 16.3 Microscopic appearance of lung with hyaline membrane.

Various degrees of periventricular and intraventricular haemorrhage occur as a finding at post-mortem examination in 70% of
these infants.

Incidence

The diagnosis of RDS during life is based on clinical and radiological findings and the varying incidence reported in different
studies therefore depends on the criteria used for diagnosis. Using
the criteria listed below RDS occurs in 10% of all preterm deliveries. In units where active measures are taken to delay delivery
following the preterm onset of labour (Chapter 9) there has been
a reduction in the incidence of preterm delivery and of its complications such as RDS.

Clinical signs

Respiratory distress syndrome can be diagnosed clinically in the
presence of two of the following three signs developing before the
age of four hours and persisting for at least one hour:

Respiratory rate greater than 60 per minute

Subcostal or intercostal retraction

Expiratory grunting

The respiratory rate steadily increases after birth to a peak of about 75 per minute at 24 hours of age.

The heart rate increases to 130 to 170 per minute.

The temperature often falls.

Central cyanosis is common. There may be pitting oedema of the hands and feet.

Crepitations may be heard in the lungs.

In addition to the tachycardia other cardiovascular signs include liver enlargement, hypotension and a ductus arteriosus murmur.

X-ray. Typically the chest X-ray shows a fine ground-glass mottling throughout both lung fields, and the contrast between this mottling and air in the bronchi accounts for the air bronchogram. Chest X-ray is of importance in excluding other conditions such as aspiration syndrome, congenital unilobar emphysema, diaphragmatic hernia and pneumothorax.

Assessment. Frequent clinical assessment of the infant's condition is imperative to detect deterioration at an early stage. This may include the Silverman score in some units.

Biochemical changes

Acidosis. The H^+ rises and may be 100 nmol/litre or higher in severe cases (the pH falls and may be 7.0 or lower in severe cases). This rise in H^+ (fall in pH) is due to a mixture of respiratory and metabolic acidosis.

Respiratory acidosis results from retention of carbon dioxide, and $Pa\mathrm{co}_2$ may reach 10.5 to 13.5 kPa (80 to 100 mmHg).

Metabolic acidosis develops because of the excessive respiratory muscle activity, low oxygen tension and the accumulation of lactic acid. The negative base excess may be 20 nmol per litre (20 mEq per litre) or more.

Oxygen tension in arterial blood falls progressively to below 8 kPa (60 mmHg) because of poor ventilatory exchange and right to left shunting of blood.

Management

Prevention. As preterm delivery is the most important single factor in the aetiology of respiratory distress syndrome, measures which reduce the incidence of preterm delivery are of major importance in the management of the respiratory distress syndrome.

Occasionally respiratory distress syndrome can be prevented in infants of under 32 weeks' gestation if labour can be delayed for at least 48 hours using uterine relaxants such as salbutamol and ritodrine during which time the mother is given betamethasone or dexamethasone. The lecithin:sphingomyelin ratio in the liquor aids antenatal prediction. An increase in the ratio indicates accelerated lung maturation, the presence of surfactant and a reduced risk of RDS. The presence of phosphatidylglycerol (PG) appears to be the most reliable predictor of lung maturity.

Hypothermia and acidosis should be corrected promptly as they interfere with the synthesis of surfactant. As infants with RDS may not travel well, mothers in premature labour should be transferred for delivery to a unit fully equipped to deal with RDS of all degrees of severity.

Observation. The diagnosis of RDS is primarily clinical and requires close observation of all newborn infants, particularly of those of low birth weight during the first few hours of life. Should there be any sign of respiratory distress frequent or constant observation of colour, activity, grunting, use of accessory respiratory muscles, respiratory rate, heart rate and temperature should be made.

Incubator. Such observations can most readily be made with the infant exposed in an incubator, preferably with constant recording of skin temperature.

X-ray. In order to exclude other causes of respiratory difficulty and help predict the severity of the disease, a chest X-ray should be arranged. In infants with RDS there is a characteristic ground-glass appearance of the lung fields with an air bronchogram.

Arterial blood gases. If the infant's condition is showing signs of deterioration, arterial blood gases should be measured (Chapter 20). A Pao_2 reading below 7 kPa (50 mmHg) in 60% or more oxygen is an indication to commence assisted ventilation as is a $Paco_2$ above 10 kPa (70 mmHg) in many units. The decision to ventilate also depends on the infant's clinical condition.

Oxygen. The environmental oxygen concentration should be raised sufficiently to maintain the infant's arterial blood Pao_2 to between 8 and 12 kPa (60 and 90 mmHg) using heated, humidified oxygen in a head box. Regular estimation of the oxygen concentration within the incubator should be made using an oxygen analyser.

In the absence of facilities for arterial $Pa\text{O}_2$ measurement the lowest inspired oxygen concentration which allows the baby to remain a good colour should be used. Because of the risk of retrolental fibroplasia (retinopathy of prematurity) due to hyperoxaemia following the use of unnecessarily high concentrations of oxygen it is most important that the oxygen concentration within the incubator be limited and carefully controlled. If this cannot be done the infant should be transferred to a unit where suitable facilities are available.

Correction of acidosis. Metabolic acidosis can be corrected by the intravenous injection of 4.2% sodium bicarbonate in doses of the order of 1 to 5 ml or more as judged by repeated blood gas analysis. The dose should be given slowly intravenously. Oral correction is seldom effective or necessary.

Cerebral intraventricular haemorrhage is found at necropsy in about 70% of infants dying from RDS. In the past it was suggested that over-rapid intravenous correction of acidosis with bicarbonate might be responsible for intraventricular haemorrhage but this is unproven. The early correction of a low $Pa\text{O}_2$ reduces the risk of metabolic acidosis and may render the use of alkali superfluous.

Respiratory acidosis is indicated by a raised $Pa\text{CO}_2$. This can only be reduced by increasing the efficiency of ventilation. With the natural improvement which takes place in many infants with RDS this can occur without further treatment than that already outlined. If the infant shows signs of progressive deterioration of respiratory function with fall in $Pa\text{O}_2$ below 7 kPa (50 mmHg) in 60% or more oxygen and rise in $Pa\text{CO}_2$ further treatment will be required.

Assisted ventilation

Continuous positive airways pressure (CPAP). The object of CPAP, also called constant distending pressure (CDP), is to prevent the collapse of alveoli on expiration by maintaining a positive pressure in the airways throughout the respiratory cycle. CPAP can be applied via face mask (Fig. 16.4), double or single nasal catheters (prongs) or an endotracheal tube. The use of the original Gregory box is now seldom indicated. The techniques are not without hazard, pneumothorax and inaccessability to the infant's airway being well recognized complications in addition to

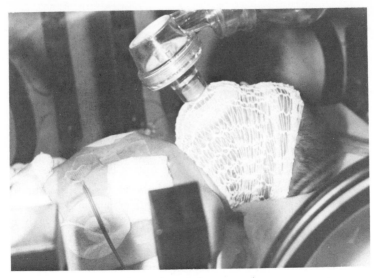

Fig. 16.4 CPAP being applied by face mask.

the hazards associated with indwelling endotracheal tubes. Use of the head box had added complications of excoriation of the neck by the seal, brachial plexus palsy and deterioration in the infant's condition during the manipulation which was required to initiate treatment. CPAP by face mask or nasal catheters is the method of choice as this is non-invasive, easily applied, and can be set up with minimal disturbance avoiding the complications associated with the head box. Infants receiving nasal or face mask CPAP should always have an open nasogastric tube in situ to prevent gaseous gastric distension. CPAP may be used for weaning infants off the ventilator. When CPAP is applied during the expiratory phase of mechanical ventilation it is described as positive end expiratory pressure (PEEP).

Following the introduction of CPAP there has been a small but significant improvement in mortality among infants weighing more than 1500 g at birth. If started early CPAP shortens the illness and minimizes the need for IPPV.

If CPAP fails to prevent clinical deterioration, the blood gases continue to deteriorate or apnoea supervenes intermittent positive pressure ventilation will be required.

Intermittent positive pressure ventilation

In general it is preferable that infants likely to require respirator management should be transferred to an intensive therapy nursery for such treatment as necessary. Most mechanical ventilators are pressure driven, time cycled machines capable of delivering heated, humidified gas at pre-set oxygen concentrations. They have controls capable of allowing fine adjustments in rate, inspiratory (IP) and expiratory pressures (PEEP) and inspiratory/expiratory time (I:E) ratios. All of these variables are important in view of the complexity of the management required for ventilator therapy. Infants receiving mechanical ventilation require intubation either by oro-tracheal or naso-tracheal tube. This must be securely fixed and a variety of suitable methods exist. The finer points of ventilation are beyond the scope of this book but preliminary settings of the ventilator are as follows:

1 Inspired heated, humidified oxygen of 80% concentration.
2 Respiratory rate of 40 per minute.
3 Inspiratory/expiratory time ratio of 1:1 (0.8 s:0.8 s).
4 Inspiratory pressure 20 cm H_2O.
5 Positive end expiratory pressure (PEEP) 4 cm H_2O.

Intensive respiratory care monitoring

Once established on ventilation the infant will require frequent reassessment of its arterial blood gas status and intensive nursing care. The latter will include careful recording of physiological data including heart rate, ECG, blood pressure and neurological state. It will also be necessary to provide regular suction of the endotracheal tube since the usual effect of ciliary action in clearing the trachea is disturbed. This should be performed with extreme care and expertise as the infant invariably develops a degree of hypoxia during the procedure.

Assessment of blood gas status. Wherever possible this should be non-invasive, and equipment exists to allow measurement of transcutaneous oxygen and carbon dioxide concentrations (Fig. 16.5). The results obtained with these sensors equate well with arterial blood gas concentrations provided the infant's skin is well perfused. These sensors utilize the principle that when the skin is heated to temperatures between 41 and 43 °C it becomes permeable to the passage of both oxygen and carbon dioxide; blood concentration of these gases can be measured by suitable sensors within the skin electrodes (Fig. 16.6). Invasive direct measurement of arterial oxygen and carbon dioxide concentrations can be made using an umbilical (or peripheral) arterial catheter. These

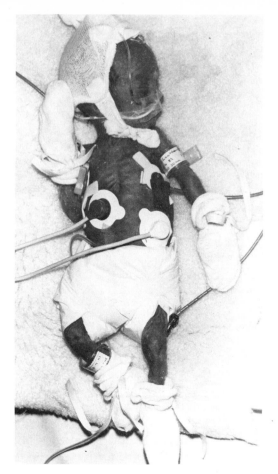

Fig. 16.5 Preterm infant with transcutaneous monitors for oxygen and carbon dioxide in position.

measurements may be obtained either continuously, using a catheter-contained electrode, or by intermittent blood sampling. Arterial samples obtained by arterial puncture are less valuable. Where neither invasive method is available capillary blood sampling from a well perfused heel site can give useful information on $Paco_2$, H^+ ion and base excess status but little information on Pao_2.

Patent ductus arteriosus. Should the infant's condition deteriorate further despite treatment with frusemide and fluid restriction then 'medical closure' should be attempted by giving a prostaglandin synthetase inhibitor such as indomethacin in a dose of 0.2 mg per

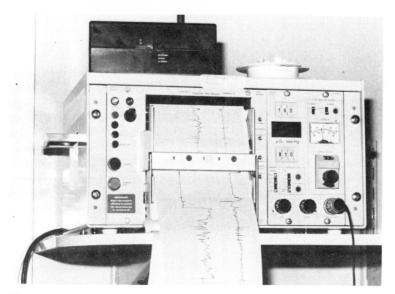

Fig. 16.6 Transcutaneous monitor showing trace of infant's TcPo$_2$ during several hours, and high/low alarm setting systems.

kg and repeated eight hourly to a maximum of three doses. It should be borne in mind that indomethacin has toxic effects on the kidneys, causes bleeding and may elevate the plasma bilirubin level. Where medical treatment has failed and in the presence of further deterioration surgical ligation of the ductus should be considered.

Complications include respiratory failure, apnoeic episodes, pneumothorax, pulmonary haemorrhage, intraventricular haemorrhage, abdominal distension following the introduction of enteral feeding and necrotizing enterocolitis. Hypotension secondary to hypovolaemia may require transfusion with blood or plasma. In infants with RDS weighing less than 1500 g at birth the ductus arteriosus remains patent in 25% of cases adding to the difficulties of management which have already been described in Chapter 9. In the same group of infants the incidence of patent ductus arteriosus increases to 35% when treated with IPPV. Where CPAP or IPPV has been used through an endotracheal tube there is a risk of pulmonary infection which increases with the length of time for which these procedures are required.

Prognosis. RDS is unfortunately a condition for which we cannot guarantee a cure. Many infants who are mildly affected will survive without specialized treatment. In the most severely affected death may occur in spite of the most sophisticated treatment.

In individual infants the response of the arterial Pao_2 to increase in the concentration of inspired oxygen gives some indication of prognosis, the poorer the response the poorer the prognosis. Acidosis which is not readily correctable by the methods outlined similarly carries a poor prognosis. Conversely an infant with a minor degree of acidosis and a Pao_2 which is easily kept within the normal range has a good prognosis.

The prognosis for infants with severe RDS will improve further as a result of preventing preterm delivery, minimizing the duration and severity of intrapartum asphyxia and ensuring a high standard of care in specialized units. Work is also proceeding to evaluate the efficacy of instilling natural or artificial surfactant materials, soon after birth, into the lungs of these babies at high risk of RDS. Preliminary reports suggest that such therapy may reduce the severity but not prevent RDS.

Recovery. Most infants who survive for three days without major disturbance of their H^+ (pH) or Pao_2 make a complete recovery free of any associated long-term respiratory problems. Less than 10% who were severely ill will, on follow-up, be found to have developed neurological sequelae or lung damage (bronchopulmonary dysplasia).

Pulmonary haemorrhage

Dyspnoea associated with the coughing up of blood-stained secretion or the aspiration of blood-stained material from the trachea is highly suggestive of pulmonary haemorrhage. This diagnosis can be suggested by radiological changes but can only be proved at postmortem examination and may then be found without any clinical evidence of its presence during life.

Pulmonary haemorrhage is often a terminal event after fulminating infection or severe RDS. It occurs most commonly in low birth weight infants, particularly in those who are small for dates. It can be a manifestation of disseminated intravascular coagulation and is found in severe hypothermia. It is thought to be due to the combination of pulmonary capillary damage and left heart failure, leading to pulmonary oedema and capillary leakage of red blood cells.

Treatment is symptomatic and supportive by giving extra oxygen when required, by antibiotic if infection is present and by correction of hypothermia, coagulation abnormality and blood volume expansion.

Pneumonia

Pneumonia is found at postmortem examination more often than any other infective disease. The source of infection in early, as distinct from strictly congenital, pneumonia may be material aspirated before, during or after birth. Alternatively, the infection may be airborne or part of a bacteraemia of antenatal or postnatal origin. The use of prophylactic antibiotics in cases of known maternal infection or prolonged rupture of the membranes is considered by some to be of value.

The newborn baby is particularly susceptible to staphylococcal pneumonia but infection by streptococci, pneumococci, *E. coli* and *Pseudomonas aeruginosa* are not uncommon. Staphylococcal

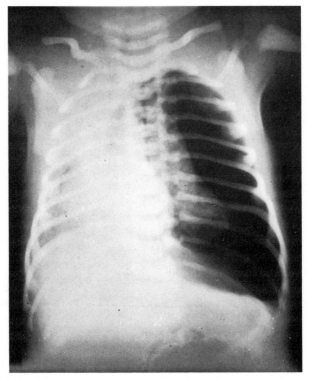

Fig. 16.7 Staphylococcal pneumonia complicated by left pneumothorax.

pneumonia is particularly dangerous because of the tendency to form lung abscesses which rupture into the pleural cavity, with resultant pyopneumothorax (Fig. 16.7).

Clinical evidence of pneumonia is frequently absent. The presence of an acute infection is suggested by anorexia, drowsiness, vomiting, pallor, irregular temperature, dyspnoea and cyanosis. Chest signs are limited to generalized crepitations, the other signs of pneumonia being rarely found. Chest X-ray (Fig. 16.8) is frequently helpful in arriving at a diagnosis.

Humidified oxygen is given in sufficient concentration to relieve cyanosis. Before starting antibiotic treatment blood culture should be arranged and swabs should be taken from the nose, throat, ears and umbilicus. The antibiotics chosen should have a sufficiently broad spectrum to cover all likely infections. Suitable combinations are penicillin and gentamicin or ampicillin and cloxacillin. These should be given intramuscularly or intravenously as oral absorption is variable and poor.

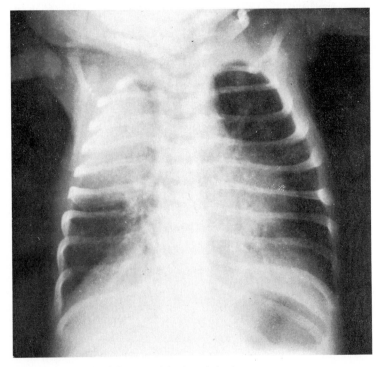

Fig. 16.8 Pneumonia right upper lobe (age 6 days).

Feeds should be given in small quantities frequently. Tube feeding or intravenous nutrition is frequently required.

Emphysema

Compensatory emphysema occurs to make up for persisting atelectasis elsewhere.

Obstructive emphysema. Massive inhalation of foreign material can give rise to impaired expulsion from, but continued air entry into, alveoli with resultant obstructive emphysema.

Pulmonary interstitial emphysema (PIE). This occurs when air escapes along perivascular spaces in the lung. It is seen most frequently in infants requiring high pressure mechanical ventilation for RDS. It can also follow rupture of alveoli from resuscitative methods employing excessive pressures. This danger is decreased in any system in which the pressure is restricted, by a blow-off valve which limits the pressure to 30 cm of water (Chapter 5). Necrosis of parenchymatous lung tissue in staphylococcal pneumonia sometimes enables air to escape from the lungs along the perivascular spaces producing interstitial emphysema.

Unilobar emphysema can give rise to signs and symptoms resembling those in pneumothorax. These are cyanosis and dyspnoea of increasing severity, hyperresonance over the affected lobe and mediastinal displacement. X-ray findings (Fig. 16.9) are characteristic. Lobectomy (Fig. 16.10) provides prompt and permanent relief and is associated with a low mortality risk.

Pneumothorax

Rupture of emphysematous areas of the lungs releases air into the pleural cavities causing a pneumothorax. The commonest causes are over-vigorous initial resuscitation or the use of excessive pressure during subsequent ventilation. Spontaneous rupture of an emphysematous lobe may occur. Pneumothorax may also be a complication of RDS.

Symptoms and signs will depend on the volume and pressure of air in the pleural cavity. Small pneumothoraces under low pressure may only be discovered on X-ray examination and require no treatment.

Pressure (tension) pneumothorax will occur if there is a valve effect at the site of the alveolar rupture which only allows air to pass outward into the pleural cavity. As the pressure rises the lung

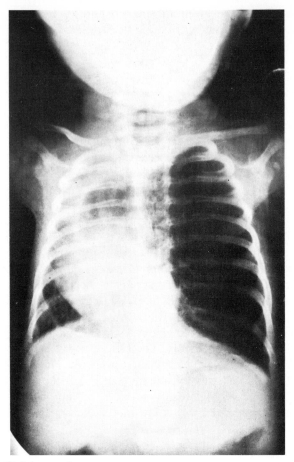

Fig. 16.9 Unilobar emphysema.

collapses and the infant shows increasing evidence of dyspnoea. The heart and mediastinum will become displaced away from the side of the pneumothorax and the contralateral lung may be compressed. As the infant finds breathing progressively more difficult cyanosis develops and the infant will die unless treated quickly.

Drainage of the pneumothorax may be carried out surgically with a catheter from the pleural cavity leading to an underwater seal. Where immediate surgery is not available life can be saved by passing a needle into the chest and connecting this to a Heimlich valve (Chapter 20).

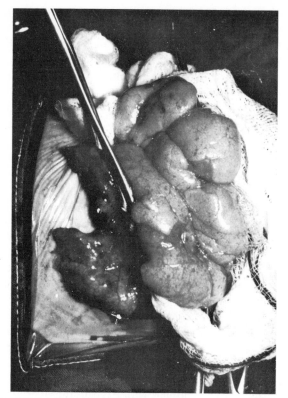

Fig. 16.10 Unilobar emphysema. Exposure of affected lobe prior to operative removal. (By courtesy of Mr D. A. Watson, F.R.C.S.)

Wilson-mikity syndrome

This condition, of unknown aetiology, is restricted to immature babies of less than 36 weeks' gestation. Affected babies are usually dyspnoeic at birth and present a clinical picture not unlike that seen in the respiratory distress syndrome. Improvement takes place within one to two weeks to be followed by the insidious onset of cyanosis and costal recession which may then persist for several months. Rhonchi are to be heard in the lungs. During this period the baby requires extra oxygen to prevent cyanosis. Other babies have no respiratory symptoms at birth, receive no added oxygen, yet some weeks later develop the symptoms described above. The condition is associated with fracture of the ribs which may be due to bone mineral deficiencies secondary to the nutritional difficulties in these infants.

X-ray of the chest is normal during the first weeks of life but later bilateral, coarse infiltration and cystic changes are seen. Complete clearing of these lung changes can take place any time up to two years. Abnormalities of pulmonary function including carbon dioxide retention, substantial right to left shunts, reduction of lung compliance and increased airways resistance have been reported.

Treatment consists of supportive measures and sufficient oxygen to relieve cyanosis.

Bronchopulmonary dysplasia (BPD)

This condition, which has increased in frequency over the past 10 years, appears to occur only in those low birth weight preterm infants who have required prolonged high pressure mechanical ventilation with high inspired oxygen concentrations. The infants usually fail to wean easily from the ventilator and remain oxygen dependent. This may continue for some weeks or months. Histology of the lung shows disruption of the alveoli and the presence of fibrous tissue. They develop radiological changes similar to those in Wilson-Mikity syndrome and frequently develop secondary respiratory infections. Their management is prolonged and despite aggressive treatment with oxygen, diuretics, antibiotics and other drugs (e.g. steroids) as many as one third of infants die.

Transient tachypnoea of the newborn (TTN)

It has been suggested that transient tachypnoea is due to delayed absorption of alveolar fluid. This condition often occurs in term babies who have been delivered by elective Caesarean section or breech delivery, and have not therefore experienced the normal chest compression in the birth canal. Within a few hours of birth the respiratory rate increases to between 80 and 120 per minute and remains high for two to five days. No signs are heard in the chest but X-ray examination may show signs of 'wet' lungs with fluid in the fissures and prominant vascular markings. The clinical and radiological signs return to normal within about five days. Cyanosis can usually be relieved by 30–40% oxygen but occasionally CPAP or ventilation is required.

Intrathoracic disorders

Developmental defects of the lungs

Developmental defects of the lung, including pulmonary agenesis and pulmonary cysts, are very rare causes of dyspnoea in the newly born infant.

Pulmonary agenesis. Failure of development of the primitive lung bud may lead to all gradations of underdevelopment of the lung ranging from hypoplasia of one segment or lobe to complete absence of both lungs. Affected babies experience great difficulty from birth with dyspnoea and cyanosis. Those who survive are prone to repeated respiratory infections.

Pulmonary cyst. Dyspnoea is usually the first recognizable sign of the presence of a pulmonary cyst (Fig. 16.11) whether of congenital or acquired origin. Signs may appear suddenly or

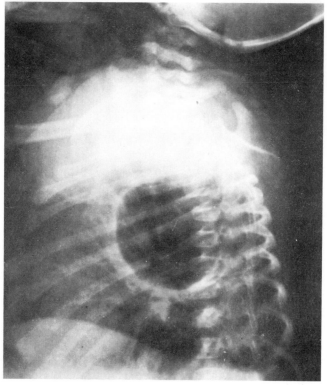

Fig. 16.11 Pulmonary cyst.

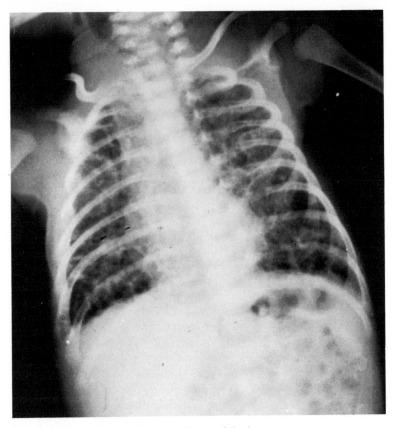

Fig. 16.12 Congenital multiple cystic disease of the lungs.

gradually and at any time in the neonatal period, dependent upon the rate of distension by air of the cyst. Cystic lesions of the lung may be single or multiple (Fig. 16.12) and are sometimes asymptomatic being discovered accidentally in the course of X-ray examination. Immediate operative intervention is an urgent necessity where tension in a cyst is increasing, and is indicated when the cyst contains pus.

Sequestered lobe. Sequestered lobes, which mainly affect the left lower lobe, rarely give rise to symptoms in the newborn period. They are usually detected on chest X-rays taken for other reasons. Sequestered lobes are the site of repeated infection so they should always be resected.

Disorders of the diaphragm

Diaphragmatic hernia usually occurs on the left and gives rise to persistent severe cyanosis from birth in most instances. There is associated dyspnoea and often a scaphoid abdomen as the abdominal contents occupy the hemithorax. To limit inflation of the gut oxygen should not be given by mask but endotracheal intubation should be carried out. Suspected dextrocardia on first examination is an indication for a chest X-ray, as the heart may be displaced to the right by a diaphragmatic hernia. Early operation is essential and continuous efforts must be made to keep the gut empty until this can be performed. The infant should also be nursed sitting or on an inclined plane, (head-up) if possible. Occasionally the hernia can occur on the right side or if the defect is less severe only become apparent some time after birth.

Diaphragmatic paralysis is an occasional complication of Erb's palsy (Chapter 13) when nerve roots C5 and 6 are damaged during delivery. Dyspnoea in such circumstances should be investigated by X-ray screening.

Elevated diaphragm. Abdominal distension due to intestinal obstruction causes dyspnoea due to pressure on the diaphragm.

Oesophageal atresia

An obstetric history of hydramnios should always raise the suspicion of oesophageal atresia.

Excessive secretion in the buccopharynx of a newly born baby, or secretion which tends to 'drool' more or less continuously should immediately raise the question of oesophageal atresia. Any fluid given overflows from the blind upper pouch of the oesophagus into the respiratory tract. Pneumonia results and is only too liable to be followed by death after, or even before, operation. If the infant is unfortunate enough to be given a feed the milk overflows into the larynx and may be aspirated into the lungs producing cough, cyanosis and dyspnoea.

Investigation. Immediate investigation is indicated. The tip of a firm radio-opaque 10–14 Fg catheter will be arrested some 10 cm beyond the alveolar margin, and on X-ray screening is found to be on a level with the fourth thoracic vertebra. The blind ending of the upper pouch of the oesophagus may be outlined by injecting contrast medium down the catheter but this is seldom warranted.

The contrast medium should always be removed on completion of the examination to prevent an aspiration pneumonia.

Management. Once the diagnosis has been made the infant should be maintained in a sitting position to prevent acid stomach contents passing through the lower oesophageal segment to the lungs. The infant should have the contents of the upper oesophageal pouch aspirated at 15 minute intervals pending operation as a minimum or continuously by a Replogle tube if available. Details of operative procedures vary according to the exact nature of the defect. In general it can be said that the operation consists of end to end anastomosis of the two segments of the oesophagus with closure of any accompanying tracheo-oesophageal or broncho-oesophageal fistula, although this may require a two stage procedure.

Intrathoracic tumours and cysts

These cause dyspnoea by compressing the lungs and airways. A large variety of solid tumours and fluid-filled cysts have been found in the chests of newly born infants. Malignant tumours occur less frequently than cysts of gastrointestinal origin, dermoid cysts and teratomatous tumours. Mediastinal lesions may arise posteriorly (neuroblastoma, duplications of the gut, bronchogenic cysts), centrally (vascular tumours) and anteriorly (enlarged thymus, teratomas). Fibrosarcomas and hamartomas may be found in the lung substance itself.

These tumours and cysts give rise to increasing dyspnoea and frequently become infected and come to light on X-ray examination of the chest. Treatment consists of excision followed by irradiation when indicated.

Pleural effusion

A massive effusion into the pleural cavity will cause dyspnoea and cyanosis with dullness on percussion and diminished breath sounds. Pleural effusions were found in babies severely affected by rhesus incompatibility. A rare cause is chylothorax which usually occurs for no obvious reason but cases have been reported in babies born with the umbilical cord tightly around the neck when the thoracic duct has been torn.

If the chylothorax persists despite repeated aspiration and the use of medium chain triglyceride feeds, then surgical intervention is indicated.

Heart failure

Dyspnoea due to congenital disease of the heart is not usually severe but increases in the presence of cardiac failure. Dyspnoea of cardiac origin is liable to be aggravated by crying and disturbance, and in the more severe cases is associated with restlessness. An infant suffering from extreme respiratory distress due to intrathoracic infection or to terminal cardiac failure frequently lies with his neck retracted, suggestive of intracranial disease. At the same time he lies panting desperately, his fixed gaze conveying the impression of extreme apprehension. The treatment of cardiac failure was dealt with in Chapter 11.

Extrathoracic causes of dyspnoea

Cerebral

Cerebral birth trauma may cause apnoeic attacks progressing to generalized cyanosis and convulsions. Following an apnoeic attack respirations are often slow and gasping or periodic in nature and of variable depth. These symptoms, which are due to raised intracranial pressure, are also found in hypoxaemia, hypoglycaemia and meningitis. When the anterior fontanelle tension is raised, and lumbar puncture has excluded meningitis, then bilateral subdural taps should be carried out to exclude an encysted haematoma (Chapter 13).

Severe anaemia

Dyspnoea is seen in the presence of severe anaemia secondary to haemorrhage or haemolytic disease. A strikingly pale and dyspnoeic infant at birth must have a haemoglobin and packed cell volume estimation carried out immediately and must be given blood when indicated. Severe anaemia may cause death within a few hours of delivery as a result of shock and cortical necrosis of the kidneys.

Febrile conditions

Dyspnoea may be seen in conditions accompanied by pyrexia, e.g. urinary tract infection, acute respiratory infections and septicaemia.

Metabolic acidosis

Dyspnoea is a feature of metabolic acidosis. In severe cases respirations are both deep and rapid.

Inadequate nutrition in the first few days of life in small immature babies leads to increased catabolism with resultant metabolic acidosis. At a later stage, when feed volumes are increased to promote growth, there is occasionally a metabolic acidosis if a high protein containing feed is used and the kidney is unable to excrete the resultant acid load.

Metabolic acidosis is a feature of RDS and also accompanies fetal hypoxia. As described earlier fetal hypoxia results in anaerobic glycolysis with the accumulation of lactic acid in the blood. In both situations the acidosis is corrected by the administration of sodium bicarbonate and appropriate respiratory care.

Nursing observations

Observations made by the midwife concerning dyspnoea are of importance in recognizing the presence of disease and in assessing clinical progress. Thus changes in the rate, rhythm and depth of respiration are of great significance in the first 48 hours of life in evaluating the trend of clinical events in a baby who has been born hypoxic or prematurely. An increase in the rate of respirations may be the first sign of disease or the spread of infection from pharynx to the trachea, bronchi or lungs. The sudden onset of dyspnoea should always suggest an emergency which may have its explanation in a pneumothorax, a fulminating infection or massive haemorrhage.

CYANOSIS

Cyanosis is a blue colour of the skin or mucous membranes which is usually due to the presence of an excessive amount of reduced haemoglobin in the small blood vessels of the tissues. Very occasionally it is due to the presence of methaemoglobin or sulphaemoglobin. There must be at least 5 g of reduced haemoglobin per dl (100 ml) blood before cyanosis occurs, consequently cyanosis does not occur in the presence of severe anaemia.

Cyanosis can be either peripheral or central. In central cyanosis the arterial blood is unsaturated whereas in peripheral cyanosis the arterial blood is normally saturated but the extraction of oxygen from the blood in the tissues is excessive. The distinction is best made by examining the buccal mucous membranes where blood flow is always good. If these are blue the cyanosis is of the central type. In cases of doubt the baby should be compared with a healthy infant. The various causes of cyanosis are detailed in Table 16.3.

Table 16.3 Causes of cyanosis in the newborn

PERIPHERAL CYANOSIS
    Poor peripheral circulation
    Traumatic cyanosis
CENTRAL CYANOSIS
    Transitory
        Primary apnoea
        Secondary apnoea
        Airway obstruction
        RDS
        Pulmonary vasoconstriction
        Intrathoracic abnormalities
        Infective
    Persistent
        Congenital heart disease
        Pulmonary hypertension
        Polycythaemia
        Methaemoglobinaemia

Peripheral cyanosis

Peripheral cyanosis occurs when the flow of blood through the superficial skin and mucous membranes is unusually slow with the result that most of the oxygen in the normally oxygenated blood passes into the surrounding tissues. This form of cyanosis is present in the hands and feet (and sometimes the face) of a large proportion of babies during the early hours of life, and in the lips and extremities of newly born babies of any age who have become chilled. In lethargic infants or in infants whose circulation has become temporarily slow (as in sleep) circumoral cyanosis may develop but disappears with a return of normal activity.

Traumatic 'cyanosis'

Traumatic cyanosis, which results from venous compression followed by extravasation of blood, is limited to the head and neck and follows when the cord has been wrapped tightly around the neck or when the head has been on the perineum for some considerable time. In addition to the cyanosis, which contrasts with the normal pink of the trunk and extremities, close inspection will reveal the presence of tiny petechiae in the scalp and skin of the head and neck. Subconjunctival haemorrhages may also be present. In the absence of a serious complicating condition traumatic cyanosis need not cause concern and does not interfere with normal progress.

In traumatic cyanosis petechiae are limited to the head and neck but where petechiae are distributed over the whole body the possibilities of congenital rubella, toxoplasmosis, cytomegalovirus infection and congenital thrombocytopenic purpura must be entertained.

Central Cyanosis

Reduction of the oxygen content of all the blood is evident as central cyanosis. The hypoxaemia may be due to lack of oxygen in the inspired air, failure to absorb oxygen in the lungs or to mixture of venous and arterial blood within the heart or great vessels.

Central cyanosis is always significant and requires immediate investigation and treatment. The causes of transitory cyanosis are in general different from those of persistent cyanosis.

Transitory cyanosis

Primary apnoea. At birth the infant will be cyanosed until respiration is satisfactorily established.

Secondary apnoea. Any cause of secondary apnoea will also result in cyanosis. This may occur in low birth weight infants due to central nervous system immaturity and in infants with RDS, patent ductus arteriosus, sepsis, hypoxaemia and hypoglycaemia. It will also occur during convulsions or as a separate manifestation of cerebral birth injury and intraventricular haemorrhage.

Airway obstruction. Aspiration of milk or secretions, blockage of the airway by the tongue in Pierre-Robin syndrome or any other form of obstruction of the airway will produce cyanosis.

The serious significance of severe hypoxaemia and cyanosis in RDS has already been discussed earlier in this chapter. Pulmonary vasoconstriction as a result of continuing hypoxia, found especially in RDS, may persist after birth accompanied by marked right to left shunting of blood through the foramen ovale, ductus arteriosus and atelectatic portions of the lung.

Intrathoracic causes include diaphragmatic hernia, pulmonary agenesis, emphysema, pneumothorax and lung cysts which have already been discussed.

Infections, whether in the lungs or in other parts of the body, may cause cyanosis.

Persistent cyanosis

Congenital heart disease. Persistent central cyanosis is the presenting sign of certain congenital heart lesions involving a right to left shunt of deoxygenated blood. Lesions include transposition of the great vessels, pulmonary atresia, tricuspid atresia and total anomalous pulmonary venous drainage. Central cyanosis of later onset is associated with Fallot's tetralogy.

Pulmonary hypertension. Persistent pulmonary hypertension resulting in early death from cor pulmonale occurs rarely and appears to be due to an abnormality in the pulmonary blood vessels. Affected infants will present with cyanosis, breathlessness and failure to thrive. More commonly, in term infants who have experienced perinatal asphyxia or in preterm infants with other severe lung disease, the fetal circulation may persist. This usually responds to oxygen or occasionally requires ventilation or drug therapy.

Polycythaemia. Cyanosis due to polycythaemia may be detected at or shortly after birth. This may be the result of antenatal transplacental maternofetal bleeding or, in a twin pregnancy, of an arteriovenous shunt from the placenta of one to that of the other twin. Infants born to diabetic mothers have a naturally high colour which may lead to suspicions of cyanosis more especially when they are crying.

Methaemoglobinaemia. Central cyanosis is an early sign in congenital methaemoglobinaemia in which a deficiency of the methaemoglobin reductase system in the red blood cells leads to an accumulation of methaemoglobin. The absence of signs of illness in the presence of deep cyanosis is diagnostic. The baby is not dyspnoeic and the cyanosis is not increased by crying or diminished by the administration of oxygen. Blood examination shows no evidence of either anaemia or polycythaemia, and methaemoglobin bands are seen on spectroscopic examination. Reducing agents in the form of ascorbic acid (200 to 500 mg daily) and methylene blue (4 mg per kg daily by mouth in three divided doses) have been used in treatment for many years without ill effects. There is risk in the use of benzocaine and related anaesthetics and of long-acting sulphonamides in these babies.

Nursing observations

Cyanosis of sudden onset requires immediate investigation and treatment. Baby's air passages must be cleared of any obstruction and the effect on respiration noted. Increased respiratory movement suggests continuing obstruction and tracheal intubation and aspiration may be required.

FURTHER READING

Auld, P. A. M., (ed.) (1980) Neonatal intensive care. *Clinics in Perinatology*, 7, no. 1.

Klaus, M. H., Fanaroff, A. A. & Martin, R. J. (1979) In *Respiratory Problems in Care of the High Risk Neonate*, 2nd edn, ed. Klaus, M. H. & Fanaroff, A. A. Philadelphia: Saunders.

Morley, C. J. (1986) The respiratory distress syndrome. In: *Textbook of Neonatology*, Ed. Roberton, N. R. C. Edinburgh: Churchill Livingstone.

Roberton, N. R. C. (1980) Problems in the management of respiratory failure in infants with hyaline membrane disease. In *Topics in Perinatal Medicine*, ed. Wharton, B. A. Tunbridge Wells: Pitman Medical.

Vyas, H. & Milner, A. D. (1986) Other respiratory diseases in the neonate. In: *Textbook of Neonatology*, Ed. Roberton, N. R. C. Edinburgh: Churchill Livingstone.

17

Convulsions and other abnormal behaviour

In this chapter consideration will be given to convulsions, hyperactivity, hypertonia, hypotonia, drowsiness and abnormal posture.

CONVULSIONS

Convulsions are repetitive jerky movements which may be accompanied by apnoea, rigidity and loss of consciousness (Fig. 17.1). They vary considerably in form and degree and occur in 2 to 10 per thousand livebirths. The majority have a biochemical aetiology. A full blown grand mal (tonic-clonic) seizure is seldom seen and in many infants, especially preterm, seizure activity is particularly subtle and difficult to identify.

Types of seizure

Tonic. These represent an attack of decerebrate rigidity but are seldom followed by a clonic (jerking) phase. They occur at any gestation and usually represent severe brain damage. They may be precipitated by any strong stimulus. During the episode the infant becomes stiff and cyanosed, and spontaneous opisthotonus and extensor plantar responses are seen. They are always associated with unconsciousness and frequently with apnoea.

Clonic. Seizures of the clonic variety are much more common. They consist of rhythmical jerking, usually of the limbs or a limb, at a rate of 1 to 3 per second. They need to be distinguished from jitteriness (see below). They may be *focal* or *localized* to a limb or side of the face, or *generalized* in which the whole body is involved. A third variety is *multifocal* in which different parts of the body are affected, sometimes at different frequencies of seizure activity. Clonic seizures are frequently metabolic or biochemical in origin.

Fragmentary (primitive). These seizures commonly occur in

451

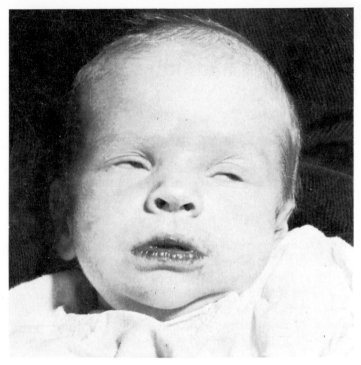

Fig. 17.1 The facies and deviation of the eyes during a convulsion. At the time this photograph was taken baby was momentarily unconscious and there were clonic movements of the extremities.

preterm infants and may be difficult to identify. They may take the form of sudden sucking, cycling movements of the limbs, tongue rolling, horizontal nystagmus or apnoea. They frequently reflect brain-stem seizures.

Jitteriness. Convulsions should not be confused with neuromuscular hyperexcitability, an exaggerated form of the startle reflex, sometimes referred to as the 'dithers' or the 'jitters'. Typical jitteriness occurs as a fast tremor, often produced on handling or startling, which can be abolished by flexion of the limb which eases tension on the stretched muscle spindles.

The clinical conditions in which convulsions occur are listed in Table 17.1, and the more common conditions with time of onset are listed in Table 17.2.

Table 17.1 Clinical conditions associated with convulsions

Cerebral disorders
    Hypoxia, haemorrhage and oedema
    Maldevelopment, Genetic disorders
Metabolic disturbances
    Hypoglycaemia
    Hypocalcaemia and hypomagnesaemia
    Hypo/Hypernatraemia
    Pyridoxine dependence/deficiency
    Aminoacidopathies
    Galactosaemia
    Organic acidaemias
    Hyperammonaemia (urea cycle defects)
Infection
    Septicaemia/Meningitis
    Tetanus
'Fifth Day Fits'
Withdrawal
    Diazepam
    Narcotic

Table 17.2 Common causes of convulsions with typical time of onset

First Day	Intracranial injury: asphyxia
Second Day	Hypoglycaemia
Fourth to Sixth Days	Hypocalcaemia
End of First Week	Meningitis
Prolonged Convulsions	Cerebral maldevelopment: genetic

Cerebral disorders

Intracranial damage

This was the commonest cause of convulsions in the newly born infant but is no longer, as a result of advances is obstetric care and prevention of hypoxia.

Hypoxia. As pointed out in Chapter 12 hypoxia is the most important factor.

Intracranial haemorrhage is less common and is usually associated with the rapid delivery of a large postmature or preterm infant.

Time onset. Convulsions due to cerebral birth trauma and hypoxia commonly occur within the first 24 hours of life, being preceded by hypotonia, then irritability, a high-pitched cry, an anxious expression and tonic or clonic seizures, and followed later in the more severe cases by neck stiffness and a bulging fontanelle.

In such cases convulsions, in association with cyanotic attacks and feeding difficulties, signify a poor prognosis and in those who survive there is a high probability of neurological handicap.

Cerebral maldevelopment

Convulsions which start within a day or two of birth and which prove resistant to anticonvulsant therapy are suggestive of gross cerebral abnormality with underdevelopment of one of both cerebral hemispheres or a genetic disorder.

Hypoglycaemia

Whenever a newborn infant suddenly has a convulsion or apnoeic episode hypoglycaemia should be suspected. A low Dextrostix or BM Test Glycemie 20/800 reading should be checked immediately in the laboratory by glucose measurements on a whole blood sample to confirm the diagnosis.

Blood glucose. Hypoglycaemia occurs particularly in infants weighing less than 1500 g at birth. This is confirmed as the cause of convulsions in the presence of a single blood glucose level below 1.2 mmol/l (20 mg/dl) during the first month of life. Asymptomatic hypoglycaemia can also occur.

In the term infant a blood glucose level of less than 1.7 mmol/l (30 mg/dl) during the first 72 hours and below 2.2 mmol/l (40 mg/dl) thereafter is an indication of hypoglycaemia.

Aetiology

In Chapter 9 it was suggested that hypoglycaemia is a direct consequence of insufficient stores of energy-producing glycogen with the possible additional factor of temporary adrenocortical hypofunction.

Predisposing factors are fetal malnutrition (small-for-dates infants), hypothermia, respiratory distress syndrome, cerebral damage and the infant of the diabetic or prediabetic mother.

Infant of diabetic mother. The infant born to the poorly controlled diabetic mother is usually heavy for dates with a typically bright red skin and chubby cheeks (Fig. 17.2). Because of the increased incidence of fetal death in late pregnancy labour is induced early at around 37 weeks. Regular blood glucose monitoring is essential as hyperinsulinaemia due to hyperplasia of the β cells in the pancreatic islets of Langerhans results in hypo-

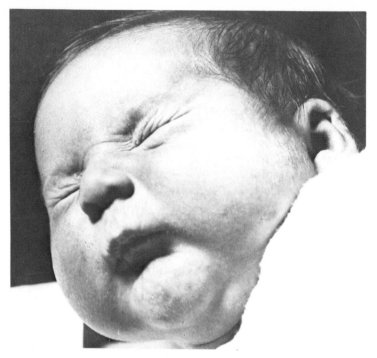

Fig. 17.2 Infant of diabetic mother.

glycaemia. There is also an increased risk of RDS, hypocalcaemia, jaundice, infection and venous thrombosis, especially renal vein thrombosis, in these babies. The abnormal features and complications described above are less likely to occur if the mother's diabetes is well controlled and she remains normoglycaemic throughout the pregnancy.

Rare causes of hypoglycaemia, occurring after the first week or so of life, are glycogen storage disease, pancreatic islet cell tumour, leucine sensitivity and nesidioblastosis (hypertrophy of the β cell mass). Amino acid disorders (e.g. maple syrup urine disease) and galactosaemia may also present as hypoglycaemia.

Clinical signs

The early signs of hypoglycaemia include apathy, refusal to feed, cyanosis, apnoeic episodes, temperature instability and tremulous or jittery movements. Later signs are severe apnoeic attacks, convulsions and deep coma. These may be mistakenly attributed to cerebral or adrenal haemorrhage.

Prevention

Early and adequate feeding of low birth weight infants and infants of diabetic mothers will prevent the onset of hypoglycaemia in most infants. All infants at risk of hypoglycaemia should have blood glucose estimations performed by Dextrostix or equivalent soon after birth and at four to six hourly intervals thereafter for 24 hours and then at 12 hour intervals till 48 hours if they remain normal. Symptomatic infants should continue to have blood glucose estimates until the blood glucose concentrations stabilize.

Treatment

Symptomatic. In the presence of symptoms, a blood glucose level of less than 1.2 mmol/l (20 mg/dl) in the preterm or 1.7 mmol/l (30 mg/dl) in a term infant is an indication for immediate treatment to prevent brain damage.

Intravenous glucose: in the presence of symptoms, the blood glucose must be elevated quickly by the intravenous injection of 10–15 ml of 20% dextrose solution. Treatment is continued with 10% dextrose solution to provide 6–8 mg glucose/minute. Oral feeding is resumed when symptoms have settled and the blood glucose has returned to normal. The intravenous fluids are progressively reduced and then withdrawn.

Steroids: very occasionally there is difficulty in maintaining a normal blood glucose. Steroids can be given as prednisolone 0.5 mg per kg two to four times daily. Occasionally glucagon, growth hormone or diazoxide may be required.

Asymptomatic. If on routine Dextrostix an infant at risk (e.g. SFD) is hypoglycaemic, additional oral feeds should be given. These should preferably be breast milk or milk formula and may require to be given by tube. The blood glucose should be checked one hour later and, if this has returned to normal, enteral feeds continued. If the blood glucose is still low treat as if symptomatic. It is important to continue enteral feeds with additional carbohydrate if necessary (e.g. Caloreen) whenever possible and to reduce intravenous dextrose slowly to prevent rebound hypoglycaemia.

Prognosis

Infants who have shown evidence of symptomatic hypoglycaemia in the newborn period should be considered 'at risk' and should be reviewed in a follow-up clinic with particular reference to neurological function.

Severe type. The prognosis for infants with severe and prolonged hypoglycaemia is poor and the majority will prove to have severe cerebral dysfunction.

Mild type. It is more difficult to assess the outlook for infants with slight symptoms but in general it is good. Careful assessment at school age may, however, show that some of these infants have learning difficulties and other forms of handicap which were not evident at an earlier stage.

Hypocalcaemia

Neonatal tetany. Fits due to neonatal tetany present with irritability followed by twitching and sometimes focal or multifocal jerking movements at a rate of one to three per second but without tonic phases. Between fits the infant remains alert. Neonatal tetany commonly occurs when the serum calcium falls below 1.75 mmol/l (3.5 mEq/l) and can be provoked by external stimulation such as lightly tapping the sternum.

Early onset. There is a significant difference in the prognosis of infants who develop hypocalcaemia in the first few days of life and in those who develop it later in the first week. Hypocalcaemia occurring in the first three days of life may be found in low birth weight babies, in babies born to diabetic mothers and in babies who have suffered cerebral birth trauma or asphyxia. These infants often have a poor prognosis.

Late onset. Hypocalcaemia occurring towards the end of the first week of life, with a peak incidence between the fifth and eighth days of life, is more common than the hypocalcaemia of early onset. It is usually associated with unmodified cow's milk feeding (Chapter 8).

Infants particularly at risk are those born to mothers of high parity, Asian mothers and mothers whose vitamin D and calcium intake during pregnancy may be deficient. The low serum calcium concentration is secondary to hyperphosphataemia which arises since the immature kidney is unable to deal with the high phosphate content of unmodified cow's milk. In addition, the low vitamin D status of the mother may lead to similar low concentrations in the fetus and infant and thus impair absorption of calcium from the gut. These infants also have a low plasma parathormone level and may be unable to release calcium from stores in their bones. Mothers who are vitamin D deficient during pregnancy develop a secondary compensatory hyperparathyroid state and this interferes with the ability of the infant's parathyroid function to cope with a high dietary phosphate load after birth. Late onset hypocalcaemia has a good prognosis.

Maternal hyperparathyroidism. Hypocalcaemia may occur in transient congenital hypoparathyroidism associated with maternal hyperparathyroidism. The mother's blood calcium should be checked if her baby develops persisting tetany.

Treatment

Treatment of tetany consists of correction of the mineral deficiency and in avoiding unnecessary disturbance.

Breast milk or a modern modified cow's milk preparation should be used (Chapter 8).

Extra calcium can be given orally as supplements of 5–10 ml of a 5% solution of calcium gluconate with feeds.

Intravenous calcium. Where oral treatment fails or is not feasible 2 ml of a 10% calcium gluconate solution should be given slowly and intravenously. Vitamin D and parathormone are required when supplements of calcium are insufficient to correct the serum calcium but hypomagnesaemia should be excluded (see below).

Prognosis

As far as is known infants who have suffered from transient hypocalcaemia develop normally without any neurological sequelae or intellectual impairment although later enamel hypoplasia and dental caries are recognized complications.

Hypomagnesaemia

Primary hypomagnesaemia may occur with hypocalcaemia and should be suspected whenever an infant with hypocalcaemia does not stop convulsing when the serum calcium returns to normal. The symptoms are identical to those of hypocalcaemia and respond

dramatically to treatment with magnesium sulphate given parenterally as magnesium sulphate (50% solution), 0.2 ml/kg by deep
intramuscular injection.

Hyponatraemia

Hyponatraemia (plasma sodium < 130 mmol/l) can occur when
infants are given excessive amounts of electrolyte free dextrose. As
a rule dextrose alone should not be given for longer than 24 hours.
Following asphyxia and septicaemia, excessive inappropriate
production of antidiuretic hormone from the posterior pituitary can
cause hyponatraemia. Treatment requires fluid restriction only.
Occasionally low birth weight infants fed exclusively on expressed
breast milk may develop hyponatraemia. This is due to the low
sodium content of breast milk and the poor sodium retention of
the preterm kidney. These infants may require additional sodium
supplements in their feeds.

Hypernatraemia

This usually occurs when inadequate attention is paid to the
sodium intake or fluid intake of sick infants. It is particularly
common in preterm infants nursed under radiant heaters and
allowed to 'dry out'.

Fifth day fits

This variety of neonatal seizures was first described in Australia
where it was observed that epidemics occurred in nurseries in
which apparently normal infants developed seizures in the first 4
to 6 days of life (peak fifth day). These were usually clonic, often
frequent but were not associated with abnormal biochemistry or
other investigations. They subside without treatment and have an
excellent prognosis. The cause has not yet been firmly established.

Meningitis

Meningitis is described in Chapter 14. The illness is part of a
septicaemia with the infection localizing in the meninges. Persistent
lethargy or drowsiness and a 'distant' expression, more rarely slight
stiffness of the neck, and occasionally associated convulsions would
suggest meningitis. There is sometimes a further hint in the

presence of slight exophthalmos. The diagnosis is confirmed by lumbar puncture. Treatment with antibiotics and anticonvulsants should be instituted immediately (Chapter 14).

Tetanus neonatorum

Convulsions also occur in tetanus. There is spasm of the muscles of the jaw, face, trunk and limbs. The conditions is rarely if ever seen in the United Kingdom. In areas where the standard of hygiene is low a sickle blade or dirty knife may be used to cut the cord with the danger that tetanus spores may be introduced. Treatment is by antibiotics, sedation with diazepam, antitetanic serum and general supportive measures. The prognosis is poor in very young infants. The importance of maternal immunization before or during pregnancy cannot be overstated.

Rare cause of convulsion

Drug withdrawal. Convulsion may precede coma in babies of mothers addicted to narcotics. Treatment consists of sedation with phenobarbitone or diazepam for a few days or weeks as necessary. It is also occasionally seen in infants whose mothers have used anticonvulsants or benzodiazepines (e.g. Diazepam) during pregnancy.

Metabolic disorders

Severe convulsions in the newborn may be a feature of such rare metabolic disorders as maple syrup urine disease, organic acid-aemias, galactosaemia, urea cycle defects, glycogen storage disease and pyridoxine dependency/deficiency.

Maple syrup urine disease is a rare condition which can give rise to a clinical picture simulating meningitis or intracranial haemorrhage within a week of birth. Failure to thrive is typical. The disorder is due to defect in the metabolism of the branched chain amino acids, leucine, isoleucine and valine. The plasma amino acid profile is typical. The urine has the typical odour of maple syrup (or burnt sugar), which on chromatography reveals a characteristically abnormal aminoaciduria. Treatment with special diet may be effective.

Organic acidaemias and urea cycle defects. These are rare inborn errors of metabolism which lead to marked metabolic acidosis and severe metabolic derangement. In the urea cycle defects there is hyperammonaemia, low blood urea and often a metabolic alkalosis initially. They often present with seizures. They require sophisticated dietary and other metabolic management.

Glycogen storage disease. Rarely Cori's type I glycogen storage disease (von Gierke's disease) may present in the neonatal period with anorexia, vomiting, convulsions due to hypoglycaemia and hepatomegaly. Treatment consists in giving a high protein, low carbohydrate diet but the prognosis is extremely poor.

Pyridoxine dependency or deficiency are disorders in which convulsions are rapidly controlled by the intravenous or intramuscular administration of 100 mg pyridoxine. Pyridoxine is important in the production of one of the brain's natural anticonvulsants (gamma amino butyric acid) and low levels of this compound lead to seizure activity. In deficiency states correction is easily achieved by single dose theapy; in dependency continuing treatment is required.

HYPERACTIVITY

Low birth-weight babies are constantly on the move even when asleep. Their abdominal muscles are constantly moving and every now and again a limb will flex and relax in a perfectly natural manner. Occasionally the most immature preterm baby shows remarkable activity during the first day or two of life after which the behaviour resembles that of other preterm babies.

Congenital thyrotoxicosis (Fig. 17.3 and 17.4) is sometimes seen for a limited period after birth following delivery of a mother with hyperthyroidism, with a history of previous thyroidectomy or with history of thyroid medication. Symptoms and signs of congenital thyrotoxicosis include tachycardia which is sometimes associated with heart failure, hyperactivity, abnormal eagerness for feeds, enlargement of the thyroid and exophthalmos. Their onset may be delayed for about a week as a result of prenatal therapy given to the mother. Treatment of the baby is by antithyroid drugs, beta blockers (propranolol), and such supportive digoxin therapy as may be indicated by signs of heart failure.

It is now known that the condition is due to the passage of thyroid-stimulating IgG immunoglobulins across the placenta from a mother with thyrotoxicosis. It resolves as the maternal antibody disappears from the infant's blood, usually in two to three months. Treatment can then be discontinued.

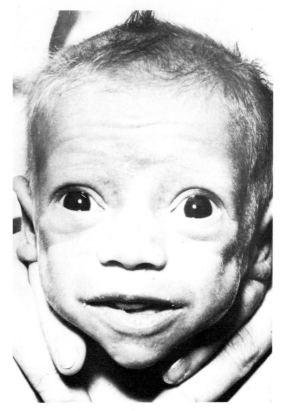

Fig. 17.3 Congenital thyrotoxicosis. (By courtesy of Professor A. G. Watkins.)

HYPERTONIA AND HYPOTONIA

Both hypertonia and hypotonia can be seen in newborn infants who have experienced hypoxia. The initial hypotonia of severe hypoxia gives way to hypertonia after some hours of life and indicates a poor prognosis. Less severely asphyxiated infants usually show hypertonicity soon after birth. This should be differentiated from stiffness due to lack of joint movement as in arthrogryposis (Fig. 17.5) or due to sclerema associated with neonatal cold injury (Fig. 17.6).

Hypotonia in the newly born infant may also be due to disorders of the spinal cord, muscles, peripheral nerves or connective tissue. Causes, both common and rare, are listed in Table 17.3.

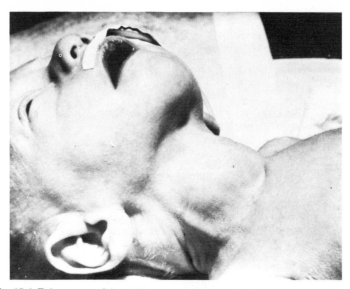

Fig. 17.4 Enlargement of thyroid in congenital thyrotoxicosis.

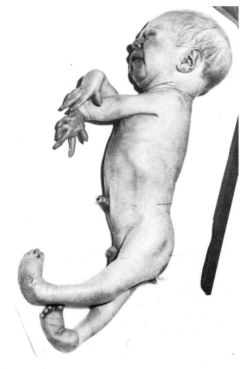

Fig. 17.5 Arthrogryposis.

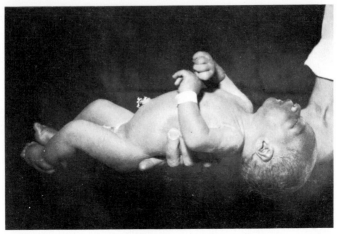

Fig. 17.6 Severe hypothermia with generalized rigidity.

Table 17.3 Causes of hypotonia in the newborn

Cerebral causes
    Birth trauma
    Maldevelopment
    Chromosomal anomaly
    Intrauterine infection
    Hypoxia
Preterm
Sepsis
Drug depression
Rarer causes
    Metabolic disturbances
    Neonatal hypothyroidism
    Myasthenia gravis
    Werdnig-Hoffman disease
    Muscular disorders
    Prader-Willi syndrome
    Familial dysautonomia

Cerebral causes

Hypotonicity is a feature of major dysfunction of the central nervous system.

Brain damage. Extensive injury to the brain whether from hypoxia, intrauterine infection, mechanical injury or haemorrhage can result in hypotonia.

Maldevelopment of the brain, particularly dysplasia, is frequently associated with poor muscle tone.

Chromosomal anomaly. Infants with Down's syndrome and other chromosomal abnormalities associated with mental retardation frequently present with hypotonia.

Preterm infants

Preterm infants have poorer muscle tone than more mature infants. This hypotonia is the basis for several of the tests which are used for the clinical assessment of maturity (Chapter 9). Hypotonia is not inconsistent with the periods of hyperactivity seen in low birth weight infants. Improvement in muscle tone is a sign of normal healthy progress.

Sepsis. Infants with sepsis often present with hypotonia. This resolves with treatment.

Drug depression. Mothers who have regularly taken diazepam and similar drugs in pregnancy often have hypotonic infants who gradually recover as the effect wanes.

Other rare causes

Persistent hypotonia in the newly born infant should bring to mind the rarer diagnoses listed in Table 17.3.

Metabolic disturbances

As described earlier in this chapter, certain metabolic disturbances produce a clinical picture not unlike that presented by the infant who survives perinatal severe hypoxia. In addition to hypotonia these babies exhibit expressionless facies, unresponsiveness to approach and normal stimuli, abnormal quietness and total disinclination to feed. The baby with glycogen storage disease will have a large heart and tongue.

Neonatal hypothyroidism occasionally presents with hypotonia.

Myasthenia gravis

There are two forms of myasthenia gravis in the newborn.

Juvenile. In the so-called 'juvenile' form signs in the baby persist throughout life, but it is altogether exceptional for them to appear in the first week of life. In these cases the mother has no signs of myasthenia.

Neonatal. The other form is called neonatal myasthenia gravis.

The mother is suffering from myasthenia but the signs which are present in the baby at or shortly after birth disappear within a few hours or days, although occasionally they last as long as six to eight weeks. It has been estimated that about 20% of babies of severely myasthenic mothers are affected. Slight delay in the initial appearance of signs in the baby could be explained by therapy given to the mother. Generalized muscular hypotonia dominates the clinical picture, with symmetrical involvement of face, trunk and limbs. In the severe case there is lack of facial expression, difficulty in sucking and swallowing and poverty of movement. If, as is unlikely with a knowledge of the mother's condition, there is doubt concerning diagnosis, confirmation is obtained by the injection of edrophonium chloride (Tensilon) 1 mg intramuscularly which will rapidly restore normal muscle tone. Maintenance with pyridostigmine is then required. Occasionally exchange transfusion to remove maternal antibody is indicated. Progress is good, with the reservation that exceptionally death follows respiratory failure.

Any apparently healthy baby born to a mother with myasthenia gravis should be kept under continuous skilled observation for some two to four days because of the risk of the delayed appearance of myasthenic signs.

Werdnig-Hoffmann disease

Werdnig-Hoffmann disease, or spinal muscular atrophy, is an autosomal recessive condition which is characterized by hypotonia and wasting of the skeletal muscles resulting from degeneration of the anterior horn cells of the spinal cord. Fetal movements are feeble or absent, and at birth the baby is limp, flaccid and areflexic. Characteristically the baby lies in a froglike position and there is fibrillation of the tongue. Muscle biopsy shows diagnostic changes and death usually occurs within the first year of life.

Muscular disorders

There are a number of such disorders which may present with hypotonia in the newborn period.

Benign congenital hypotonia improves spontaneously as the infant grows. The number of infants labelled with this disorder has fallen steadily as improved methods of diagnosis have become available.

Muscular dystrophies usually become apparent well after the neonatal period but affected babies are occasionally noted to be hypotonic at birth.

Myotonic dystrophy. This is an autosomal dominant disorder with muscle weakness and myotonia. The myotonia causes delayed release of muscle activity which can easily be detected by shaking hands with mother, who is often unable to release her grasp. The infant has a droopy (myopathic) facies and often respiratory difficulties which may be fatal.

Prader-willi syndrome

Infants with this syndrome are particularly hypotonic and may be unable to cry or suck. In the male child the scrotum is hypoplastic, the testes undescended and the penis small. As they grow older they become obese but this can be prevented by careful control of the diet. A chromosomal deletion (15) is found in approximately 50% of these children.

Familial dysautonomia

Familial dysautonomia, or the Riley-Day syndrome, is an autosomal recessive condition almost exclusively confined to the Jewish race. The condition is transmitted as an autosomal recessive trait and is thought to be a disorder of the autonomic nervous system. Affected infants are hypotonic and areflexic, have difficulty in feeding and swallowing and suffer repeated respiratory infections. In addition there is defective or absent lacrimation, loss of corneal sensation leading to ulcer formation, impaired temperature control, and eventual physical and mental retardation. Treatment is symptomatic and some infants reach adult life.

The floppy infant

The differential diagnosis of the hypotonic infant must include consideration of the causes described above. It is often difficult to reach a firm diagnosis in the early stages. The urgency to establish a diagnosis depends upon the severity of the hypotonia and the risk which this implies to the infant's well-being.

Close observation is required and rapid resuscitative measures will be required if a hypotonic infant aspirates mucus or milk. An assessment of change in muscle tone is a most important observation as the final diagnosis may well depend on the recognition of signs of improvement which will eventually appear in a condition such as benign muscular hypotonia.

Investigation. Nerve conduction studies, electromyography, serum enzyme studies and muscle biopsy may be necessary before a final diagnosis and prognosis can be made.

Genetic advice. Accuracy in diagnosis is essential before genetic advice is given.

DROWSINESS

Drowsiness is an indication of poor cerebral function which may occur in small preterm infants, after cerebral injury, with raised intracranial pressure and following sedation. It may also occur with infections, severe hypothermia and in some metabolic disorders.

Cerebral dysfunction

Preterm infants. The smallest preterm infants, although showing episodes of hyperactivity, periodically tend to be drowsy and inactive, particularly after feeds.

Cerebral damage whether due to mechanical trauma, hypoxia or haemorrhage, may cause profound drowsiness and inactivity.

Raised intracranial pressure. Infants with hydrocephalus or subdural haematoma become increasingly drowsy as the intracranial pressure rises.

Oversedation. Infants whose mothers have been treated with sedatives or hypnotics shortly before delivery may be very drowsy and difficult to resuscitate at birth. If one of the morphine group of drugs has been used an injection of naloxone should be given. Infants who have been sedated following a convulsion will also become drowsy.

Infection

Persistent drowsiness and lethargy in association with a 'distant' expression suggests the possibility of widespread infection probably involving the meninges. Lumbar puncture, blood and urine cultures should be arranged and antibiotic treatment given.

Neonatal cold injury

Severe hypothermia with fall in central temperature is associated with progressive drowsiness as well as the other features already described in Chapter 9.

Metabolic disorders

Earlier in this chapter mention was made of the drowsiness which forms part of the clinical picture of some metabolic disorders such as maple syrup urine disease, the organic acidaemias and urea cycle defects.

ABNORMAL POSTURE

The normal posture at birth is one of generalized flexion which involves both the spine and the limbs. In the course of normal development the primary flexion curve of the spine is modified by secondary extension curves in the cervical and lumbar regions as the baby first acquires head control and later sits, stands erect and walks. Immediately after birth, flexion of the limbs is of such a degree that it is frequently impossible to fully extend the limbs. This inability to straighten the legs makes accurate measurement of length at birth both difficult and unreliable. It is important that no attempt is made to extend the limbs or trunk forcibly, whether for measurement or any other purpose.

Abnormal postures result from peripheral nerve palsies, abnormal fetal positions and fractures (Chapter 13).

Peripheral nerve palsies

Dropped wrist is a feature of radial nerve and Klumpke's palsy. In Erb's palsy the arm is rotated internally and hangs limply from the shoulder, the elbow is extended, and the hand is partially closed with the palm directed outwards and posteriorly in the typical 'waiter's tip' position. Obturator nerve palsy results in full external rotation and abduction of the leg with flexion of the knee. Sciatic nerve palsy resulting from unskilled intramuscular injection or mistaken injection into the obturator branch of the umbilical artery causes weakness of the leg with a dropped foot.

Fractures

Fracture of limb bones can cause deformity and pseudoparalysis.

Epiphyseal injuries, usually of the upper epiphyses of the femur and humerus, produce swelling of the part with immobility.

Abnormal fetal positions

Fetal positions responsible for abnormal postures at birth were described in Chapter 11.

Genu recurvatum is a deformity consisting of abnormal hyper-extension of the knee joint. It may involve one or both limbs and is sometimes complicated by posterior dislocation of the knee. Spontaneous improvement is usual and splinting for a limited period is necessary only in severe cases.

Arthrogryposis. The congenital stiffness of one or more joints together with hypoplasia of related muscles as seen in arthrogryposis congenita multiplex has already been mentioned earlier in this chapter.

Breech delivery. Where the baby has presented at the breech with extended legs the abnormal posture of the legs is maintained for some days after birth. From the clinical point of view it is wise to remember that breech presentation favours congenital dislocation of the hip.

Talipes. Flexion deformities of the wrist and talipes calcaneo-valgus are not infrequently associated with oligohydramnios. These abnormal postures usually disappear spontaneously within the neonatal period.

Hyperextension of the neck, or opisthotonos, is a worrying sign in the neonate. Possible causes, all of which have already been fully described, include face presentation, meningitis, tetanus, vascular ring and kernicterus.

FURTHER READING

Brown, J. K. & Turner, T. L. (1977) Fits in the neonate. *The Journal of Maternal and Child Health* 2, 11. Richmond: Barker Publications.

Cornblath, M. & Schwartz, R. (1976) *Disorders of Carbohydrate Metabolism in Infancy*, 2nd Edn. Philadelphia: Saunders.

Dubowitz, V. (1980) *The Floppy Infant*. Suffolk: Spastics International Medical Publications.

Horwitz, S. J. & Arneil-Tison, C. (1979) Neurological problems. In: *Care of the High Risk Neonate*, 2nd Edn. ed. Klaus, M. H. & Fanaroff, A. A. Philadelphia: Saunders.

Wald, M. K. (1979) Problems in metabolic adaptation: glucose, calcium and magnesium. In: *Care of the High Risk Neonate*, 2nd Edn, ed. Klaus, M. H. & Fanaroff, A. A. Philadelphia: Saunders.

18

Pallor, polycythaemia, haemorrhage and purpura

PALLOR

The skin of a healthy newborn European infant is sufficiently 'pink' for pallor to be readily recognizable as an abnormal physical sign. Similar lack of coloration from capillary blood in nailbeds and mucous membranes can be seen in pigmented races. In any infant pallor must be considered as a serious sign and the cause sought out and treated urgently.

Pallor of recent onset

This is likely to have arisen from one or more of the following: peripheral vasoconstriction, anaemia following haemolysis, anaemia following haemorrhage.

Each of these may occur independently but are often interrelated.

Blood loss may cause immediate peripheral vasoconstriction and be followed by the pallor of anaemia as plasma volume is restored.

Haemolysis, purpura and circulatory collapse may occur together or in quick succession in infants with severe infection.

Several causes of pallor have already been dealt with in previous chapters. The circulatory collapse associated with damage to the brain in Chapters 12 and 13, the pallor of severe infection in Chapter 14, the anaemia of haemolytic disease in Chapter 15.

Physiological anaemia

Marrow inactivity

Pallor of slow onset occurs most frequently in preterm infants and is due to a progressive fall in haemoglobin associated with relative inactivity of the bone marrow (Chatper 5). The resulting 'physiological anaemia' is less marked in more mature infants and does not require treatment. The fall in very small infants is such that by 8 to 9 weeks of age the haemoglobin may have fallen to 7 g per dl (7 g per 100 ml) and in addition to pallor the infant may have tachycardia with difficulty in feeding. A sick preterm infant has frequent small blood samples taken for analysis. Each time blood is taken a helpful and sometimes salutary practice is to record the volume removed on a chart kept on the infant's incubator. It does not require too many samples to remove 10 ml blood which is 15% of a 900 g infant's blood volume.

Marrow activity improves slowly during the first two to three months, and provided sufficient haemopoietic factors including iron, folic acid, vitamin C, thyroxine and trace elements such as copper and cobalt are available the haemoglobin rises. If there is deficiency of any of the necessary dietary factors anaemia may persist for many months.

Haemopoietic factors

Recognition of any deficiency of haemopoietic factors is essential to the planning of appropriate therapy.

Iron and vitamin C. In practice iron and vitamin C are the factors most commonly involved, and it is generally considered advisable to give preterm infants supplements of these factors from the second month of life. Some feeds are fortified with iron, but where these feeds are not being used a preparation such as ferrous sulphate mixture for infants NF 5 ml a day should be given together with ascorbic acid 25 mg a day. Iron supplements should not be given before 6 weeks after birth as iron may reduce the infant's immune capabilities and precipitate vitamin E deficiency anaemia, especially in preterm infants.

Folate deficiency is difficult to recognize clinically, and measurement of blood folate is necessary to establish the diagnosis. It has been demonstrated that folate deficiency is more common in preterm infants as a cause of continuing anaemia than was previously realized. Deficiency is particularly likely to occur following infection. The routine prophylactic administration of folate to preterm infants is not generally accepted but the need for treatment of incipient or established deficiency is clear. A therapeutic dose of folic acid in the newborn period would be 0.5 mg per day. Where there has been significant haemolysis (e.g. Rh isoimmunization), there is often folic acid deficiency and these infants benefit from regular supplements during the first three months of life.

Vitamin E deficiency. In some preterm infants, especially those under 34 weeks and fed a diet high in polyunsaturated fats, a haemolytic anaemia develops at about two months. This is usually associated with peripheral and facial oedema. Diagnostic tests include a raised hydrogen peroxide haemolysis test and low plasma tocopherol levels. Treatment is with either intramuscular tocopherol acetate, 25 mg daily for two to three weeks, or oral tocopherol succinate, 25 mg daily for six weeks.

Blood loss

Infants may lose blood for one or more of the causes shown in Table 18.1.

Table 1.1   Blood loss in newborn infants

BEFORE OF DURING DELIVERY
   Fetomaternal transfusion
   Feto-fetal transfusion in twins
   Rupture of placental vessels
     Placenta praevia, vasa praevia
     Surgical incision
   Rupture of cord vessels
     Precipitate delivery
AFTER DELIVERY
   External blood loss
     Cord stump
     Gastrointestinal tract
     Menstruation in females
     From skin injury
     From nose
   Internal blood loss
     Brain, lung, adrenals — often fatal
     Liver and spleen
     Kidney and muscles

Antenatal

Blood loss from the fetus before labour begins is difficult to detect and may only be suspected because of a change in fetal activity or heart rate. Occasionally mothers may experience a mild shivering attack and episode of discomfort if a considerable fetomaternal haemorrhage occurs.

Recognition. Fetal blood can be recognized in the maternal circulation by the acid elution technique of Kleihauer and an estimate made of the volume of blood lost by the fetus.

Twin pregnancies. Bleeding from one twin to another occurs through a communicating vessel between the placentae. If this is from the artery of one twin to the vein of the other, blood transfer will occur, the one twin becoming progressively more anaemic until intrauterine death may occur. The other twin will be plethoric and is generally the larger of the two at birth. Figure 18.1 shows a fetus papyraceus alongside the placenta of the healthy surviving twin — which may have been the result of an early feto-fetal transfusion. If both twins are born alive both may require treatment, blood transfusion for the anaemic twin and removal of blood from the plethoric twin (Fig. 18.2). Blood loss from the placental vessels, vasa praevia or cord generally occurs as the result of trauma but abnormal vessels may rupture with minimal injury. Fetal blood loss

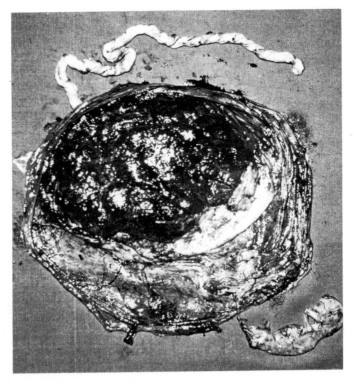

Fig. 18.1 Twin pregnancy with fetus papyraceus.

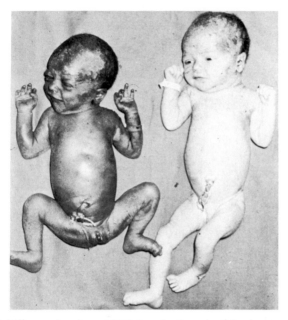

Fig. 18.2 Difference in colour at birth in uniovular twins following prenatal twin to twin transfusion.

can be recognized in the presence of maternal vaginal blood loss by the Apt's test (p. 476).

Postnatal blood loss

After delivery blood loss may be recognizable by direct observation, as when it comes from the cord stump, skin or nose.

Cord blood loss from the cord stump is less frequently seen since plastic cord clamps were introduced. Such blood loss can, however, be overlooked in infants who are fully dressed and wrapped up. The cord stump should be the first site inspected when an infant becomes pale and blood loss is suspected.

Gastrointestinal tract. Blood loss from the gastrointestinal tract is easy to recognize when it occurs in the form of vomiting of blood. Melaena is more difficult to recognize when the infant is still passing meconium. By examining the edge of the stool and thinning it out on the napkin the green colour of meconium can be readily distinguished from the reddish brown colour of melaena.

Swallowed maternal blood. Blood in the stool of an infant does not necessarily come from the infant and may be swallowed

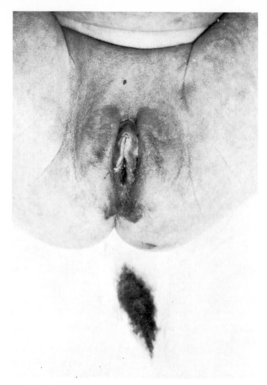

Fig. 18.3 Vaginal bleeding.

maternal blood. Fetal blood can be recognized by its ability to resist denaturation by 1% sodium hydroxide solution. If maternal blood is present the solution turns a brownish yellow colour (Apt's test).

Vaginal blood loss (Fig. 18.3). Vaginal bleeding may occur in female infants on the second to fourth day of life as the withdrawal of transplacental maternal oestrogens produces the equivalent of menstruation. In female infants it is not always clear whether blood on the napkin is coming from the bowel, vagina, urethra or skin. Careful observation after the perineum has been thoroughly cleaned will generally resolve the issue. Confusion can occur when the napkin shows a pink discoloration due to urate crystal deposits.

Internal haemorrhage

Haemorrhage into the organs of the infant may prove rapidly fatal and this is more likely to occur where the brain, lungs or adrenal glands are the organs involved. Infants may, however, survive less extensive haemorrhage into any of these organs but are likely to be ill with signs of circulatory collapse, cyanosis and possibly convulsions.

Liver and spleen. Haemorrhage into the liver and spleen appears to be more common following breech delivery and tends to occur under the capsule of these organs, producing palpable swelling in the abdomen associated with pallor and collapse. Should the subcapsular haematoma rupture, death may occur very rapidly but some infants survive long enough for surgical repair to be undertaken.

Kidneys. Bleeding into the kidneys and muscles is less frequent and generally follows local trauma.

Internal or external haemorrhage will be more marked where there is any failure of coagulation as occurs in any of the group of conditions which can be termed the haemorrhagic disorders of the newborn.

Treatment of acute anaemia

The management of acute anaemia, usually due to blood loss, is a neontal emergency which requires urgent action. The diagnosis may be difficult to confirm immediately from the haemoglobin and PCV as they may not fall for some time. However, the infant will be pale, vasoconstricted and hypotensive with a tachycardia and air hunger. In addition, the central venous pressure (CVP) will be low or negative. This can be confirmed when the umbilical venous catheter is inserted. The immediate treatment if the infant is obviously shocked is the infusion of 20 ml/kg of group O −ve blood over 5–10 minutes. This uncrossmatched blood is always available in a maternity unit. The infant will also benefit from oxygen therapy and the correction of the acid-base status. If the infant responds, repeat the Hb or PCV and reassess the infant. If the infant remains shocked a further 20–30 ml/kg can be given over 20–30 minutes with diuretic cover. The aim is to achieve a normal blood pressure and CVP.

Where the blood loss has been less acute prenatally (e.g. feto-fetal transfusion) or haemolysis is the cause, exchange transfusion with semi-packed red blood cells of a single blood volume (80–90 ml/kg) usually corrects the anaemia. The haemoglobin concentration after both forms of replacement should be approximately 16 g/dl or greater, and the PCV 40–50%.

Treatment of anaemia of prematurity

Apart from providing adequate haematinics it may be necessary to transfuse with packed red cells some preterm infants who, apart from a moderately low Hb, show clinical signs of anaemia (e.g. reluctance to feed, failure of weight gain, recurrent apnoea). Some clinicians depend on clinical acumen to decide on a transfusion policy, others use the concept of available oxygen. Whatever the method of decision, it is usual to give 20 ml/kg packed cells slowly over four to six hours with diuretic cover. The formula (4 ml packed cells raises the Hb of a 1 kg infant by 1 gm/dl) can also be used to calculate the blood volume for replacement transfusion.

POLYCYTHAEMIA

Polycythaemia occurs when the venous packed cell volume exceeds 70%. It occurs in infants who have been the recipient of twin-twin or materno-fetal transfusion, those who are postmature, small for dates and infants of diabetic mothers. Down's syndrome children are often affected.

As the viscosity of the blood increases the blood flow diminishes and ischaemia and thrombosis occur in vital organs. To prevent this, plasma exchange may be necessary to haemodilute the infant. It is usual to perform an exchange transfusion using 20 ml plasma per kg body weight.

THE HAEMORRHAGIC DISORDERS OF THE NEWBORN

The chief causes of haemorrhagic disorders in the newborn are shown in Table 18.2.

Table 18.2   The haemorrhagic disorders of the newborn

Vitamin K_1 deficiency
Disseminated intravascular coagulation
Deficiency of other clotting factors
Thrombocytopenia

Haemorrhagic disease of the newborn

It has been recognized from very early times that some newborn infants were prone to bleed excessively during the first week of life, and the Laws of Moses made allowance for this in their ordinance in relation to circumcision which was to be deferred until the eighth day. It was not until the end of the nineteenth century that the term haemorrhagic disease of the newborn was coined. This was at one stage thought to be entirely explicable by deficiency of vitamin K_1. As the limitations of treatment with vitamin K_1 became evident it was clear that more than one condition was involved.

Vitamin K_1 deficiency

Vitamin K_1 is essential for the synthesis of four of the factors necessary for the clotting process — factors II (prothrombin), VII, IX and X. These factors are present in the newborn but at lower concentration than in the adult, falling to their lowest level on about the third day of life. The subsequent rise depends upon the provision of vitamin K_1 in the diet or as a result of bacterial action in the bowel producing vitamin K_1. Breast milk contains only one quarter of the vitamin K_1 of cow's milk formula.

'Haemorrhagic disease of the newborn' due to lack of dietary vitamin K_1 is virtually confined to those infants who have been breast fed, or have not received oral feeds. It can also occur when mothers have been on anticonvulsants in pregnancy as these lower the maternal vitamin K concentration.

Bleeding most commonly occurs from the gastrointestinal tract, but bleeding from other sites may occur. The diagnosis is confirmed by finding the infant's prothrombin time prolonged (normal 14–16 seconds) or the Thrombotest low (normal 40–60%).

Treatment is with parenteral vitamin K_1 (Konakion) 1 mg combined occasionally, if the bleeding has been severe, with blood transfusion or fresh frozen plasma.

Other haemorrhagic disorders do not respond to treatment with vitamin K_1.

Prevention

Haemorrhagic disease of the newborn can be prevented by providing all infants with vitamin K_1 (Konakion) after birth. This can be provided as Konakion 1 mg intramuscularly or orally after birth (0.5 mg for preterm). Additional vitamin K_1 can be provided to breast feeding mothers (20 mg orally per week) or during labour to those on anticonvulsant therapy.

Disseminated intravascular coagulation (DIC; secondary haemorrhagic disease)

Intravascular coagulation, by using up clotting factors including platelets, causes a haemorrhagic state by a process of consumptive coagulopathy.

Aetiology

The common causes of DIC are severe hypoxia, sepsis, hypothermia and hypotension.

Signs

Clinically, disseminated intravascular coagulation is evident as widespread bleeding, which often involves the brain and lungs as well as the skin and which is frequently fatal. The liver and spleen are often enlarged. The platelet count is low as is the plasma fibrinogen concentration. The prothrombin time and partial thromboplastin times are prolonged and the blood film contains fragmented red blood cells.

Fibrin degradation products. As a result of inappropriate coagulation taking place in the blood vessels, the body's fibrinolytic system produces excessive quantities of fibrin degradation products.

Treatment

The treatment of haemorrhagic disorders in the newborn period must be related to diagnosis of the specific cause of the bleeding tendency. Where bleeding is occurring and a haemorrhagic disorder is suspected a prothrombin time or thrombotest and a platelet count are essential investigations. When specimens have been taken 1 mg of vitamin K_1 by slow intravenous injection should be given. This will prove effective only in haemorrhagic disease of the newborn but will do no harm in other conditions and will not obscure the diagnosis. The management of thrombocytopenia and of disseminated intravascular coagulation are discussed later in this chapter.

Investigation of deficiency of other clotting factors will be necessary in the absence of thrombocytopenia and if bleeding continues after vitamin K_1 has been given and DIC excluded.

Facilities for detailed investigations are usually available in a regional centre to which it may be advisable to transfer the affected infant.

PURPURA

Purpura in the newly born infant may be produced by:
Thrombocytopenia
Capillary damage
   (a) Venous obstruction
   (b) Hypoxia.

Thrombocytopenia

Thrombocytopenia (platelet count less than $100 \times 10^9/l$) may occur for the reason shown in Table 18.3.

Maternal idiopathic thrombocytopenia (ITP). Purpura, which may be temporary, occurs in about half of the infants of mothers suffering from idiopathic thrombocytopenic purpura at the time of delivery and is apparently due to transplacental transmission of the maternal platelet IgG antibodies. It may also occur even when the mothers' platelet count has returned to normal. Such infants may be better delivered by Caesarean section because of the risks of intracranial haemorrhage during passage through the birth canal.

Table 18.3   Causes of thrombocytopenia in the newborn

MATERNAL FACTORS INVOLVED
   Maternal idiopathic thrombocytopenic purpura
   Iso-immune thrombocytopenia
   Transplacental infection
   Severe rhesus incompatibility
   Thiazide diuretics given to mother
   Inherited thrombocytopenia
OTHER CAUSES
   Infection acquired postnatally
   Disseminated intravascular coagulation
   Marrow hypoplasia
   Giant haemangioma

Iso-immune thrombocytopenia. This is due to the transplacental passage of platelet antibody from a platelet antigen negative mother, who has been immunized either by blood from her platelet antigen positive fetus or previous blood transfusion, to a platelet antigen positive fetus. The result is analagous to Rhesus immunization. Ninety-eight per cent of all individuals are platelet antigen

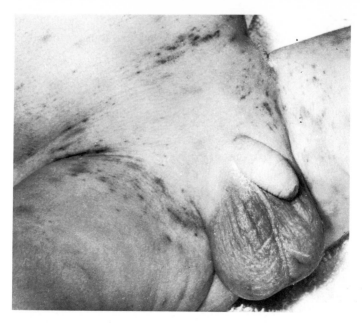

Fig. 18.4 Purpura in infant with congenital rubella.

positive, only 2% antigen negative. The mother will have a normal platelet count.

Antenatal infection. Syphilis, toxoplasmosis, rubella (Fig. 18.4), cytomegalovirus and herpes virus infection acquired antenatally are frequently accompanied by thrombocytopenic purpura in the infant.

Thiazide diuretics. Thrombocytopenia has been described in a small number of infants of mothers who had been on prolonged courses of thiazide diuretics. It is not certain that the diuretic is responsible for the low platelet count.

The inherited thrombocytopenias are only rarely manifest in the newborn period.

Other causes of thrombocytopenia in the infant do not involve maternal factors. Severe postnatal infection, bacterial or viral, may be accompanied by purpura due to platelet deficiency and this is generally a poor prognostic sign. In such situations thrombocytopenia may be a manifestation of disseminated intravascular coagulation. Marrow depression from any cause such as drugs, congenital leukaemia and bone disorders may present as purpura due to thrombocytopenia. The platelet consumption which occurs

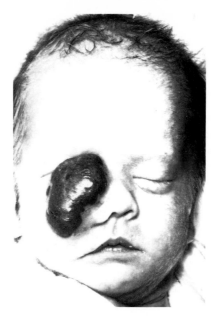

Fig. 18.5 Giant haemangioma with thrombocytopenia (Kassabach's syndrome).

in giant haemangiomas (Fig. 18.5) may rarely be a cause of purpura in the newborn period.

Non-thrombocytopenic purpura

Purpura not associated with thrombocytopenia is frequently due to a local cause such as constriction of the neck veins producing purpura over the head and neck. More extensive purpura occurs with persistent hypoxia and as the brain is often involved death is frequent (Chapter 12).

Treatment

Treatment of purpura is generally that of the underlying condition. Where the platelet count is above $40 \times 10^9/l$ treatment is seldom required. Below this level platelet transfusion may be indicated, especially if there is bleeding. Where the cause is maternal ITP, platelets will be consumed rapidly by the antibody and may required to be given frequently. Occasionally exchange transfusion can be used to wash out the maternal antibody. In cases of isoimmune thrombocytopenia any platelets transfused must be platelet antigen negative. These can be obtained from the mother, and washed prior to transfusion, or from other family members who are antigen negative. Steroid therapy is controversial but is often used.

The place of heparin and of exchange tranfusion in the treatment of disseminated intravascular coagulation has not been firmly established but there are several reports in favour of the controlled use of heparin. This requires very close supervision and should be carried out in an intensive therapy unit to which the infant should be transferred.

FURTHER READING

Gross, S. (1979) In *Haematologic Problems in Care of the High Risk Neonate*, 2nd edn. ed. Klaus M. H. & Fanaroff, A. A. Philadelphia, Saunders.
Oski, F. A. & Naiman, J. L. (1982) *Hematologic Problems in the Newborn*, 3rd edn. Philadelphia: Saunders.
Turner, T. L. (1986) Coagulation disorders in the newborn. In: *Textbook of Neonatology*, Ed. Robertson, N. R. C. Edinburgh: Churchill Livingstone.
Willoughby, M. L. N. (1977) *Paediatric Haematology*. Edinburgh: Churchill Livingstone.

19

Weight loss and other important signs

Many of the signs of disorders which are commonly found in the neonatal period have already been discussed in the preceding four chapters. This chapter will deal with weight loss and a variety of other different signs which, although some may occur less frequently than others, are all nonetheless of importance.

WEIGHT LOSS

Most babies lose weight for a few days after birth. This drop in weight is normally less than 10% of the weight at birth and may be termed physiological.

Physiological weight loss

Physiological weight loss is the result of loss of fluid by evaporation from the skin, and in the course of normal micturition, defaecation and respiratory exchange. The term artificially fed baby begins to gain weight about the fourth day of life and the breast fed and preterm baby between the seventh and tenth day of life. Infants vary greatly in the rate with which they gain weight, and fluctuations in weight progress are consistent with normal growth and development. A weekly gain of 175–240 g is usual in healthy babies. Some infants increase in weight more rapidly, but periods of exceptional progress are apt to be followed by phases of relatively slow gain in weight. Too much significance should not be attached to the results of successive weighings carried out at short intervals. After the first week of life weekly weighing provides all the necessary information.

Excessive weight loss

Weight loss may be described as excessive when it amounts to more than 10% of the birth weight.

The causes of excessive weight loss are listed in Table 19.1.

Table 19.1 Causes of excessive weight loss

Inadequate intake
  Underfeeding
  Difficulty in feeding
Vomiting
  Intestinal obstruction
  Functional disturbance
Diarrhoea
Excessive surface evaporation
Excessive urine loss

Inadequate intake

Underfeeding

Underfeeding must always be considered in the assessment of the infant with excessive weight loss.

Test weighing. If the baby is breast-fed an estimate can be made of mother's milk production. Weighing the baby before and after a feed gives an indication of the volume of milk taken. It is important that no change of clothing or napkin be made between the two test weighings. Test weighing is considered by many to be of dubious value. The mere knowledge that a test weight is to be performed may be sufficient to inhibit lactation. A series of test weighings is more valuable than a single examination.

Nutrition. In artificially fed infants the qualitative as well as the quantitative adequacy of the feed being offered must be reviewed. The fluid requirements of the very active baby are greater than those of the placid infant of comparable weight and age. The nutritional requirements of the newborn infant were considered in Chapter 8.

Difficulty in feeding

Difficulty in feeding may be the cause of underfeeding. The infant may be incapable of taking feeds because of some form of physical handicap such as nasal obstruction or cleft palate. He may be disinclined to accept feeds because of discomfort (e.g. thrush). Infants with cerebral dysfunction due to brain injury, congenital abnormality or infection are poor at sucking and swallowing. The preterm infant may not have the strength to feed from the breast or bottle.

Vomiting

Vomiting may be mechanical and due to obstruction in the gastrointestinal tract, may follow a disturbance of function or be due to over-feeding. The character of the vomitus (Table 19.2) is usually a good guide to the probable diagnosis.

Table 19.2   Types of vomitus

Frothy mucoid
  Oesophageal atresia
Bile-stained
  High intestinal obstruction
  Swallowed meconium
  Intracranial injury
  Low birth weight
Blood-stained
  Swallowed maternal blood
    During delivery
    Cracked nipple
  Trauma to pharynx
  Haemorrhagic disease
  Hiatus hernia
Milk, with or without mucus
  Gastritis
    Infective
    Non-infective
  Infections
    Enteral
    Parenteral
  Feeding problems
  Low intestinal obstruction
  Raised intracranial pressure

Alimentary tract malformations

Vomiting is an important sign of intestinal obstruction. The timing and character of the vomiting are of importance in diagnosis.

Early vomiting

Vomiting within the first day of life usually signifies the presence of a potentially fatal malformation of the upper alimentary tract which requires immediate surgical intervention.

Oesophageal atresia. Continuous dribbling of frothy mucus, coughing, spluttering and cyanosis on feeding and a preceding history of hydramnios are highly suggestive of oesophageal atresia. In 10% of cases there is associated small bowel or anal atresia.

Clinical diagnosis should be made before the first feed and confirmed by radiological examination. Pending surgical treatment the baby should be propped up and the upper oesophageal segment sucked out continuously or at 15 minute intervals to prevent inhalation pneumonia.

Bile-stained vomiting

Vomiting of bile-stained fluid in the first 24 hours of life is due to high intestinal obstruction, usually duodenal atresia, until proved otherwise. All such babies require immediate investigation and treatment.

Duodenal atresia. A preceding history of hydramnios would suggest the possibility of duodenal atresia which is confirmed by the typical double gas bubble seen on X-ray examination (Fig. 11.42). Surgical treatment consists in duodenoduodenostomy. With careful preoperative preparation and expert postoperative care the mortality rate is low. Duodenal atresia and annular pancreas are often associated with Down's syndrome.

Other surgical causes of bile-stained vomiting after the first 24 hours of life include atresia, stenosis, volvulus or reduplication of the small bowel, meconium ileus, peritonitis with ileus and Hirschsprung's disease.

Non-surgical causes. Apart from surgical causes early bilestained vomiting may be associated with intracranial injury, and in immature preterm babies because of associated ileus. It frequently follows the swallowing of meconium at birth.

Blood-stained vomiting

Maternal blood. The vomiting of blood always causes concern, particularly to parents. Most of the blood vomited on the first day of life is of maternal origin and has been swallowed during delivery. Infants who are breast fed may swallow blood from cracks in mother's nipple and later vomit the blood. The adult haemoglobin in maternal blood can be differentiated from fetal blood by the alkali denaturation test which was described in Chapter 18 (Apt's test).

Infant's blood. Injury to the mouth or pharynx during resuscitation or feeding may lead to bleeding and subsequent vomiting of swallowed blood. Rarely bleeding may take place from a tear of the oesophagus or ulceration of the gastric mucosa.

Disturbances of function

Vomiting may be caused by conditions which disturb gastro-intestinal function such as gastritis, enteral and parenteral infections, ingestion of drugs, raised intracranial pressure and the adrenogenital syndrome.

Gastritis

Vomiting due to gastritis may be of infective or non-infective aetiology.

Escherichia coli and *Candida albicans* are examples of infective causes of gastritis while drugs and swallowed meconium are non-infective causes of gastritis leading to vomiting.

Swallowed meconium. Gastric irritation caused by meconium, liquor amnii and swallowed blood is treated by gastric lavage.

Infection

Enteral and parenteral infections causing the newly born baby to vomit include gastroenteritis, urinary tract infection, neonatal hepatitis, meningitis and septicaemia.

Raised intracranial pressure

Raised intracranial pressure due to intracranial injury, subdural effusion, hydrocephalus and meningitis is a not uncommon cause of vomiting.

The adrenogenital syndrome

The presenting sign of the adrenogenital syndrome, which was discussed in Chapter 11, is commonly vomiting.

Overfeeding

Overloading the stomach with a volume of feed greater than the stomach can hold often results in some of the excess being returned in the form of a vomit. Provided that the infant continues to thrive this does not matter.

Frequency of feeds. If such vomiting is associated with poor weight gain or weight loss the volume given at each feed must be reduced. This will involve increasing the frequency of feeds by introducing additional feeds during the night or reducing the time interval between feeds.

Low birth weight. This problem is most likely to arise in the first two or three weeks of life of preterm infants when, in order to reduce the volume at individual feeds, feeding may have to be at two hourly or hourly intervals. In the smallest infants continuous infusion may be required as described in Chapter 9.

Management

Primary cause. Diagnosis and correction of the primary cause of the vomiting is the basis of management. Where a surgical cause is suspected early consultation with a paediatric surgeon is indicated.

Fluid, electrolyte, energy. The loss of fluid, electrolyte and energy which occurs because of vomiting has to be replaced and this generally implies intravenous therapy. It is not easy to supply sufficient nutrition by this route without using intravenous fat preparations. As experience with such preparations in the newborn is limited their use should be confined to specialist units.

Gastric lavage. When vomiting is due to irritation of the gastric mucosa by swallowed foreign material, gastric lavage is often the only treatment which will relieve symptoms.

Propping up the infants after feeds may prevent vomiting.

Diarrhoea

Causes of diarrhoea in the first month of life are shown in Table 19.3. The commonest causes are dietary and infective.

Dietary

Volume overload. If intake of an excessive volume of feed has not been relieved by vomiting, the amount of food passing the pylorus may exceed the digestive capacity of the bowel and diarrhoea follows.

Disaccharide overload. If more disaccharides such as lactose or sucrose are present in the diet than can be split by the intestinal disaccharidases (the sugar-splitting enzymes) then undigested sugars remain in the bowel and are fermented by bowel organisms. Water is drawn into the bowel by osmosis and the extra bowel content together with the lactic acid and other breakdown products

Table 19.3   Causes of diarrhoea in the first month of life

DIETARY
   Volume overload
   Disaccharide overload
ENTERAL INFECTION
   Bacterial
   Viral
   Necrotizing enterocolitis
PARENTERAL INFECTION
   Septicaemia
   Pneumonia
   Urinary tract infection
   Otitis media
   Neonatal hepatitis
RARER CAUSE
   e.g. Cystic fibrosis

produce a watery diarrhoea. The stool fluid contains acid reducing substances which excoriate the buttocks. Reduction of the disaccharide content of the diet gives relief from symptoms.

Alactasia. Lactase, the enzyme which splits lactose, is relatively deficient in the first few days of life particularly in the preterm infant. Rarely the enzyme is absent because of inherited deficiency. Temporary alactasia may occur after a bowel infection. Where the enzyme is deficient or absent diarrhoea occurs when there is lactose in the diet. Treatment consists of arranging a lactose-free diet. This requires the withdrawal of milk feeds and their substitution by special preparations some of which are based on soya bean flour.

Enteral infection

In communities with a high standard of hygiene, bowel infection is now a relatively uncommon cause of diarrhoea in the newborn. Where standards of hygiene are not adequate diarrhoea is a common and serious problem among bottle-fed infants.

Breast feeding protects infants against many of the infections which affect bottle fed infants (Chapter 8). The IgA of breast milk protects infants against viral and *E. coli* infection. The protein lactoferrin combines with iron which is then unavailable for the metabolism and multiplication of *E. coli*. The acid stool of breast fed infants predisposes to the growth of bacillus bifidus which inhibits the growth of pathogenic *E. coli*. Breast milk also contains active phagocytic cells and lysozymes which are effective against staphylococcal infection.

Breast feeding is therefore a prophylactic measure which should be strongly encouraged in any situation where there is doubt about the standard of hygiene.

Epidemics. Outbreaks of diarrhoea and vomiting due to pathogenic *E. coli* or salmonella organisms occur from time to time in newborn baby nurseries, the organism being carried by a mother or attendant. The disease is potentially very serious when it affects low birth weight babies and babies with congenital abnormalities. Less frequently diarrhoea and vomiting may be due to infection with other organisms including viruses.

Clinical signs. Reluctance to feed is the first sign of an enteral infection followed by occasional vomiting and the explosive passage of frequent loose watery stools. Dehydration with loss of skin elasticity, depressed fontanelles, sunken eyes, dryness of the lips, tongue and buccal mucous membranes, and rapid weight loss soon follow. If untreated there is progression to circulatory collapse with tachycardia and generalized grey cyanosis.

Treatment. Isolation is essential to prevent spread to susceptible infants. The newly born infant withstands salt and water loss badly hence replacement of water and electrolytes is an urgent necessity. In most cases scalp vein infusion, starting with 0.45% sodium chloride in 5% dextrose solution and changing to 0.18% sodium chloride with added potassium once urine has been passed, is essential. In less severe cases replacement fluid (oral rehydration fluid containing sodium 35 mmol/l, potassium 20 mmol/l, chloride 37 mmol/l, bicarbonate 18 mmol/l and glucose 200 mmol/l) can be given by mouth followed later by the gradual introduction of milk feeds. When recovering from an attack of severe diarrhoea and vomiting some infants are unable to tolerate breast milk, cow's milk or even any of the specialized formulas and require intravenous nutrition. Antibiotic therapy must be very carefully assessed, taking into account the infant's general condition and the type of organism isolated. Parenteral treatment is indicated if there is evidence of bloodstream spread.

Cross-infection

Only in about 20% of cases will stool bacteriological culture produce a pathogenic organism. Diarrhoea and vomiting in many cases is of viral aetiology (e.g. Rotavirus) whereas in others it may be due to non-infective causes such as dietary intolerance. If two or more infants develop diarrhoea at the same time, cross-infection must be presumed and the babies isolated and barrier-nursed. Depending on the severity of the symptoms and the number of babies involved it may be necessary to close the ward to new admissions.

Necrotizing enterocolitis

Necrotizing enterocolitis occurs most commonly in low birth weight infants who are not breast fed. No single cause for the condition has been found but the association with the respiratory distress syndrome, umbilical catheterization, sepsis, PDA and recent blood transfusion suggests that hypoxia leads to ischaemic lesions of the gastrointestinal tract. Other suggested aetiological factors include cow's milk feeding, the use of polyvinyl catheters for feeding and *Clostridium difficile*. The condition is characterized by vomiting, abdominal distension, gastrointestinal bleeding, irregular temperature and peritonitis in some cases. Typically plain radiological films of the abdomen show dilated loops of bowel in which there are intramural bubbles of gas. Symptoms develop within a few days of birth and treatment is symptomatic consisting of resting the intestine, treatment of shock, intravenous fluids and antibiotics unless perforation of the gut occurs, when surgical intervention is indicated.

Parenteral infections

Parenteral infections such as septicaemia, pneumonia, urinary tract infection, otitis media and neonatal hepatitis, which are associated with diarrhoea, have all been discussed elsewhere.

Cystic fibrosis of the pancreas may present in the first month of life with large, bulky, fatty and offensive stools. Occasionally the stools are numerous and of fluid consistency.

Hirschsprung's disease usually presents with constipation but occasionally diarrhoea may be the earliest manifestation of the condition signifying the presence of a complicating enterocolitis.

Morphine withdrawal in babies whose mothers are morphine addicts is typified by vomiting and diarrhoea. In addition to the diarrhoea and vomiting there is extreme irritability, high-pitched cry, thirst and sometimes convulsions and coma. Treatment consists in sedating the baby with phenobarbitone or diazepam for a few days or weeks.

Adrenal insufficiency, with or without adrenocortical hyperplasia, may be associated with bouts of severe diarrhoea in addition to the more common sign of vomiting.

Hypersensitivity to cow's milk or soya protein may cause diarrhoea in the early days of life of infants fed on cow's milk or soya preparations.

Excessive surface evaporation

A natural body covering of oils enables the newly born infant to conserve water. If this natural barrier is removed by the ritual bath at birth then the infant may lose excessive amounts of fluid through the skin. We recommend that bathing be delayed for at least 48 hours.

Excessive loss of fluid may also take place from the respiratory passages if an infant is nursed in an excessively hot, dry atmosphere. Such a situation may occur naturally in certain countries. In temperate climates similar situations may arise if infants are nursed in too hot an incubator, too near to a radiator, in direct sunshine or if they are over-clothed. In most instances there will be a rise in central temperature. Treatment is by removing the infant to a cooler environment and giving extra fluid such as 0.18% sodium chloride in 5% dextrose until the infant is back to normal. Extremely preterm infants are particularly prone to water loss through their skin in the first few days of life.

Excessive urine loss

Polyuria calls for the exclusion of temporary congenital diabetes mellitus and nephrogenic diabetes insipidus. Both conditions are exceedingly rare.

Temporary congenital diabetes mellitus (Fig. 19.1) disappears spontaneously within weeks or months but treatment with insulin may be necessary for a period.

Nephrogenic diabetes insipidus is a sex-linked recessive condition in which the male infant's renal tubule is unresponsive to antidiuretic hormone. The infant's brain is damaged by hypernatraemia if water loss is not made good

Loss of oedema. The oedematous infant who gets rid of his oedema does so by increasing his urine output whether this be done naturally or as the result of treatment.

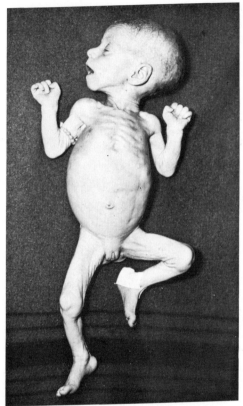

Fig. 19.1 Dehydration and weight loss in infant with temporary congenital diabetes mellitus.

EXCESSIVE WEIGHT GAIN

Excessive weight gain is not a common sign in the newborn period. When rapid excessive weight gain is associated with the retention of fluid it is commonly manifest as oedema and is therefore to be expected in such conditions as heart failure, hypoalbuminaemia and congenital nephrosis.

Oedema

Oedema may be classified into generalized and localized, the causes being listed in Table 19.4. In the presence of oedema the skin and

Table 19.4   Causes of oedema

GENERALIZED
  Immaturity
  Cardiac failure
  Renal disease
  Cold injury
  Hypoproteinaemia
  Protein overload
  Fluid overload
  Sodium overload
LOCALIZED
  Birth trauma

subcutaneous tissues look and feel spongy or puffy, due to the excess of fluid which they contain. Pitting on pressure is a common but not invariable finding (Fig. 19.2). Oedema should be regarded as potentially serious when it is both gross and generalized, more especially when it develops in generalized form at an interval of some days after birth. In such circumstances possible causes are cardiac failure, kidney disease, cold injury, hypoproteinaemia and sodium overload. The potential seriousness of oedema is increased when there is associated hypothermia.

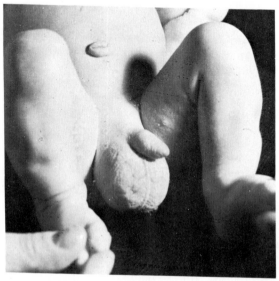

Fig. 19.2 Pitting oedema of lower legs.

Low birth weight

Many small preterm infants show oedema of the face, limbs, pubis and external genitalia during the first few days of life. Pitting on pressure can be demonstrated in the pubis and legs but not in the face. Oedema of any considerable extent in the very small infant results in the skin having a characteristically shiny appearance. In the absence of renal disease, and provided it begins to disappear gradually within 48 hours of birth, oedema in the newly born preterm infant need not cause undue concern.

Cardiac failure

The infant in cardiac failure from congenital heart disease presents with tachypnoea, tachycardia, hepatomegaly and oedema with unexpected weight gain. Hydrops fetalis is a severe form of heart failure in haemolytic disease. Treatment was dealt with in Chapter 11.

Renal immaturity

As mentioned in Chapter 9 the presence of oedema in the preterm infant is generally accepted as evidence of immature renal function which is usually associated with sodium retention. It will also be recalled that the immature kidney is unable to deal effectively with urea and phosphate. Apart from these physiological handicaps kidney disease proper, including urinary tract infection, and congenital nephrosis, are both associated with oedema.

Hypoproteinaemia occurs in congenital nephrosis and cystic fibrosis, may be found in immature infants, and may result from feeding a protein deficient milk or rarely from placental chorangioma.

Congenital nephrosis may be transmitted as an autosomal recessive condition, be secondary to cytomegalovirus infection, renal vein thrombosis or syphilis, or may be due to maternofetal antibody transference following a previous fetal death. The placenta is usually large and pale, weighing up to 50% of the infant's birth weight. Oedema may be present at birth with albuminuria, hypo-albuminaemia and hypercholesterolaemia and death due to infection is invariable. Renal biopsy is useful as a guide to prognosis of the two main pathological varieties. Infants with the Finnish type congenital nephrosis who have immature glomeruli and cystic dilatation of the proximal tubules die early whereas those with the glomerulosclerotic type of congenital nephrosis may survive into their teens. Antenatal diagnosis is possible by finding a high alpha-fetoprotein level in the amniotic fluid affording the opportunity of terminating an affected pregnancy.

Mineral overload. Oedema is also associated with the mineral overload which results from use of an unmodified or overconcentrated feed.

Localized oedema

The infant born at term rarely shows evidence of oedema other than that occurring locally as a result of trauma. The caput succedaneum is one example, and it should be remembered that oedema of the scalp sometimes changes position under the influence of gravity. Other causes of oedema of the extremities include Turner's syndrome (Fig. 19.3) and idiopathic hereditary lymphoedema.

Oedema of the brain was discussed in Chapter 12, which dealt with birth asphyxia.

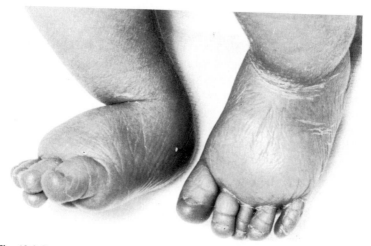

Fig. 19.3 Lymphoedema in infant with ovarian dysgenesis. (Bonnevie-Ullrich variant of Turner's syndrome.)

PYREXIA

Definition

Pyrexia is present when under normal environmental conditions the rectal temperature exceeds 37.5 °C. It may or may not be of serious significance and an attempt should be made to determine the cause even in the absence of other signs.

Temperature recording. Twice-daily recordings of temperature should be a routine in all maternity hospital nurseries to detect both hyper- and hypothermia. This may be taken either in the axilla or, with the greatest care, rectally. The temperature chart of a baby due for discharge should always be carefully scrutinized. Pyrexia may be the first detectable sign of infection.

A distinction must be made between a fluctuating body temperature, which usually signifies a high environmental temperature, and the permanently elevated body temperature commonly associated with infection. Exposure to the sun, excessive clothing and nursing in an overheated incubator are all factors in promoting a high environmental temperature (Chapter 5).

Common causes of pyrexia

Infection, stress of labour or delivery and dehydration are the commonest causes of an elevated temperature. Infection has been considered in Chapter 14.

Dehydration fever may result from the baby receiving inadequate fluid. In units where newly born infants are given adequate fluids dehydration fever is rarely encountered.

ABDOMINAL DISTENSION

The common causes of abdominal distension are listed in Table 19.5.

Table 19.5 Causes of abdominal distension

Gaseous distension
Intestinal obstruction and peritonitis
Enlarged intra-abdominal organ
Absent or weak abdominal muscles
Ascites

Gaseous distension

Air swallowing is a frequent finding in infants who are greedy feeders or who are constantly crying. Unless the swallowed air is returned by eructation gaseous distension of the bowel follows.

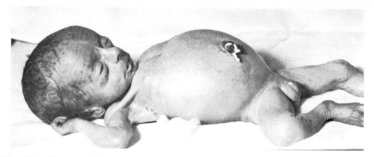

Fig. 19.4 Gaseous abdominal distension.

Bad feeding technique using a teat with too small a hole encouraging air swallowing is another cause of gaseous distension. Gaseous distension is also a complication of feeding carbohydrate-rich milk preparations.

Infection. Gaseous abdominal distension can complicate serious illness of any kind in the newborn (Fig. 19.4). It is a common complication of septicaemia and of intrathoracic infection, more especially in low birth weight infants. The resultant pressure on the diaphragm increases respiratory and cardiac embarrassment and adds to the seriousness of the prognosis.

Management. Treatment of infection and attention to feeding techniques are necessary. In many situations there is no treatment other than waiting for the gas to be passed from the anus. Trial should be made of keeping the baby supported in his cot in a sitting position. If oral feeds are given they must be small and frequent.

Intestinal obstruction

Intestinal obstruction is accompanied by distension. The more important causes of intestinal obstruction (principally mechanical) were discussed earlier in this chapter when dealing with vomiting. In some cases paralytic ileus may be a complication of hypoglycaemia, hypoxaemia, severe sepsis or hypothermia. Correction of the primary condition relieves the ileus but frequently not without the aid of intravenous therapy.

Milk plug syndrome. Rarely, in infants receiving large volumes of cow's milk, thick curds may obstruct the small bowel, especially the terminal ileum near the ileocaecal valve. The syndrome usually occurs between the second and tenth days of life and in 50% of cases is heralded by rectal bleeding. Abdominal X-rays are diagnostic showing low small bowel fluid levels, replacement of the normal gas pattern in the right lower quadrant of the abdomen by a faecal mass containing bubbles and the presence of gas in the rectum. In medical treatment with a gastrografin enema (which is also diagnostic) fails then surgical treatment will be necessary, when at laparotomy the bolus will be broken up through the bowel wall.

Peritonitis. In the presence of peritonitis, distension is characterized by limited or absent abdominal movements, shiny tautness of the skin and sometimes exaggerated protrusion of the umbilicus. Abdominal distension is a feature also of postnatal perforation due to peptic ulceration or very rarely to appendicitis or Meckel's diverticulitis. Bacterial peritonitis supervenes.

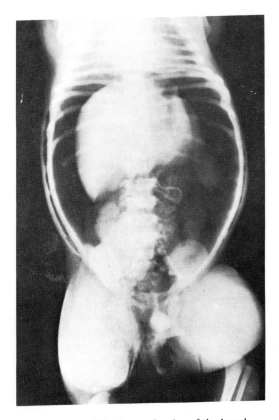

Fig. 19.5 Pneumoperitoneum following perforation of the bowel.

Spontaneous perforation of the bowel with peritonitis occurs as a rare but early complication of exchange blood transfusion (Fig. 19.5). There may or may not be signs of intestinal obstruction, and in a significant proportion of cases distension is accompanied by melaena. On occasion, there may be features indicative of necrotizing enterocolitis. Treatment consists of immediate laparotomy and broad-spectrum antibiotic therapy, although recently paediatric surgeons have recommended simple drainage in extremely low birth weight infants.

Enlargement of an intra-abdominal organ

Enlargement of an intra-abdominal organ, most commonly the kidney (see later), causes distension of the abdomen. The causes of hepatosplenomegaly will be discussed later. Distension of the bladder can also be the cause of an enlarged abdomen.

Stomach. In immature preterm infants temporary distension is a common finding after feeds. The outline or pattern of the stomach or bowel is often easily recognizable and there may be visible peristalsis.

Meconium. Persistent distension in low birth weight babies may be associated with delay in passing meconium which has been

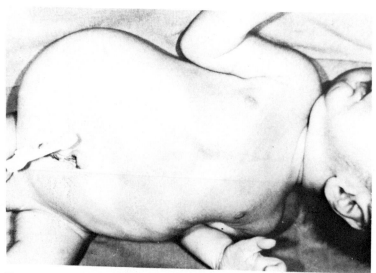

Fig. 19.6 Prune belly syndrome.

related to the thin abdominal wall and weak abdominal musculature. If delay in passing meconium extends beyond three or four
days, a per rectum examination may produce evacuation. A test for
undigested protein in meconium such as the appropriate BM test
should be performed on the meconium passed following the examination to exclude cystic fibrosis.

Prune belly syndrome. Congenital absence of the abdominal
musculature in association with hydronephrosis, hydroureter and
cryptorchidism is a feature of the prune belly syndrome (Figs 19.6
and 19.7).

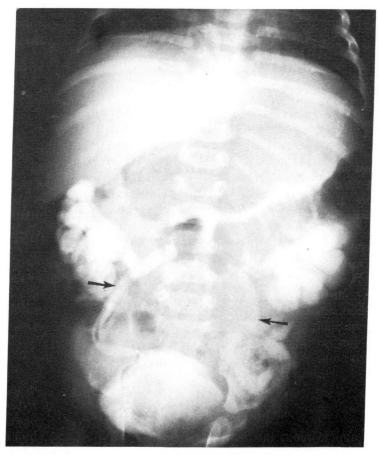

Fig. 19.7 Hydronephrosis and hydroureters in a baby with prune belly
syndrome.

Ascites

Ascites is a feature of haemolytic disease (hydrops fetalis), the nephrotic syndrome, cardiac failure and occasionally its presence is unexplained. An even rarer finding consists of chylous ascites due to anomalies of the lymph channels. At first clear, the abdominal fluid becomes cream-like in colour and consistency after milk feeding has been established.

ABDOMINAL MASSES

The majority of abdominal masses are palpable kidneys. During the early days of life it is usually possible to palpate the lower poles of the kidneys. Occasionally the kidney is displaced downwards and it is easily felt in the ectopic position.

Enlarged kidneys

The causes of an enlarged kidney are listed in Table 19.6. Renal vein thrombosis and renal infarction are the only conditions likely to make the infant ill.

Renal vein thrombosis occurs as a result of severe perinatal hypoxia and is also related to infections and severe dehydration. Affected infants present with albuminuria and haematuria. The resulting haemorrhagic infarction of the kidney causes palpable enlargement. Bilateral renal vein thrombosis is fatal. Nephrectomy is indicated for unilateral renal vein thrombosis if there is resultant hypertension.

Infarction of the kidney. As already mentioned, renal vein throm-

Table 19.6 Causes of enlarged and palpable kidney

Normally palpable
Downward displacement of a normal kidney
  Ectopic
  Adrenal haemorrhage
  Adrenal tumour
Hydronephrosis
Cystic kidney
Renal vein thrombosis
Renal infarction
Duplex kidney
Horseshoe kidney
Wilm's tumour

bosis leads to infarction of the kidney. Other causes are severe dehydration, severe asphyxia and as a terminal event in the presence of a failing circulation. Renal infarction is accompanied by haematuria and palpable enlargement of the kidney. Sometimes after severe perinatal hypoxia there can be considerable enlargement of the kidneys without evidence for renal vein thrombosis and with apparent recovery of function and return to normal size after a few days.

Hydronephrosis. A smoothly enlarged kidney would favour a diagnosis of hydronephrosis.

Polycystic kidneys. An irregular mass is a feature of polycystic kidneys and Wilm's tumour. In the case of Wilm's tumour the mass is firm and hard whereas in polycystic disease the surface of the kidney is finely nodular. The former is amenable to surgical excision, the latter usually fatal in a few months if it is truly polycystic rather than multicystic.

Multicystic kidneys. This developmental defect may be unilateral or bilateral and is the result of a failure of the embryonic glomeruli and tubules to unite properly.

Duplex and horseshoe kidneys are firm and smooth on examination whilst and adrenal tumour merely displaces a normal kidney downwards thereby rendering it palpable.

Adrenal haemorrhage. In Chapter 13, when dealing with injury, it will be recalled that severe hypoxia, breech delivery and a combination of these favour massive haemorrhage into the adrenal glands. Death is the usual outcome but should the infant survive the glands are subsequently calcified and easily demonstrated on X-ray examination.

Urine examination may be helpful in diagnosis. Gross haematuria is found in renal vein thrombosis and may also occur in renal infarction, hydronephrosis and Wilm's tumour. Albuminuria is a feature of polycystic kidney and renal vein thrombosis. Pus cells and casts are found with infarcted kidneys and are present in the other conditions only in the presence of secondary infection.

The blood urea concentration is increased and plasma electrolytes may be abnormal in renal vein thrombosis, hydronephrosis and polycystic disease and whenever the renal tract becomes infected.

Renal ultrasound, intravenous pyelography, cystoscopy and retrograde pyelography usually provide sufficient evidence on which to base a definite diagnosis.

Surgical treatment is carried out where indicated.

Hepatosplenomegaly

The liver and spleen may be just palpable in the healthy newborn infant. The thin abdominal wall of the low birth weight baby makes for easy palpation of the liver and spleen.

Causes

Hepatosplenomegaly is a feature of haemolytic disease, septicaemia, congenital syphilis, virus diseases, including rubella, cytomegalovirus disease and hepatitis, and toxoplasmosis. Haemolytic disease is usually due to ABO group or rhesus incompatibility. Less commonly, incompatibility of the fetus and mother for the Kell or other rare group may be the cause. Other less common causes of haemolytic disease in this country are congenital spherocytosis (acholuric jaundice), sickle cell anaemia, thalassaemia and G6PDH deficiency. Haemolytic disease has been described in Chapter 15.

Delay in passage of meconium

The first meconium stool in passed by 95% of normal infants within 24 hours of birth. Failure to pass a stool within the first 24 hours must be regarded with suspicion if meconium has not been passed before or during birth. Delay in passage of meconium (Table 19.7) may be associated with congenital abnormalities of the gut, abnormal consistency of the meconium and weak musculature. Meconium will not be passed when the baby has an anal or rectal atresia and passage will be delayed in Hirschsprung's disease.

Absence of abdominal musculature in the prune belly syndrome and paralysis of these muscles due to spina bifida may account for delay in passage of meconium.

Table 19.7 Causes of delayed passage of meconium

Congenital abnormalities of the gut
  Anorectal abnormalities
  Hirschsprung's disease
Abnormal consistency of meconium
  Meconium ileus
  Meconium plug syndrome
Weak, absent or paralysed muscles
  Immature preterm infants
  Prune belly syndrome
  Spina bifida

Anorectal abnormalities

Anal atresia should be recognized at the time of the first examination of the baby after birth (Fig. 19.8). Meconium staining is no assurance of the presence of a normal anus. Absence of the anus and atresia of the anus due to the persistence of a septum are sometimes associated with a rectourethral or rectovaginal fistula. In these circumstances the meconium is voided via the urethra or vagina. Alternatively the fistula may be more in the nature of a sinus and open to the exterior in the perineum of boys or between the fourchette and introitus in girls. Meconium may also be voided via a patent vitellointestinal duct.

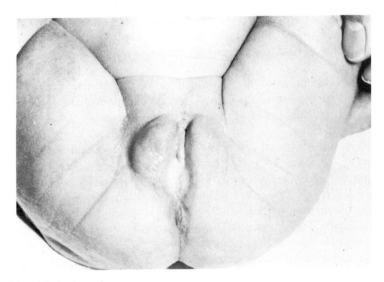

Fig. 19.8 Anal atresia.

Hirschsprung's disease

Hirschsprung's disease occurs when segments of the lower bowel have an incomplete nerve supply. The affected segments do not share in the normal peristaltic activity of the gut and remain narrow and collapsed. Segments of the gut proximal to the abnormal bowel are distended as a result of efforts to propel the contents to the colon beyond these abnormal segments. Distension together with diarrhoea and vomiting often first present within days of birth, when the diagnosis should be made. Hirschsprung's disease must always be considered in the differential diagnosis of intestinal obstruction in the newborn. The diagnosis is confirmed by biopsy of the affected bowel and demonstration of the absence of ganglion cells. Definitive surgical treatment is the excision of the aganglionic segment. Emergency treatment consists of making a temporary colostomy.

Meconium ileus

Infants with cystic fibrosis may present at birth with meconium ileus. In this condition, dry inspissated meconium may cause total intestinal obstruction at or even before birth. Meconium ileus occurring before birth may lead to intestinal perforation and meconium peritonitis. Ultrasonic examination of the fetal abdomen can detect the echogenic inspissated meconium and help in the prenatal diagnosis of cystic fibrosis. In meconium ileus the failure to pass meconium is absolute. X-ray examination of the abdomen shows tiny bubbles of gas trapped in the meconium contained in the small bowel.

The BM (meconium) or Albustix test on the meconium is positive. In the absence of proteolytic enzymes the meconium protein content is high and accounts for the positive test. The obstruction may be relieved by gastrograffin enemas but if they fail to relieve the obstruction within a short time, surgical decompression is indicated. Measurement of immunoreactive trypsin in a blood sample obtained at the end of the first week of life will help confirm the diagnosis of cystic fibrosis if the values are elevated. Many countries now include routine screening for cystic fibrosis in the metabolic screen performed on the capillary blood samples collected for phenylketonuria and hypothyroidism screening (see p. 321).

Meconium plug syndrome

Intestinal obstruction due to the meconium plug syndrome occurs in the absence of enzymatic and ganglion cell deficiency. The meconium is unusually thick and hard and rectal examination induces the passage of a firm plug of meconium. Thereafter normal bowel movement supervenes.

Failure of or delay in passage of urine

Micturition before delivery. It must be remembered that urine may have been passed unnoticed during delivery and so account for apparent failure to pass urine after birth.

Renal agenesis is a cause of failure to pass urine. Congenital absence of one kidney causes no symptoms but absence of both kidneys is incompatible with life. Lack of passage of urine into the amniotic cavity results in oligohydramnios with amnion nodosum. Fetal compression leads to altered facies (Fig. 19.9), abnormal positioning of the hands and feet and breech presentation. There is frequently pulmonary hypoplasia causing early death. Almost all affected infants are small-for-dates infants who possess certain pathognomonic features of the squashed baby syndrome first described by Potter. There include widely separated eyes, prominent epicanthic folds which run downward and then laterally below the eyes, flattened bridge of nose, receding chin and large, floppy, low-set ears.

Ureteral obstruction leading to hydronephrosis, hydroureter (but without megacystis) is rare. If bilateral it causes fetal or early post-natal death.

Bladder neck obstruction is evident as an enlargement of the

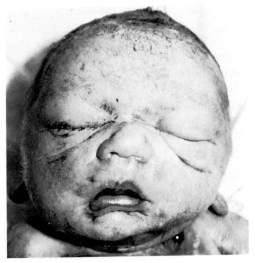

Fig. 19.9 The squashed facial appearance of an infant with renal agenesis (Potter's facies).

bladder, ureters and kidneys and difficulty in passing urine. It is commonly brought to light by the development of urinary tract infection. Obstruction at the bladder neck may be due to valves of redundant mucosa arising in the region of the verumontanum in males, stenosis or muscular hypertrophy of the bladder neck. Irrespective of the cause most infants are symptomless until infection develops and the kidneys have been seriously damaged. It is therefore imperative to exclude this remediable cause of renal damage by early investigation of infants with a persistently palpable bladder. In males the quality of the urine stream should also be visually confirmed before discharge, in an attempt to identify posterior urethral valves at an early stage. Careful ultrasonic examination of the fetus can detect many of these renal tract abnormalities prenatally. Results of fetal surgery to relieve ureteric obstruction have so far been disappointing.

CARDIAC MURMURS

At initial examination

Patent ductus arteriosus. A cardiac murmur is frequently heard during the initial routine examination after birth. Despite the murmur the baby is symptom-free and the usual explanation is a ductus arteriosus which is still patent. Normally the ductus arteriosus undergoes spontaneous closure shortly after birth with disappearance of the murmur. The ductus becomes converted gradually into a fibrous cord.

Small ventricular septal defects (VSD) may also produce a pansystolic murmur and they become more noticeable towards the end of the first week of life when the normally high right ventricular pressure falls, thus increasing the left to right shunt. The majority of these murmurs disappear in a few months as the VSD closes.

At later examination

Surprisingly, cardiac murmurs which signify congenital heart disease (Chapter 11) are not usually heard until after the first few days of life. Such murmurs may be accompanied by other signs and symptoms such as failure to thrive, tiring easily, reluctance to feed with panting respiration, constant or sporadic respiratory embarrassment of varying degree, sudden periods of distress suggestive of pain, and changes of colour which may be characterized by pallor, a grey cyanosis or intense blueness. Any of these signs can occur alone or in combination and may be present at birth or only develop gradually. Additional to the midwife's observations the doctor will note any deformity of the chest, tachypnoea, oedema, enlargement of the liver, position of the apex beat, presence or absence of the femoral pulses, exhaustion following examination and murmurs on auscultation. Such late signs and symptoms occur around the second to third week of life and are found particularly in cases of ventricular septal defect, Fallot's tetralogy and patent ductus arteriosus.

Cyanosis resulting from congenital heart disease has been discussed in Chapter 16. The anatomical and functional abnormalities likely to cause cyanosis were discussed in Chapter 11.

Diagnosis depends principally on the total clinical picture, as murmurs are frequently of little help at this early age. Chest X-ray and ECG often provide important information. Now that surgical treatment is possible in a considerable number of congenital heart lesions an accurate diagnosis is essential at an early age. This will generally involve echocardiography, cardiac catheterization and angiography. For this, transfer to a specialist unit is generally indicated.

SKIN RASHES

The skin of the newly born infant is extremely sensitive to rapid changes of environmental temperature, clothing and chemicals, so that rashes are a common finding. It is useful to separate them by cause into non-infective and infective groups (Table 19.8).

Non-infective

Urticaria neonatorum (also known as erythema toxicum) is an eruption which resembles papular urticaria or nettle rash. It is extremely common and is usually seen in the first week of life. The eruption appears as irregular blotchy red spots, each of which has a pale central papule or wheal. These erythematous spots are not raised above the level of the skin, but the central papules can be readily felt if a finger is drawn gently over the skin. Although the erythema is sometimes extensive, it often consists of only a few isolated spots. Development of the condition may be associated with overheating. Cases of urticaria neonatorum require no

Table 19.8 Skin rashes

NON-INFECTIVE
  Urticaria neonatorum
  Sweat rash
  Milia
  Seborrhoea of the scalp
  Seborrhoeic eczema
  Ammoniacal dermatitis
  Epidermolysis bullosa
  Petechiae
    Traumatic cyanosis
    Congenital thrombocytopenic purpura
  Drug rashes
INFECTIVE
  Pustules, infected vesicles and dermatitis
  Pemphigus neonatorum
  Exfoliative dermatitis
  Infected ammoniacal dermatitis
  Petechiae
    Rubella
    Toxoplasmosis
    Cytomegalovirus infection
  Vesicles
    Chickenpox
    Smallpox
  Granulomata

---

treatment. The condition is not infective and does not interfere with the baby's general progress.

Sweat rashes may be erythematous or vesicular.

The erythematous form is usually seen in the flexures after the first week of life and occurs most commonly in babies who have been nursed in a warm atmosphere with excessive clothing and who have had inadequate hygiene. Prevention and treatment are dependent on cleanliness, efficient drying of the skin and on the provision of clothing which should be light, airy and of suitable texture. Powders and lotions are no substitute for attention to the infant's personal hygiene.

Vesicular sweat rash appears as collections of very small vesicles on the head and chest of a baby who has been sweating as a result of illness or overheating. Each vesicle is related to a sweat gland, the duct of which has been obstructed and occluded. The vesicular rash differs from milia in that it is more gross in character and lacks the white opacity of the latter. Sweating in small preterm babies is less profuse than in larger infants, but occasionally minute colourless seed-like spots can be seen on the forehead of a prema-

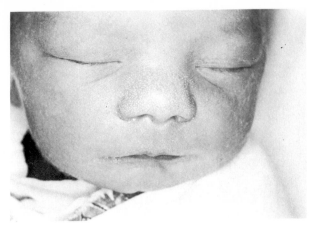

Fig. 19.10 Milia.

ture baby and these correspond to the vesicular rash of other babies.

Milia (Fig. 19.10) is a common finding and is the appearance on the nose and surrounding structures of large numbers of minute yellowish-white opalescent spots. If the tip of a finger is gently passed over these spots they can be felt as extremely small, firmly defined spots. The spots are not pustules but cysts consisting of obstructed sebaceous glands. They disappear without treatment and contrast with a vesicular sweat rash in not being due to excessive sweating.

Seborrhoea of the scalp (cradle cap) (Fig. 19.11) is not uncommon towards the end of the neonatal period and results from lack of attention to local hygiene. The normal secretion of the sebaceous glands of the scalp accumulates as a grey, rather greasy, crusted layer of irregular thickness. Many mothers are hesitant about washing their baby's scalp because of doubts concerning the risks attached to handling the open fontanelle. Soap and water suffice to remove the crust in most instances. In severe cases cleansing can be facilitated by gently rubbing olive or nut oil into the scalp. This loosens the crust. Where sebaceous secretion is more extensive and persistent than usual and after the crusts have been removed, washing the head with a solution of sodium bicarbonate, 5 g per 500 ml of warm sterile water is a valuable simple measure. Alternatively, Hibitane as a shampoo can be used.

Seborrhoeic dermatitis. Scales of scurf on the scalp and forehead

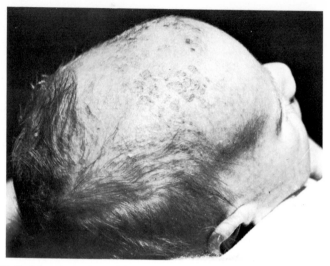

Fig. 19.11 Seborrhoea of the scalp.

are sometimes accompanied by a seborrhoeic condition behind the ears. This form of seborrhoeic dermatitis is milder than infantile eczema and responds rapidly to treatment. For mild cases bathing with sodium bicarbonate solution is adequate. Where the condition is more pronounced, benefit will result from the use of an ointment containing a very dilute steroid after first cleaning the affected areas with liquid paraffin, olive oil or a neutral soap.

Ammoniacal dermatitis is not seen so frequently in babies in the first week or two of life as it is in older infants. In its mildest form the dermatitis consists of no more than an erythema. Excoriation and ulceration may occur. Characteristically the skin involved corresponds to the area covered by the napkin, and, where there are folds in the skin, the raised margins are affected while the depressions between are not. The dermatitis results from irritation of the skin by ammonia liberated from the urea of the urine by the action of organisms excreted in the faeces.

Napkin changing. Attention to napkin changing is of first importance in the matter of local treatment. Napkins must be changed as soon as they are wet or soiled. The numbers of changes involved in the 24 hours is considerably in excess of that expected by most mothers. Destructable napkins are valuable but expensive. Ordinary napkins, if used, should be treated with a chemical disinfectant after initial rinsing, and if they have been washed with soap or detergents they must be thoroughly rinsed until all the soap or detergent has been removed. Occasionally the disinfecting compound may produce skin irritation if there is insufficient rinsing, and its use may have to be discontinued.

Epidermolysis bullosa is a rare condition which may be mistaken for pemphigus. It is an inherited condition characterized by the appearance of vesicles and bullae in parts of the skin subjected to pressure or trauma. There is sometimes malformation of the nails. Occasionally involvement of the buccal mucous membrane creates a critical feeding problem. Secondary infection is a constant risk. Treatment is limited to evacuation of the bullae, the use of a mild antiseptic ointment and the giving of antibiotics if infection develops.

In traumatic cyanosis petechiae are limited to the head and neck and result from compression during the process of delivery. Usually the cord has been wrapped tightly around the neck or the head has been on the perineum for some considerable time. The petechiae disappear spontaneously and no treatment is necessary.

Drug rashes is the form of bullous eruptions are sometimes found in the newly born infant after the mother has been taking anti-mitotic or cytotoxic drugs during later pregnancy. When administered in relatively high doses during the first months of pregnancy these drugs may cause fetal death or multiple malformations.

Infective

Skin infections may present as pustules, secondarily infected vesicles, or dermatitis with or without exfoliation. They may occur in any site, but should be looked for particularly where skin surfaces are normally opposed as in the axillae, the groins, the folds of the neck and the perineum. Any of the lesions may occur singly, in local crops, or simultaneously in a number of situations. They may spread locally, become generalized and diffuse, or assume the form of frank furunculosis. In its most severe forms spread gives rise to cellulitis or deep abscess formation. There may be difficulty in differentiating an early pustule from an uninfected papule or even from urticaria neonatorum.

Pemphigus neonatorum is now a rare condition. Large bullous eruptions with hyperaemic margins and raw moist surfaces after exfoliation are associated with systemic disturbance.

Exfoliative dermatitis. A more severe form of pemphigus is exfoliative dermatitis (Ritter's disease), which constitutes an emergency requiring isolation, antibiotic therapy and frequently intravenous fluids. The organism responsible is usually *Staphylococcus aureus* phage type 71.

Treatment of minor skin lesions consists in the application of spirit and a mild antiseptic powder, having first obtained a swab of the lesion for culture of the organism (Chapter 14). More extensive and more advanced lesions require systemic antibiotic therapy in addition to local treatment.

Secondary infection of an ammoniacal dermatitis by staphylococci, *E. coli* and *Candida albicans* is not uncommon. Where infection is due to staphylococci or *E. coli* treatment consists in the application of an antiseptic or antibiotic cream followed by the regular use of a barrier cream. Whenever a napkin rash does not respond to treatment and there is a history of oral thrush, especially if the infant has been in receipt of oral antibiotics, then the possibility of a *Candida albicans* infection must not be forgotten. The affected area

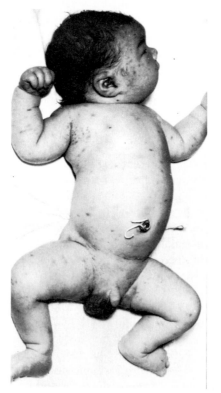

Fig. 19.12 Generalized petechiae.

is usually intensely red with numerous satellite lesions away from the main area of infection. In addition, the skin folds are not spared as in ammoniacal napkin rash. Treatment consists in giving Nystatin 100 000 units (contained in 1 ml) by mouth four times daily after feeds for at least five to seven days, and the local application of a Nystatin-containing cream until the infection has cleared.

Petechiae (Fig. 19.12) distributed over the whole body are a feature of congenital rubella, toxoplasmosis and cytomegalovirus infection.

Transplacental infections. A baby may show evidence of chickenpox and smallpox at birth having contracted the disease from his mother in utero. Other diseases contracted during pregnancy and marked by a rash at birth include syphilis, measles and typhoid fever (Chapter 14).

Granulomata of the skin are a feature of infection with *Listeria monocytogenes* contracted by the baby during delivery. The more usual presentation of *Listeria monocytogenes* infection is meningitis. Treatment consists in the administration of both penicillin and ampicillin when survival is now to be expected.

20

Practical procedures

Any book on the care of the newborn infant would be incomplete without some guidance on nursing and medical aspects of practical procedures as applied to the newborn. Some procedures such as umbilical artery or vein cannulation will only be of significance at this period but others such as lumbar puncture are essentially similar at all ages but require modification for the newborn. Similarly the general nursing and medical principles of preparation of the necessary materials and of asepsis and antisepsis apply to all ages but may require modification for use at this age.

General principles

No attempt will be made here to give guidance on those general principles which are taught as part of basic nursing and medical training but attention will be concentrated on those aspects which require particular attention when applied to a small helpless infant.

Central sterile supply. As most hospitals in developed countries have some form of central sterile supply with prepared packs for nursing procedures we shall not give lists of the materials required for each procedure. Some indication of any special instruments likely to be required will, however, be given.

Prevention of heat loss

The very small size of the newborn infant is the most obvious difficulty to be encountered in undertaking practical procedures at this age. Less obvious is the need to protect the infant against heat loss. This can be done by reducing exposure to the minimum, maintaining a high environmental temperature (above 25 °C) — avoiding draughts and moisture on skin surfaces and by the provision of extra warmth from radiant heat sources or by an electrically heated mattress. Precautions must equally be taken to prevent burns. Many procedures can be carried out in incubators if necessary.

Immobilization

Whereas the small sick infant may be inactive and immobile, healthy mature infants can be surprisingly active and will require immobilization. The success of many procedures is largely dependent on the way the infant is held. We shall describe the immobilization and positioning for each procedure as appropriate.

Protection of the infant

Gentleness and reasonable speed are requirements common to all procedures.

Inhalation of vomit. Protection of the infant from harmful side effects of all aspects of any procedure must be kept constantly in mind. This includes protection of the infant against the risk of inhalation of vomitus.

Feeds. Although an infant may be quieter after a feed major procedures are safer if left for one hour or more after a feed. If this delay is not justifiable the stomach should be emptied before any procedure, such as lumbar puncture, in which the infant is held with the spine flexed, which might provoke vomiting.

Suction. Facilities for suction of the pharynx and for tracheal intubation should be immediately at hand for the resuscitation of any infant who develops respiratory problems during a procedure.

Equipment. All equipment likely to be required must be checked before the procedure is started.

Training. Because of the potential risks involved no procedure should be carried out by those who have not had full training in the techniques involved.

Preparation

It is the responsibility of the senior nursing and medical staff present to make sure that all preparations have been completed and that all the equipment is ready before allowing the procedure to start. If any of the staff have not been present at a similar procedure previously it is essential that instruction be given beforehand about the part that each member of the staff is expected to take particularly any emergency action that might be expected of them.

Records. One member should be given the express duty of keeping a record of what has been done, of any drugs administered and of instructions about further observations or treatment. Such detailed action may seem unnecessary for simple procedures but it is only by being prepared for complications that even simple procedures can be made absolutely safe.

COLLECTION OF SPECIMENS

Of the procedures likely to be carried out on newborn infants collection of specimens for microbiological or biochemical examination are the most common and therefore probably the most time consuming. Skill in these minor procedures is just as important as ability to carry out major procedures and attention to detail will save unnecessary disturbance of the infant and avoid wasting the operator's time.

Microbiology of superficial sites

As discussed in Chapter 14, knowledge of the organisms acquired by an infant during or after delivery is essential to the management of potential or open infection in the individual infant in the nursery as a unit.

Microbiological samples

Microbiological samples, should be taken from those sites known to have the highest chance of colonization. These are shown in Table 20.1.

Table 20.1 Sites from which swabs should be taken for microbiological examination in suspected infections

Nose
Throat
Ear
Umbilicus
Groin

Swabbing. When taking specimens from these sites it is generally most convenient to use a sterile cotton wool pledget on the end of an orange stick in a sterile test tube or some similar type of 'swab'. The swab should come into contact with the area concerned but undue pressure which might cause local injury and promote entry of organisms to deeper tissues must be avoided.

Plating. Special arrangements for the immediate plating of a conjunctival discharge suspected of being due to the gonococcus may be required by the microbiologist. Similarly special arrangements may be required for viral cultures. Consultation with the laboratory concerned is therefore advisable before taking any specimens requiring special studies.

Labelling. All specimens must be accurately labelled with both the infant's name and the site from which it was taken. It is also useful to record in the infant's notes that the specimens have been taken.

COLLECTION OF BLOOD SAMPLES

Samples of blood are generally only required in healthy infants for routine procedures such as the Guthrie test. Very small and ill infants may, however, require repeated blood samples for biochemical and microbiological testing. It is essential that those involved in sample collection thoroughly wash their hands to the elbow before the procedure.

Volume

In some infants the amounts withdrawn, unless strictly controlled, can soon accumulate to surprisingly large volumes, sufficient to require replacement by transfusion. Always keep in mind the infant's blood volume is 80 ml/kg.

Micromethods. Infants likely to require repeated investigations should not be treated in units where there are no facilities for biochemical investigations using micro or ultra-micro methods.

Record. Where such methods are available the medical staff must be constantly aware of the volume of blood being taken for investigations and a record should be kept of the volume of all specimens withdrawn. Such a record often has a salutary effect in keeping the number of investigations down to the level necessary to the proper management of the infant involved.

Consultation. An insufficient specimen may prove of no use to the laboratory and a further larger specimen be demanded. Before taking blood the volume required by the laboratory should be checked, bearing in mind the possibility of a high PCV and low plasma volume in the first few days of life and where there is dehydration. Prior discussion with the biochemist will often lead to a more rational and economical form of investigation.

Capillary samples

Capillary blood is suitable for many biochemical investigations and, except in shocked infants, is easy to obtain.

Sites. Several sites may be used; those most commonly employed being the heel, the finger and the ear lobe. Because of the risk of transfer of infection disposable sterile lancets should be used. The skin must be warm and pink, indicating an adequate peripheral blood flow.

Technique for heel prick. When the heel is used it should be held as shown in Figure 20.1. The skin is sterilized with surgical spirit and allowed to dry. Smearing the surrounding area with sterile white paraffin helps to prevent dispersion of the blood when it

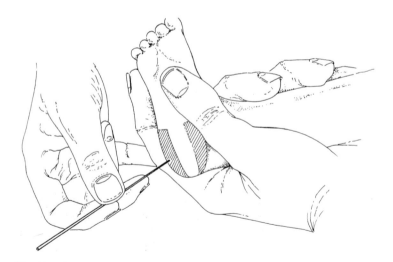

Fig. 20.1 Capillary blood being obtained from heel stab. The puncture site should not be on the plantar aspect but on the lateral or medial aspects of the heel.

begins to flow and is used in some units. A firm stab into the lateral border of the heel with the lancet is preferable to a tentative scratch which may have to be repeated several times. In most infants at least 1.0 ml of capillary blood can be obtained readily.

Specimen tubes. Capillary tubing, heparinized where necessary, is suitable for collecting capillary blood samples but specimens may also be taken into small containers. Wide containers are not in general suitable for small volume specimens.

Control of bleeding. When the specimen has been collected, care must be taken to ensure that bleeding has ceased completely and a small protective dressing should be applied to prevent abrasion of the site and possible further bleeding. If blood does not flow freely from the original site another site should be chosen and the procedure repeated or the specimen should be taken by venepuncture.

Arterialized capillary blood

The technique for taking 'arterialized capillary blood' for blood gas analysis is as given above. Particular attention must be paid to the state of the local circulation, and unless the skin is throughly warm and pink the specimen taken is more likely to represent venous capillary blood.

Venous blood

When the infant's circulation is too poor to allow adequate capillary samples, or where larger volumes than 1 ml are required, blood should be taken from a vein except in those particular situations where arterial blood is required as discussed below. Individual doctors have their own particular preference as to which vein to try first. Although it is a good thing to acquire expertise in one method it is also advisable to have experience of venepuncture at more than one site.

Hand veins. By using a hypodermic (size 21–23 gauge) needle in a small vein on the back of the hand and allowing the blood to drip directly into the specimen tube small volumes of blood, e.g. 2 ml, can often be obtained with minimum disturbance of the infant.

Larger veins are advisable where specimens are to be withdrawn into a syringe.

Preparation

Position. In each case careful preparation is required with immobilization and accurate positioning of the infant. Such procedures are therefore more likely to distress the infant, and every effort should be made to limit the time of the procedure and to ensure that an adequate specimen is obtained at the first attempt especially in sick preterm infants where apnoea may be induced.

Heat loss. As in all procedures, precautions should be taken to prevent heat loss.

Two people are required, one to hold the infant and the other to take the specimen.

The skin should be cleaned and treated with a local antiseptic such as 70% alcohol.

The syringe should not be larger than is required to hold the specimen.

The needle. Gauge 21 is generally suitable for most purposes. Some clinicians prefer to use 'Butterfly' type needles but this is more expensive. Special short shaft and short bevelled needles are required for puncture of the superior sagittal sinus.

Antecubital fossa veins

Both the medial basilic and cephalic vein can usually be identified in the antecubital fossa.

Position. The nurse holding the infant should fix the upper limb by a gentle but firm hold on the upper arm and below the wrist. Gentle pressure should be applied above the elbow to distend the veins. The veins are visualized or palpated and the skin cleaned efficiently.

Puncture. Blood can be readily obtained using a 21 or 23 gauge needle and syringe by the method commonly used in older children and adults. Gentle local pressure is applied following removal of the needle and a sterile adhesive patch applied. This is the site of choice for blood culture and most venous blood collection procedures (Fig. 20.2).

External and internal jugular vein

The positioning for puncture of the external/internal jugular vein (Fig. 20.3) is not comfortable for the infant and may require the assistance of a third person to hold the head if the infant objects violently.

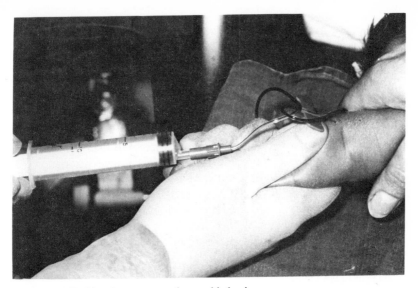

Fig. 20.2 Position for puncture of antecubital veins.

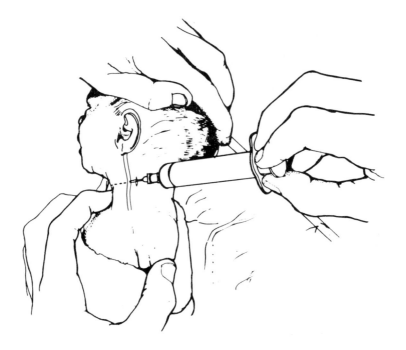

Fig. 20.3 Position for external jugular vein puncture.

The external jugular vein can most readily be identified when the infant is crying or the vein has been obstructed by pressure just above the clavicle. The internal jugular vein, although not visible, is readily located with experience.

Position. When the most suitable side has been chosen the wrapped infant is held supine with its shoulders at the table edge. The neck is then rotated to look over the opposite shoulder and the head depressed.

Puncture. As the vein is most obvious where it crosses the sterno-mastoid muscle it is advisable to insert the needle through the skin in the line of the vein but nearer the angle of the mandible. The needle is then advanced to enter the vein as it lies over the sternomastoid muscle and blood is withdrawn. After the procedure local pressure should be applied if there is any bleeding but often all that is required is to sit the baby up.

Femoral vein

Skin preparation. Because of the probability of bacterial colonization of the skin in the inguinal region particular attention must be taken in cleaning the skin. The site is not satisfactory for taking blood for culture as contamination by skin organisms is difficult to avoid. Many clinicians avoid its use because of the danger of introducing infection into the underlying hip joint.

The femoral vein lies immediately medial to the femoral artery and the femoral artery must be identified before attempting to enter the vein.

Position. For right-handed people it is generally easiest to keep a finger of the left hand on the infant's right femoral artery and to hold the syringe and needle in the right hand. Nurse, or whoever is holding the infant, places the buttocks near the edge of the table and partially abducts the infants thighs holding them steady with her hands and immobilizing the infant with inward pressure from her forearms. This is made easier if the infant's arms have been immobilized by being wrapped in a small blanket or towel. Having ensured that the infant is comfortably held the inguinal region is carefully sterilized and the femoral artery identified.

Puncture. The puncture is then made vertically slightly medial to the line of the artery and 0.5 to 1.0 cm distal to the inguinal ligament. The fingers of the left hand can now be used to steady the syringe and needle while the right hand is used to withdraw the plunger of the syringe slightly to maintain a small negative

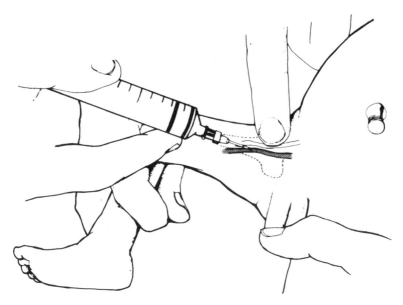

Fig. 20.4 Position for femoral vein puncture.

pressure in the syringe as the needle is slowly advanced. If blood is not obtained after the needle point has been advanced 1.0 cm, the needle should be slowly withdrawn, maintaining a negative pressure. Provided the site has been correctly chosen blood should be obtained readily (Fig. 20.4).

Problems. If blood is not obtained the needle should be withdrawn, and no further attempt made. After withdrawal of the needle firm pressure should be applied over the vein until it is quite certain that bleeding from the vein whether superficial or subcutaneous has ceased. A sterile occlusive dressing should be applied.

Risks of femoral vein puncture include haemorrhage and thrombosis of the vein. The artery may be entered accidentally. Infection may be introduced. For those reasons the femoral vein should be avoided wherever possible.

Superior sagittal sinus

Precautions. Injections or infusions should never be given into the superior sagittal sinus because of the risk of thrombosis or the possibility of the needle moving out of the sinus. There appears to be very little, if any, risk associated with removal of blood from the sinus provided that certain precautions are observed. This method should not be used in dehydrated infants or those with a suspected bleeding problem.

Training. It should only be used by those who have been competently trained in the technique and this applies particularly to the person holding the infant.

Needle. The normal long shaft, long bevelled needle used for other venepunctures must not be used for this procedure. Gauge 22 needles, with the shaft cut down to 2 cm length and with a short bevel, have to be prepared locally and sterilized. No other special equipment is required.

Fontanelle. As the superior sagittal sinus is larger and has a greater blood flow at the posterior as opposed to the anterior fontanelle, and as the posterior fontanelle is generally open during the first month of life, the procedure in relation to the posterior fontanelle will be described.

Position. Before positioning the infant the posterior fontanelle should be palpated to make sure that there is no difficulty in its identification. Both operator and nurse should be sitting on chairs or stools facing one another. The infant is wrapped and placed on nurse's knee in the sitting position with his back towards the operator. Nurse steadies the trunk with her forearms resting her elbows on her knees. With her hands she holds the infant's head with the neck slightly flexed. By applying traction with her palms and fingers she draws the infant's scalp forward and downward so that the area over the posterior fontanelle becomes tense and the sutures are separated to their maximum extent. At the same time nurse must hold the head absolutely steady. The technique of holding the infant is essential to the success and safety of posterior fontanelle tap and should always be rehearsed with each infant before puncture is made.

Technique. When a satisfactory position has been achieved the hair over the posterior fontanelle is shaved and the skin sterilized. The operator should hold the syringe as shown in Figure 20.5 using the forefinger of the right hand as a guide to the depth to which the needle is inserted. The fingers of the left hand can be used to check on the suture lines and aid in the spreading effect. As the needle is inserted through the skin the syringe should be lowered so that the needle is pointing towards the anterior fontanelle. Resistance will be felt as the external dura mater is entered and a short push will be required to enter the sinus. It is because of the risk of perforating the opposite wall of the sinus during this push

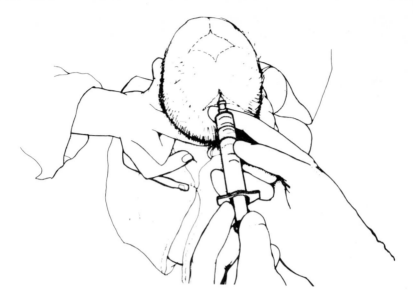

Fig. 20.5 Position for sagittal sinus puncture through the posterior fontanelle.

that short shaft, short bevelled needles are essential. When the sinus has been entered blood can be easily withdrawn and care must be taken not to exceed the volume required.

After removal of the needle firm pressure over the fontanelle should be maintained until bleeding has stopped.

More space has been spent on describing this method of venepuncture because, if correctly carried out, it is easy and rapid to perform, causes less distress to an active infant and will readily provide larger volumes of blood should these be necessary.

Umbilical vein cannulation

In situations where continuous intravenous therapy is required umbilical vein cannulations will provide a route for treatment and venous blood specimens can also be withdrawn from the cannula with suitable precautions to ensure that they are not contaminated by fluid being given.

Equipment. Apart from suitable towels, swabs and antiseptic solution the equipment required is as follows (Fig. 20.6):

1 pair Spencer-Wells forceps
2 mosquito artery forceps

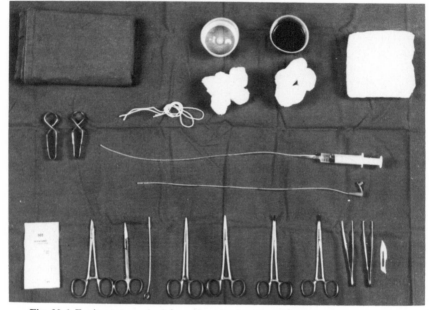

Fig. 20.6 Equipment required for catheterization of umbilical vessels.

1 pair small dissecting forceps
1 pair small toothed forceps
1 pair dressing scissors
1 pair ophthalmic scissors
Black silk and needle
Needle holding forceps
Umbilical catheters sizes 4.5 to 9.0 fg (these should be side hole)

Preparation. The clamp or ligature used to prevent bleeding from the cord may have to be moved distally or removed to allow about 2 cm of cord to be exposed. The cord over this area and the surrounding skin is prepared with antiseptic and the area draped with a sterile towel.

Incision. The cord is transected approximately 1 cm from the abdominal wall. The vein is easily recognizable as being much the larger of the three vessels. It usually lies open in the exposed cord. The arteries are usually smaller, thicker walled, whiter and closed.

Introduction of catheter. The exposed and transected vein is held by one or two mosquito forceps applied to grip the edges of the vein. If closed, slight traction on these forceps will create an opening into which the catheter can be introduced and advanced

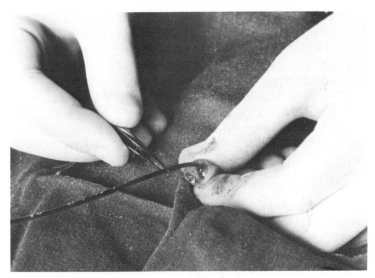

Fig. 20.7 Introduction of catheter into umbilical vein.

(Fig. 20.7). Some obstruction may be encountered when the catheter reaches the point at which the vein passes through the abdominal wall. Pressure above the umbilicus may help to overcome this. The catheter is advanced gently to a distance of about 8 to 12 cm according to the infant's size until blood flows back freely. It is useful to note the distance the catheter has been advanced or to mark it. Radiological confirmation of the catheter tip position is recommended.

Management. The catheter is then connected to the giving set or syringe according to the procedure intended by a two- or three-way tap. If the catheter is to be left in place but no immediate transfusion is to be undertaken it should be filled with 0.9% saline containing 1 unit heparin per ml to prevent clotting or a slow transfusion of dextrose/electrolyte, begun at 1–2 ml per hour, to maintain patency. The forceps are removed and the catheter held in place by a black silk 'purse-string' suture. If there is bleeding around the catheter a ligature should be placed around the cord stump but this must not be sufficiently tight to occlude flow through the catheter.

Complications. Umbilical vein catheters provide a possible entry for infection into the portal circulation. Hyperosmolar solutions given by this means may cause thrombosis. These complications must be borne in mind when using this route for intravenous infusions. Other veins may be equally suitable and less open to risk. If the umbilical vein is used the catheter should be left in for as short a time as possible and seldom more than 48 hours.

Withdrawal of the catheter. It is advisable to arrange for microbiological examination of the tip of the catheter so that the appropriate antibiotic can be prescribed should the infant subsequently develop septicaemia. Local pressure should be applied to the umbilical stump after withdrawal until any bleeding stops; the stump is then left exposed to reduce the risk of infection.

Arterial blood specimens

Arterial blood samples are required for accurate measurement of the blood gases and in particular of oxygen (Pao_2). Cannulation will also be necessary if arterial infusions are to be given.

Puncture or cannulation. As specimens are likely to be required on several occasions at relatively short intervals an early decision has to be made as to whether to attempt repeated arterial puncture or to insert an umbilical artery cannula. As these techniques are likely to be required only in infants requiring intensive therapy the decision therefore becomes whether the infant requires transfer to an intensive therapy unit. This book is not intended to cover the work of intensive therapy units and only brief mention will be made of the techniques involved.

Arterial puncture. The radial, temporal and femoral arteries are suitable for arterial puncture. A small gauge needle should be employed. The procedure is, however, likely to disturb the infant considerably because of the pain, rendering assessment of the arterial Pao_2 less accurate.

Umbilical artery cannulation

Umbilical artery cannulation is essentially similar to cannulation of the umbilical vein (see above) but made more difficult by the contractility and much smaller size of the arteries. These can, however, be dilated by a suitable reamer although this is best avoided and a 3.5 or 5 fg catheter inserted once the artery is gently opened by fine ophthalmic forceps. The arterial catheter is end-holed. Some clinicians, instead of transecting the cord, incise over an umbilical artery 1 cm from the abdominal wall and having made a small incision in the artery wall insert the catheter. Either technique can be successful. If both arterial and venous catheters are to be inserted the former should be attempted first. In order to simplify the subsequent withdrawal of specimens a disposable two-way tap should be inserted between the open end of the catheter and the syringe.

Difficulty is sometimes encountered in advancing the catheter more than a few centimetres. This is sometimes overcome by waiting several minutes before attempting to advance the catheter further.

The tip of the catheter will require to be advanced into the internal iliac artery or beyond before an adequate flow of arterial blood can be maintained. The tip of the catheter should be advanced either to the level of T12 or L3–4 to avoid the coeliac axis and renal vessels. Its position should be checked by X-ray examination or ultrasound.

Precautions. Care must be taken to ensure that no air enters the syringe as the specimen is taken, and the nozzle of the syringe must be sealed with a suitable cap before the syringe containing the blood is sent to the laboratory. If the catheter is not to be used for continuous infusion it must then be filled with heparinized saline (1 unit heparin per ml saline) contained in a separate syringe attached to the other arm of the two-way tap. The volume of heparinized saline used should be limited to that required to clear the catheter.

The greatest care must be taken during use to ensure that air does not enter the catheter or blood leak from it by careless closure of taps. Like the umbilical vein, the catheter is a direct portal to the vascular system, so strict aseptic precautions should be taken during any precedure involved in either blood withdrawal or infusion.

Risks. The risk of haemorrhage after arterial puncture is greater the larger the needle or catheter used. With small needles, however, bleeding is generally easily controlled by local pressure. Withdrawal of an umbilical arterial catheter should be done progressively, withdrawing not more than 1 cm at a time at intervals over about 5 minutes. Pressure should then be applied to the stump.

Thrombosis or emboli of the internal iliac or other arteries may occur with resulting ischaemia of a lower limb or section of the bowel, or the catheter act as a source or entry of infection. The tip should be sent for culture after removal.

Urine specimens

Collecting bags

Urine specimens required for biochemical testing only are most readily collected by using one of the disposable collecting bags (Fig. 20.8) which can be stuck onto the infant's perineum and left until urine has been passed. Such urine specimens are almost certain to be contaminated by skin organisms and, even if plated out immediately after urine has been passed, often give a misleading indication of organisms present. Bags are therefore not a suitable method for collecting urine for bacteriological analysis.

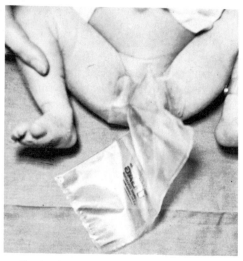

Fig. 20.8 Urine collecting bag.

Clean-catch specimens

Where urinary tract infection is suspected it is essential to obtain an uncontaminated specimen of urine for culture before treatment is considered. 'Clean-catch specimens' are adequate for this purpose if the urine can be caught in a sterile container in mid stream without the urine having dribbled over the perineum. This can be achieved by holding the infant in a suitable position according to sex and by being patient (Fig. 20.9). A suitable time is shortly after the completion of a feed. Mothers can be taught the technique. It is essential that the penis or vulva should not come

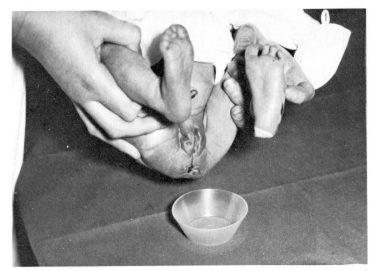

Fig. 20.9 Position for collecting 'clean catch' specimen of urine.

into direct contact with the sterile container. This unfortunately is often allowed to occur and the specimen may be contaminated.

Suprapubic aspiration

Suprapubic aspiration of urine from the bladder is the only satisfactory method of preventing contamination. Mothers, when given the choice of attempting a 'clean catch' or allowing suprapubic aspiration, generally prefer the latter when they realize how little the infant is upset.

Preparation. If a mother is not aware of the method, careful explanation of the advantages and of the safety of the technique must be given beforehand. When a urine specimen is required, mother or a nurse should prevent urine being passed by pressure over the distal urethra. In the male the penis can be held and in the female the labia can be displaced laterally.

Position. With the infant lying in the supine position and the legs held in extension the operator then confirms by palpation and percussion that the bladder is easily definable and contains urine.

Puncture. After cleaning the skin in the suprapubic region a gauge 21 needle attached to 10 ml syringe is advanced through the skin in the midline about 1.0 cm above the symphysis pubis and over the bladder, which is easily entered (Fig. 20.10). About 5 ml

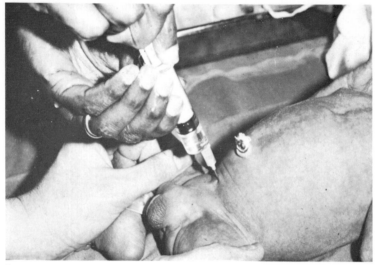

a

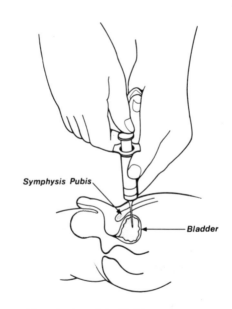

b

Fig. 20.10 Suprapubic aspiration of the bladder.

of urine are aspirated gently, the syringe and needle withdrawn and local pressure applied over the puncture site. The needle is removed and the urine transferred to a suitable microbiological container.

Specimen. It is most important that the microbiologists are informed that urine has been taken by direct aspiration of the bladder as small growths of organisms which might otherwise be ignored may be of significance in such specimens.

Risks. Experience has shown that the risk of causing haematuria is very small and that if it does occur it is of short duration and self-limiting.

In infants who are ill and who may have infection of the urinary tract suprapubic aspiration of the bladder urine is the method of choice for obtaining the initial microbiological specimen.

Cerebrospinal fluid

Cerebrospinal fluid (CSF) may be obtained from the lumbar route, from the lateral ventricles of the brain or, under special circumstances, from the cisterna magna.

Lumbar puncture

Lumbar puncture is the method of first choice unless local deformity, as in spina bifida, makes this difficult. As the spinal cord ends at a relatively lower level in relation to the lumbar vertebrae during early fetal life and as it still extends to the level of the body of the third lumbar vertebra in a term infant at birth, this difference in anatomy when compared to the older child or adult must be kept in mind.

Preparation. Fine gauge short lumbar puncture needles incorporating stilettes are advisable. As infants requiring lumbar puncture are generally ill the procedure should be carried out gently but as rapidly as possible and with minimum disturbance to the infant.

Position. The infant should be held by the nurse at the edge of the table nearest to the operator, with the spine as fully flexed as possible and the infant in the true lateral position (Fig. 20.11). Some prefer the infant to be held in the sitting position but this may be difficult to maintain steadily. As the intervertebral spaces are relatively large in the newborn, and as the vertebral canal is narrow, accurate localization is necessary before the puncture is

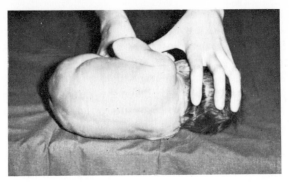

Fig. 20.11 Position of infant for lumbar puncture.

attempted. The skin is sterilized with an appropriate agent and sterile towels are applied.

Puncture. Using the junction of the line of the vertebral spines and a line drawn between the highest points of the iliac crests (supracristal plane) the fourth lumbar vertebra can be identified. Lumbar puncture may be carried out between the bodies of the third and fourth lumbar vertebrae, as in the adult, or, in low birth weight infants, between the fourth and fifth lumbar vertebrae. The needle should be advanced slowly and the stilette withdrawn frequently as it is often difficult to feel when the vertebral canal has been entered. Perforation of the longitudinal vertebral sinuses will result in contamination of the CSF with blood. This occurs readily if the needle is advanced too far. CSF should be allowed to drop slowly into the appropriate container and only the volume required by the laboratory should be removed. The stilette should be replaced before the needle is withdrawn and the puncture site sealed.

Ventricular tap

Ventricular tap is indicated where it is not possible to use the lumbar route or where it is specifically necessary to obtain ventricular CSF.

Position. The infant is wrapped and held supine with the crown of the head at the edge of the table. After identification of the edges and angles of the anterior fontanelle the skin is prepared and the infant's head draped.

Puncture. A lumbar puncture needle is inserted at the lateral angle of the anterior fontanelle and directed in the plane which would meet the internal canthus of the opposite eye. Once the skin and the external dura have been penetrated the stilette should be withdrawn to check on the possibility of a subdural collection of fluid. The shaft of the needle must then be held very steadily within a gauze swab held by the fingers of the operator's left hand so that the plane of advance of the needle remains constant. With the right hand the needle is advanced slowly and the stilette withdrawn frequently while the needle is stationary. If no CSF has been obtained after the tip of the needle has been advanced 3 cm, the needle should be withdrawn continuing with frequent withdrawal of the stilette.

Repeated ventricular taps are not advisable.

The risks associated with tapping the cisterna magna are high and this procedure is best left to those with training in neurological techniques.

THERAPEUTIC PROCEDURES

Temperature control

The commonest problem affecting newborn infants requiring treatment is inadequate control of body temperature. For a discussion of the physiological principles involved readers are referred to Chapter 5. Two lines of therapy are available, the first aimed at controlling heat loss and the second at providing a source of extra warmth or cooling as required. As fall in body temperature is the commonest problem attention will be focused on prevention of heat loss and provision of extra heat.

Prevention of heat loss

For the healthy term newborn infant, dryness, clothing, a suitable cot and bedding and a room temperature of about 20 °C described in Chapter 6 are all that is required. Low birth weight and ill infants may require to be nursed in an incubator with no or minimal clothing to allow adequate observation. Heat loss, however, still occurs when the infant is nursed naked even in a warm incubator.

Radiation loss can be reduced by covering the infant with a transparent perspex heat shield, preferably with one end blocked off to prevent draughts from the room air or incubator recirculation fan.

The head should be covered by a thick gamgee hat, the extremities with mittens and bootees. If total body observation is not essential a thick layer of heated gamgee or similar material can be wrapped round the body to reduce radiant heat loss. This can also be used during transportation. There is considerable doubt surrounding the value of silver swaddlers. In a heated incubator they may in fact reflect heat from the baby. Sick infants and all but the largest preterm infants should be transported in a heated incubator. *Remember, hypothermia kills!*

Convection loss can be reduced by limiting opening of the incubator port-holes and other apertures to an absolute minimum. Oxygen or other gas being given should be warmed before entering the incubator and should not be given by direct mask except for brief periods of crisis. The room temperature should also be maintained at between 80 and 85 °F (26–29.5 °C) when nursing preterm infants. The air temperature at the baby will be 1 °C less than the incubator inside wall temperature for every 7 °C the room is cooler than the incubator. This high environmental nursery temperature makes it important that staff have appropriate clothing and easy access to drinks.

Providing extra heat

Incubators are not entirely satisfactory means of providing heat, relying as most of them do on the circulation of heated and moistened air within the hood.

Overhead heaters. Radiant and conductive heat can be provided from overhead infrared heaters (Fig. 20.12) or from heated mattresses. When using a servocontrolled infant warmer it is important to tape the temperature probe firmly to the infant's trunk out of the direct line of heat and if possible to cover the tip with reflective material. Failure to fix the probe correctly may lead to overheating if the probe is not in contact with the skin. If the probe is directly irradiated by the heater insufficient extra heat will be delivered.

Servocontrol mechanisms can be incorporated in the type of apparatus shown in Figure 20.13, which is suitable for carrying out special procedures or for intensive care of preterm low birth weight infants provided a heat shield is used. Incubators remain the most suitable method for aiding temperature control in the less sick preterm infant. Many low birth weight infants are, however, nursed in incubators longer than is probably necessary or advisable.

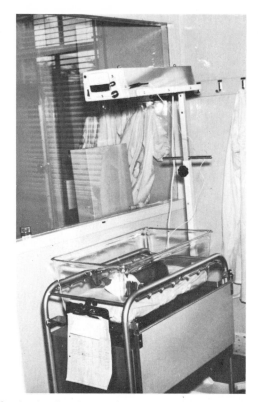

Fig. 20.12 Overhead radiant heater with servocontrol mechanism.

Oxygen

Control

Under a number of circumstances in which lowered levels of blood oxygen occur in the infant increased concentrations of inspired oxygen are required.

Arterial Pao_2. Ideally oxygen therapy should be controlled by measurement of the infant's arterial Pao_2. This is not necessary where oxygen is being given for short periods but is essential when treatment is being given for more than 30 minutes.

The umbilical artery may be used for continuous monitoring of Pao_2 levels of infants with RDS. Disposable presterilized umbilical artery catheters with a bipolar oxygen electrode at the distal end are now available, which when attached to a monitor, provide a direct continuous reading of oxygen tension. Such catheters have

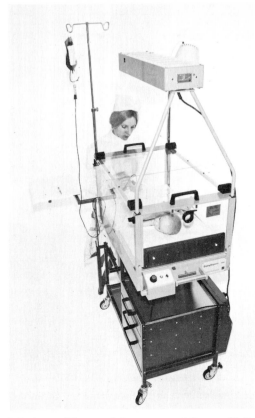

Fig. 20.13 Babytherm. (Photograph by courtesy of Draeger Medical Ltd.)

remained in place and functioned normally for several weeks but monitoring is usually only necessary for 48 to 72 hours (see Chapter 16).

Transcutaneous Pao_2 measurement of the oxygen tension in 'arterialized capillary' blood is a less invasive method of continuous monitoring.

The object should be to maintain a satisfactory level of oxygenation (Pao_2 of 8 kPa to 12 kPa [60 to 90 mmHg]) and to prevent higher levels being reached because of the risk of retinopathy of prematurity, and possible damage to the lungs.

Transcutaneous arterial oxygen saturation. Monitors have been recently developed to allow non-invasive measurement of oxygen saturation. This technique is of value in identification of hypoxia.

Clinical assessment of arterial oxygenation can be extremely difficult and at times misleading. Cyanosis is the most obvious clinical sign of hypoxaemia and requires treatment with the minimum added oxygen which will restore a normal colour.

Oxygen concentration

If there is no clinical cyanosis the concentration of inspired oxygen should not be allowed to exceed 40% and preferably should be kept at 30%.

Oxygen analyser. Sampling of the environmental oxygen concentration by an oxygen analyser (Fig. 20.14) is the only satisfactory method of estimating the inspired air concentration of oxygen. The settings given on incubators for oxygen concentrations at a given rate of flow are only guides relating to ideal conditions which are seldom achieved in practice.

High concentrations. If high concentrations of oxygen are required it may be found difficult to achieve these in an incubator unless a small headbox is placed over the infant's head (Fig. 20.15).

Arterial oxygen concentration. Prolonged use of concentrations of inspired oxygen greater than 40% should be controlled by arterial oxygen concentration measurements. These can be made intermittently by repeated arterial blood sampling or continuously by an intra-arterial electrode (Fig. 20.16) or transcutaneous monitor.

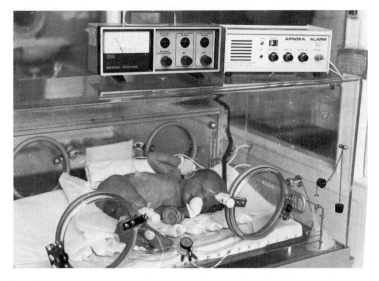

Fig. 20.14 Oxygen monitor and apnoea alarm.

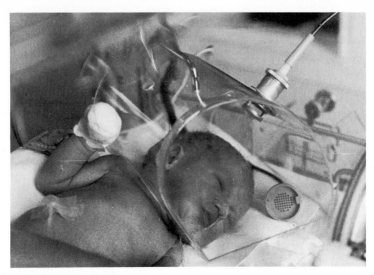

Fig. 20.15 Oxygen headbox.

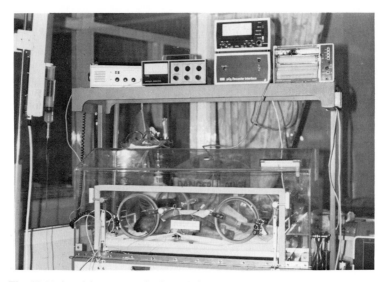

Fig. 20.16 Arterial oxygen and other monitors.

Temperature and humidity. The necessity to warm the oxygen and air being given has already been mentioned. Dryness of the oxygen and air should be avoided but there appears to be no advantage in the very high levels of humidity previously recommended unless the infant is extremely preterm, when transcutaneous water losses through the skin are extremely high in the first week of life if nursed in a warm dry environment. Oxygen and air mixtures given through the mixer valve of incubators are adequately moistened by the incubator humidifier. Many units run their incubators with no water in the humidification chamber of the incubator to reduce the risks of infection and supply warmed humidified air/oxygen mixtures separately when required.

CPAP

This has already been discussed in Chapter 16 to which reference can be made for the indications for use of CPAP and the methods available for its application.

Tracheal intubation

If adequate oxygenation cannot be achieved by spontaneous respiration of an oxygen-enriched air, some form of artificial ventilation will be required. It is not intended in this book to discuss in detail ventilation management but all, whether midwives or doctors, who are involved in the care of the newborn should understand and practise the technique of tracheal intubation and intermittent positive-pressure ventilation (IPPV).

Equipment

An infant-type laryngoscope with a straight infant blade is used (e.g. Magill, Wisconsin).

Endotracheal tubes. For the oral route endotracheal tubes of varying sizes should be available — 2.5, 3, 3.5 mm (10, 12, 14 fg). These may be of the disposable type (Fig. 20.17) with a broader section to prevent the tube being advanced too far or they may be of the simple anaesthetic type. A soft metal probe or introducer which can be inserted into the tube aids in positioning and is sometimes helpful. For nasopharyngotracheal intubation, either Jackson-Rees tubes (Fig. 20.18) or straight endotracheal tubes are required together with special forceps (Magill) for guiding the catheter from the pharynx into the trachea.

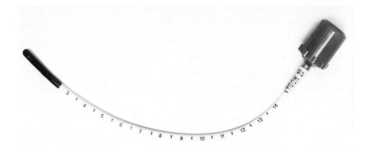

Fig. 20.17 Disposable endotracheal tube. (Photograph by courtesy of Vygon Ltd.)

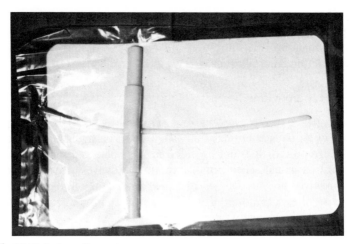

Fig. 20.18 Jackson-Rees tube.

Suction apparatus with a suitable sterile catheter 5–6 fg should be held in readiness by an assistant. Suction pressure should not exceed 150 mmHg (20 cmH$_2$O) but mucus extractors are particularly useful for clearing the pharynx.

A source of air, or oxygen-enriched air, limited to a maximum pressure of 30 cm of water and with a side hole or Y tube to allow expiration must be available together with suitable connectors for attachment to the endotracheal tube. The rate of flow does not need to be higher than that required to ensure a maximum pressure of 30 cm H$_2$O. This is generally about 3–4 litre per minute. Intermittent closure of the side hole allows IPPV to be applied.

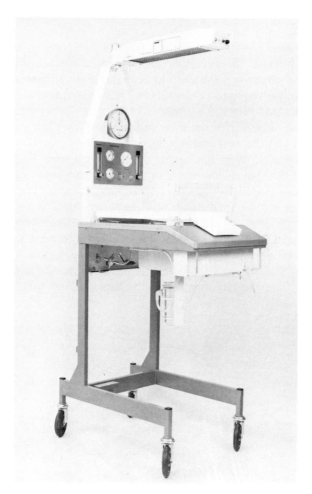

Fig. 20.19 Resuscitation trolley with overhead heater. (Photograph by courtesy of Vickers Medical.)

Resuscitation trolleys. The necessary apparatus is most conveniently available if already assembled and on a mobile trolley with a suitable area for the infant. Such resuscitation trolleys are available commercially but some have the disadvantage that no arrangement for providing local heat is available and a separate heat source is also required (Fig. 20.19). There is a major risk of fall in superficial temperature followed by fall in central temperature during tracheal intubation unless adequate precautions are taken to prevent heat loss.

Technique

Preparation. As the oral route is the easier to perform it will be described. Once the necessary expertise has been acquired this procedure is relatively simple. The beginner should, however, learn the technique required on a stillborn infant or on one of the artificial dolls made for this purpose.

Position. The infant is laid supine with the head partially extended and the neck slightly flexed.

Laryngoscopy. With the handle of the laryngoscope held in the left hand the blade is inserted gently at the left angle of the infant's mouth and passed forward over the infant's tongue (Fig. 20.20). The blade is then used to depress the tongue until the epiglottis comes into view. By sliding the tip of the laryngoscope into the glossoepiglottic fold and pulling the epiglottis forward the vocal cords come into view (Fig. 20.21). Suction is applied as necessary to clear the airway and to allow unimpeded vision. With the right hand holding the proximal end, the endotracheal tube is then

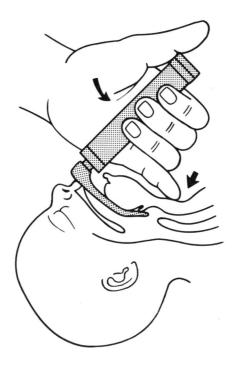

Fig. 20.20 Position for inserting laryngoscope.

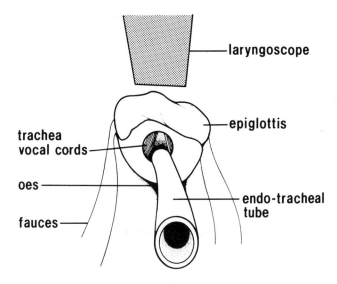

Fig. 20.21 Diagrammatic representation of view of vocal cords during laryngoscopy.

passed under direct vision into the larynx and upper trachea making sure that the tip of the tube lies above the origin of the main bronchi. Further suction through the tube may then be required.

Intermittent positive-pressure ventilation

After laryngoscopy and tracheal intubation the proximal end of the endotracheal tube is connected to the IPPV apparatus and air allowed to flow for approximately 1 second followed by a similar period for expiration resulting in about 30 to 40 respiratory cycles per minute. By observing chest movement and listening over both lungs with a stethoscope the operator must check that air is entering both lungs. If not, the situation must be reassessed and, if necessary, laryngoscopy be repeated to make certain that the tube is in the trachea and not in the oesophagus. This situation can be confirmed by listening by stethoscope over the stomach. Gas will be heard to gurgle in the stomach if the tube is in the oesophagus. Should one lung only be adequately ventilated the tip of the endo-tracheal tube may have passed into a main bronchus and should be withdrawn until both lungs are adequately ventilated. If the tube is in a good position but air entry is poor further suction is

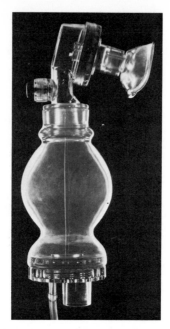

Fig. 20.22 Mask and bag.

required. Once the tube is in a satisfactory position and if further IPPV is required the tube should be strapped to the angle of the mouth to prevent further movement. Where apparatus for tracheal intubation is available without a source of gas under pressure IPPV can be applied by an anaesthetic or resuscitation bag attached to the tube (Fig. 20.22). If a suitable bag is not available in an emergency situation air can be blown into the tracheal tube from the operator's mouth.

Bag and mask ventilation. This method was described in Chapter 12 and can be effective in the short term if carefully applied. A round face mask is most easily applied in the newborn infant.

For *mouth to nose insufflation* the infant is conveniently supported by the thorax in the palm of the right hand with the fingers palpating the apex beat and chest movement. With the left hand the head is supported and the neck extended. By placing his mouth over the long axis of the infant's nose and across the infant's mouth the operator is now ready to blow small volumes of air from his puffed out cheeks into the infant's lungs. The pressure required can be learned from practice with a water manometer and should not exceed 30 cm of water. This is readily exceeded with a hard puff from the chest which will also be of too large a volume. The fingers of the right hand which are wrapped round the infant's chest give an indication of the respiratory movement being produced and also show whether the heart rate is returning to normal.

Risks. Mouth to nose insufflation and blowing directly into an endotracheal tube naturally carry a risk of virus and bacterial contamination of the infant's respiratory tract. These methods should therefore only be used where no better method is available and they should only be continued as long as they are necessary for the infant's well-being. More detailed descriptions of ventilation procedures can be found in books dealing with neonatal intensive care.

INJECTIONS AND INFUSIONS

Intradermal, subcutaneous and intramuscular injections

These injections are given to infants by the same techniques as apply to older patients. Smaller gauge needles are required and greater care is necessary to ensure that the injection is correctly placed and that no injury is done. Volumes injected must be limited preferably to not more than 0.5 ml in low birth weight infants. Because of the difficulty in measuring small volumes accurately graduated 1 ml syringes (as used for Mantoux tests) are required for doses less than 1.0 ml.

Risks. Particular care must be taken in choosing the site of the injection in order to avoid important structures such as the sciatic nerve. The margin for error in choice of site is very little in the smallest infants. Too superficial an injection may result in local tissue reaction. Too deep an injection may cause neurological or vascular damage. It is preferable to place intramuscular injections in the vastus lateralis muscle of the thigh.

Intravenous infusions

Veins

Mention has already been made of the use of the umbilical vein for giving intravenous therapy. This route is not generally available after the first week of life, and in the first week is not recommended as the vein of choice if it is not also to be used for obtaining samples of venous blood. Any peripheral vein including those of the hand and forearm may be used but many find the veins of the scalp are the most suitable.

Scalp vein infusion

Disposable scalp vein needles with a wing attachment for holding the needle and with a length of tubing and adaptor for Luer fitting attached are available in several sizes. Use of such sets has simplified the technique of scalp vein infusion. Intravenous polyvinyl or silastic cannulae can also be used with the advantage that in the absence of damage to the vein by a sharp needle the infusion is likely to run longer.

Choice of site. Before starting the procedure the operator should examine the whole scalp to identify several suitable sites. The Y junction of two veins is a useful place to make an attempt as the tributary veins steady the larger vein produced by their junction. The position and size of veins can best be judged after the flow of blood has been temporarily obstructed by pressure over the vein lower down its course (Fig. 20.23). It is advisable to make first attempts near the vertex so that further attempts can be made 'downstream', should the original attept fail. If a limb vein is selected, pressure should be applied proximally to the limb to encourage mild venous engorgement.

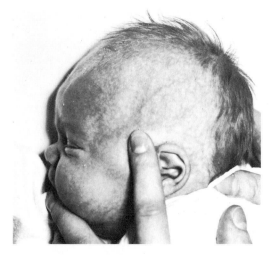

Fig. 20.23 Demonstration of scalp veins by occluding flow distally.

Preparation. After the infusion fluid and giving set have been assembled the infant is lightly held in a suitable position and the skin of the scalp or limb prepared. The scalp vein set should then be filled with sterile normal saline or similar clear fluid and the stopper removed from the adaptor.

Puncture. The needle point should be inserted through the skin about 0.5 cm proximal to the Y junction selected. The distal part of the vein is occluded by pressure and the needle passed into the vein at the Y junction. The passage of blood back into the tubing indicates that the vein has been entered. With the needle carefully held in that position the drip set is connected, pressure over the distal vein removed and the flow of infusion fluid checked. If intravenous cannulae are to be used, once the introducing trochar needle is removed it must not be reintroduced for fear of damaging the cannula tip.

Fixture. When this has been established the wings of the needle are used to fix the needle to the scalp or arm with adhesive strapping (Fig. 20.24) or by a small plaster of Paris protective covering, and the remainder of the tubing is secured so that accidental movement of the needle is prevented.

Observations. The rate of flow of the infusion is then checked and written instructions given about the total volume to be given and the time to be taken for this. It is important that those attending the infant report immediately if there is swelling near the infusion site indicating that the needle has been displaced. The

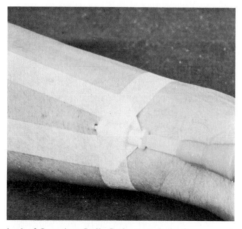

Fig. 20.24 Method of Securing Quik-Cath cannula in forearm vein. (Photograph by courtesy of Travenol Laboratories Ltd.)

infusion must be stopped and assistance sought. Minor correction of the needle position may restore flow but often a new site has to be chosen and the procedure repeated.

Control of infusions

As it is easy to overburden an infant's circulation if excessive volumes of fluid are infused, or if he infusion takes place rapidly, both the rate of flow and the total volume to be given must be carefully regulated.

Giving sets. This is made easier by using giving sets designed for infants and containing a subsidiary graduated chamber containing, for example, 30 ml which is filled from the main infusion bottle by a valve which is normally kept closed.

Electronic drop counters, with a servomechanism designed to maintain a constant number of drops per minute, are available.

Infusion syringe pumps (Fig. 20.25) which are controlled electronically to deliver a specified volume per minute have replaced the more complicated roller pumps previously used for this purpose.

Regulation. A combination of regulating the drops per minute in the drip chamber combined with repeated observation of the fluid being removed from the graduated chamber provides a sufficient degree of control in most situations.

Rate of flow. As the total volume to be given and the rates of flow required vary so considerably with the condition of the individual infant no absolute figures can be given. Except for the correction of severe blood loss not more than 20 ml per kg of body weight of any plasma expander such as whole blood or reconstituted plasma should be given without assessment of central venous pressure. Except for shocked infants at least 3 hours should be taken to give this volume. Should the heart rate increase to over 160 per minute the infusion should be stopped temporarily and if the heart rate does not return to normal within 30 minutes no further plasma expander should be given without careful clinical assessment of the cause.

Maintenance fluids are given at slower rates and for volumes of the order of 50 to 75 ml per kg per day require rates of 2 to 3 ml per kg per hour in very low birth weight infants.

Regulation. As a check on the accuracy of the flow rate the volume delivered from the graduated chamber in the giving set or the syringe should be checked regularly and recorded.

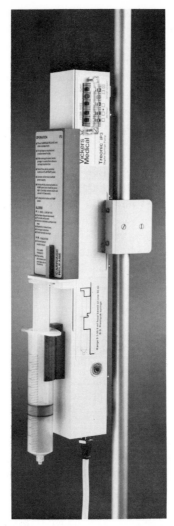

Fig. 20.25 Syringe pump with digital control. (Photograph by courtesy of Vickers Medical.)

Intravenous drugs

Drugs to be given intravenously at stated intervals can be injected into an intravenous infusion provided that there is no pharmacological contraindication. Some drugs may be added to the infusion fluid, in which case it must be made clear whether the drug is to be added to the infusion bottle, bearing in mind the length of time over which this will be administered, or into the graduated drip chamber which will be emptied in a shorter period of time.

Instructions. In either case written instructions should be given and a record made on the donor bottle or graduated chamber of the drug, the dose and the time at which it was added to the infusion fluid. Should the infusion fluid require to be changed, further instructions with regard to drugs incorporated with the previous fluid must be sought.

Precautions. Certain preparations given intravenously are irritant to veins and tissues because of their chemical or physical properties. Typical of these are 4.2% sodium bicarbonate and 50% glucose. It is safer to give these only into large veins, but in an emergency situation they may have to be given through smaller peripheral veins in which case the vein should immediately be flushed through with normal saline or 5% glucose, a record being kept of the volume used.

Exchange transfusion

The general principles of exchange transfusion have been discussed in Chapter 15. A variety of techniques may be employed some using both an artery and a vein. We shall confine this description to the use of a single catheter in the umbilical vein.

Equipment

The simplest equipment is that required for cannulation of the umbilical vein plus two two-way taps in series (Fig. 20.26) and sterile tubing to connect one side arm with the donor bottle, and the other to lead to a waste blood collecting bag.

Prepacked sterilized disposable exchange transfusion sets are available but are more expensive than the simple equipment described.

Heparinized saline. Some sets contain three- or four-way taps to allow a bottle of heparinized saline to be connected to the system. A simple system using disposable taps and syringes is not likely to become obstructed by clot, and it is no longer essential to incorporate heparinized saline into the system. It is useful, however, to prepare a bottle of 0.9% saline with 1 unit heparin per ml saline. This can be used to fill the system during any temporary halt during the procedure.

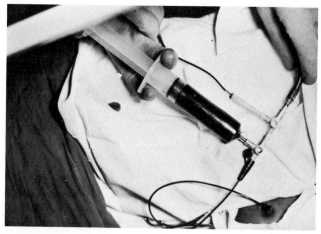

Fig. 20.26 Simple apparatus for exchange transfusion.

The donor blood should be cross-matched with the infant's blood but in the case of rhesus isoimmunization should be Rh-negative. It is inadvisable to use blood more than 48 hours old as the potassium level begins to rise rapidly over that age. As the haematocrit of phosphate citrate dextrose donor blood is generally below 40% withdrawal of 100 ml of plasma is often arranged to increase the packed cell volume.

The blood should be warmed slowly to blood heat. Rapid heating causes haemolysis. A water-bath with regulated heater coil is useful.

Time for preparation. Exchange transfusion is only an emergency procedure in infants with severe anaemia from haemolysis or blood loss. In other situations time is better spent ensuring that all preparations are complete and that the donor blood is at appropriate temperature before starting the procedure.

The infant

Some immobilization, particularly for the limbs of an active infant, is desirable during an exchange transfusion. Whatever method is used, access to the mouth must be allowed so that the pharynx can be aspirated and the trachea intubated if necessary. A variety of frames or crucifixes have been devised to which the infant can be lightly strapped.

Heat. Extra heat should be available from an electrically heated

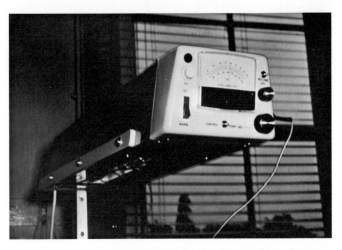

Fig. 20.27 Temperature monitoring on overhead servocontrolled radiant heater.

mattress or from an overhead infrared heater. Both sources are available in the Baby-therm (Fig. 20.12). Incubators can be used but often present problems of suitable access.

Monitoring. Recording of heart rate is most conveniently made by ECG electrodes on the limbs with the trace visible on an oscilloscope. If apparatus for this is not available a stethoscope should be strapped over the apex so that the heart rate can be monitored constantly. A permanent temperature record should also be available and can be combined with a radiant heater controlled by the infant's temperature (Fig. 20.27).

Records of volume of blood exchanged, heart rate, temperature and drugs given should be kept and it is useful to have a prepared sheet on which these observations can be recorded. Containers required for any specimens to be taken should be available.

Preparation

As will be appreciated from the foregoing remarks, preparation for an exchange transfusion takes some time. Where there is a possibility that exchange transfusion will be required rapidly after birth, as in severe haemolytic disease of the newborn (Chapter 15), all the necessary preparations must be completed before delivery is expected. In such circumstances group O, Rh-negative donor blood should be cross-matched against mother's blood and be available suitably warmed so that there is no delay in starting the transfusion should the infant's condition at birth justify immediate treatment.

Staff

At least two people should be constantly available during an exchange transfusion. The physician who is to carry out the transfusion should scrub up as for a surgical operation and wear sterile gown, cap and gloves. A senior nurse or another doctor is required to supervise the infant's condition and to keep records of the procedure. It is not necessary for them to be in sterile gowns unless they are to assist with the cannulation.

Technique

When the equipment has been checked and the infant prepared, the area is covered with a sterile towel with a central aperture, and the two-way taps and syringe connected to the donor bottle and to the waste tube. Blood is drawn into the syringe from the donor bottle and expelled down the waste tube to check that the apparatus is functioning properly. The infant's umbilical vein is then cannulated with a closed-end side-hole tube of gauge 4.5 to 9.0 fg as described earlier. When the blood flows back freely the venous pressure is measured and the catheter connected to the taps.

The exchange may then proceed by withdrawal of a carefully measured quantity of blood, generally 10 ml but varying from 5 ml in very small infants to 20 ml in large infants. As the efficiency of the exchange is reduced by using smaller volumes at each cycle the largest volume which does not upset the infant should be used. By suitable arrangement of the taps this blood is either used for collection of specimens or disposed of. The same volume of blood is withdrawn from the donor bottle into the syringe and then slowly injected into the infant.

Heart rate. The effect on the infant's heart rate of withdrawal of blood or of giving blood should be noted. Heart rates rising to greater than 160 per minute indicate stress. If this occurs only when blood is given there is probably circulatory overload and the effect of removing an extra 10 or 20 ml of blood should be assessed. Similarly, if tachycardia occurs on withdrawal of blood, extra blood may be required.

Venous pressure. Serial measurements of venous pressure will help in the decision with regard to blood volume adjustments.

An exchange proceeds by repeated cycles of the withdrawal and replacement of blood. Constant supervision is necessary to ensure that no air is injected. The total volume to be exchanged and the time involved were discussed in Chapter 15.

Completion. At the end of an exchange transfusion the umbilical vein catheter should be withdrawn unless required for other purposes. Bleeding from the umbilical stump is generally readily controlled by pressure at the site or immediately above the umbilicus. It is seldom necessary to ligate the vessel. The area should be inspected regularly for signs of bleeding.

Blood pressure

In severly ill infants requiring intensive care, blood pressure can be monitored continuously by intra-arterial catheters and transducers. For less urgent and intermittent monitoring of blood pressure, appropriately sized cuffs can be used together with recorders such as those produced by Dinomapp or Critikon. However, these are less accurate than direct intra-arterial monitoring.

Relief of tension pneumothorax

A tension pneumothorax may prove rapidly fatal unless relieved. It is essential therefore that all special care and intensive therapy baby units should have at least one set of apparatus constantly available for the treatment of pneumothorax.

Equipment. The provision of sterile disposable Heimlich valves (Fig. 20.28) has greatly simplified this procedure particularly if

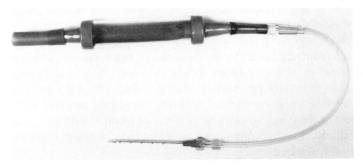

Fig. 20.28 Disposable Heimlich valve and trochar. (Photograph by courtesy of Vygon Ltd.)

combined with a trocar and cannula set of suitable size. The cannula should be firmly secured using black silk and the site covered with a protective dressing. For temporary use until more satisfactory drainage can be established wide gauge needle with facilities for connection to an underwater seal by narrow bore tubing through a two-way tap may be used.

The site at which the cannula is introduced depends upon the clinical and radiological findings but the preferred site is the 4th intercostal space in the mid-axillary line to avoid unnecessary scarring.

Marrow aspiration

Site. Marrow is most conveniently taken from an iliac bone or tibia in the newborn period. Suitably small marrow puncture needles are necessary.

Technique. After suitable preparation the infant is placed in the lateral position and held steadily. The needle is inserted into the iliac bone about 1 to 2 cm behind and below the anterior superior iliac spine and with the needle perpendicular to the flat surface of the bone. Less pressure is required than in older children to penetrate the outer table. Once the marrow cavity has been entered marrow is aspirated as in older children or adults. The tibia can be entered at the junction of its upper and middle thirds through its medial subcutaneous surface. In both methods great care must be taken not to pass right through the marrow cavity. Care and gentle persistence are required.

FURTHER READING

Auld, P. A. M. (Ed) (1980) Neonatal intensive care, *Clinics in Perinatology*, **7**, 1.
Cockburn, F. & Drillien, C. M. (1974) *Neonatal Medicine*, Oxford: Blackwell.
Wilkinson, A. & Calvert, S. (1986) Procedures in neonatal intensive care. In: *Textbook of Neonatology*, Ed. Roberton, N. R. C. Edinburgh: Churchill Livingstone.

21

Continuing care

In Chapter 1 and 2 of this book we looked at the challenge which faces midwives, doctors and all others associated with the care of mother and her child during pregnancy and the newborn period, and in particular we considered perinatal mortality as an index of failure in meeting that challenge. Stillbirth or neonatal death is clearly a failure in that the pregnancy has not resulted in a live healthy child. However, it is essential that parents of a stillborn child or one that has died after birth are not left with an empty feeling of failure. Over twelve thousand parents in the UK 'lose' a baby each year because it is stillborn or dies in the first month after birth. They must be given every opportunity to discuss with the nurses and doctors involved the reasons for their loss; when a postmortem examination has been performed the results, even when negative, must be clearly explained and a further opportunity taken to discuss any remaining uncertainties, anxieties and feelings of anger or guilt. An excellent booklet entitled 'The loss of your baby' is produced by the Health Education Council in conjunction with the National Association for Mental Health and National Stillbirth Study Group and gives helpful and practical advice to parents.

Growing up

Survival cannot, however, be equated with success unless the child is able to pass through a happy childhood and adolescence to maturity and independence. The title of this book would appear to limit our interest to the newborn period but it is foolish to consider this extremely important but limited period of our lives in isolation. Delivery and adaptation to the external environment are phases in the development of a mature adult. The problems which may arise because of difficulty in the perinatal period are not necessarily confined to infancy or even childhood and may have a profound effect, physical or emotional, on the adult.

Quality of survival

To the midwife and doctor looking after a low birth weight infant the immediate problems are so obvious that it is difficult to keep the thought of quality of adult life for that infant in mind. We have now reached the stage of development of maternity and paediatric services where this thought of the future must play a major part in the assessment of our service. It is no longer satisfactory to count survival of the infant as the only criterion of success. Quality of life for the survivor should now be our parameter of success. How does one measure quality of survival?

Quality of life means such different things to different people under different circumstances that no simple quantitative measure can be expected. The severely handicapped child with spina bifida but with understanding and loving parents may have a much happier life than the physically normal child in a broken home.

Environmental factors

Environmental factors and how they may be improved will not be discussed here beyond the newborn period. It is most important, however, to appreciate that the environment in the newborn period may have a profound and possibly life-long effect on the intimate relationship between a mother and her baby and this is a factor well within the control of midwives, doctors, hospital administrators, social workers etc. (Chapter 7). This is not a factor which can be appreciated easily or measured during the newborn period.

The home. The effects are likely to become obvious when mother is trying to look after her baby at home. Unless the midwifery department and newborn nursery staff know of such problems remedial measures cannot be put into effect.

Feedback of information about the subsequent development and happiness of mothers and babies is therefore essential to any assessment of the effectiveness of a maternity department. What has been said about emotional problems applies equally to physical problems. Mothers are perhaps more willing to have their infants re-examined to exclude physical abnormality and it is on this basis that follow-up clinics are generally arranged.

Comprehensive child health services

As it has become increasingly clear from experience gained in varying parts of the world with differing socioeconomic problems care for the health and welfare of the growing and developing child is a major factor in promoting adult health and happiness. Most health services have, however, so far been largely adult oriented and inadequate attention has been given to the importance of the health services for children. Two major reports have been published recently in the UK dealing with the need to establish adequate child health services. The first, published in 1973 by the Scottish Home and Health Department, is entitled *Towards an Integrated Child Health Service*. In 1976 the English counterpart *The Report of the Committee on Child Health Services — Fit for the Future* was published. These are often referred to by the name of the chairman of the committee involved as the Brotherston Report and the Court Report. The recommendations of the Court Report contain much that was in Brotherston's earlier report and there is therefore a considerable consensus of agreement between their recommendations. (Reference has already been made in Chapter 2 to the reports of the 'Short' Committee on Perinatal and Neonatal Mortality, 1980 and 1985.)

Integration

Both reports look to an integration of the therapeutic and preventive services for children with primary care being given by general practitioners with a special interest and' training in paediatric medicine. They are to be assisted by health visitors and other nursing staff with similar paediatric training and experience. The hospitals would continue to provide more specialized paediatric services including those for the newborn. There would be more regular links between the primary-care teams and the hospitals with hospital paediatricians being more involved in community work and primary-care doctors having closer links with hospitals. Although it will be some time before staff can be adequately trained to provide such integrated services the prospect is hopeful for improvement in our child health services. There is the likelihood that follow-up services for the newborn will become more comprehensive.

Records

Provided that an adequate data retrieval system is established there should be an increased feedback of information with regard to the later development of handicap which can be related to perinatal problems and the type of management used.

Clinics

General practitioners will increasingly become involved in the regular assessment of well infants and children. The school health service will also at least in part be staffed by general practitioners in consultation with hospital paediatricians. It is hoped that this system will avoid some of the problems which arose when there was a tripartite system with staffing and management of infant welfare clinics and school health services provided by the local authority health service.

Acceptability

The most important test of the proposed services will be the proof of their acceptability by those who are in most need of such services. At present those with the greatest need are those least likely to take advantage of the services offered. It is particularly important that thought and effort be devoted to providing services which are compatible with the needs of the community, whether it be predominantly in the deprived inner city or immigrant areas or in the well-to-do middle class areas. Each area has its special needs. The child health services must rise to each as an individual challenge. It is likely, however, that unless the new service can concentrate its activity on the deprived sections of the community it is unlikely to prove any more effective than its predecessors.

Co-ordination

Much time and effort can be wasted if there is inadequate passage of information between the various personnel involved in the child health services. Co-ordination of information is closely related to co-ordination of recording and retrieval systems. The ideal of a continuous record of a patient's health from cradle to the grave is becoming nearer to reality but has not yet been achieved. Further effort in this field should prove very rewarding.

The benefit

The individual infant and child can hope to gain from regular medical examination, including developmental assessment, if illness or minor abnormality is detected at a stage when treatment can be applied with minimal disturbance of normal life and activity.

The community can also gain from such a service. In time it is to be hoped that the regular feedback of information to maternity units about the progress of children will allow a medical audit of the relative advantages and disadvantages of procedures being employed. This would be the long-term equivalent of the shorter-term assessment of immediate results in the newborn period. Without such information the harmful effects on the low birth weight infants of high concentrations of oxygen would not have been recognized.

Reassessment. With more refined methods of serial examination, as in developmental screening, it could well be that some of our most cherished theories of management in the newborn period will be called into question. We must be prepared to abandon a policy which is shown in the long term to be harmful to the child as readily as we abandon policies which are not in the best short-term interest of the infant.

'At risk' register

So far no mention has been made of selectivity in advocating the advantages of long-term supervision of children's development. The reason for this is that we cannot as yet be certain which infants may justifiably be considered as being at risk. By selecting in the newborn period a limited number of infants for follow up and by placing these on an 'at risk' register it had been hoped that a higher quality of service could be given to those who were most in need. Experience has shown, however, that not only do many of the children on the present 'at risk' registers prove to have no special requirements but a considerable number of those who do require special facilities or education were not included on the 'at risk' register after assessment in the newborn period. Improving standards of assessment in the first month of life may improve the usefulness of 'at risk' registers.

Delivering care

Many general practitioners have established regular periodic assessment of children in their practices. This is a welcome step but more information is required as to the type of patient being brought to such clinics for periodic assessment. There is the fear that only those who come from families who are health orientated will take advantages of this service and that those children from less well educated families who are generally those most in need will not take advantage of such services. It is probable that more would be gained if it were possible to persuade parents in the deprived groups to attend such follow-up clinics so that health services could be concentrated where they are most required. In countries such as France financial inducements are used to encourage parents to take advantage of such services but this is a method which has not been tried in the UK.

The first month of life is the basis on which we build the remainder of our physical, emotional and intellectual development. This places a great responsibility on those who care for us during that formative period. The authors hope that this book has helped to provide some insight into the problems involved and the remedies available.

FURTHER READING

Black, J. (1985) *The New Paediatrics: Child Health in Ethnic Minorities*. British Medical Journal Publication, London.

Doxiadis, S. (Ed.) (1979) *The Child in the World of Tomorrow*, Oxford: Pergamon Press.

Lobo, E. de H. (1978) *Children of Immigrants to Britain*. London: Hodder & Stoughton.

Mitchell, R. G. (1980) *Child Health in the Community*, 2nd edn. Edinburgh: Churchill Livingstone.

Report of the Committee on Child Health Services (1976) *Fit for the Future*, London: HMSO.

The Loss of your Baby — produced by The Health Education Council in conjunction with the National Association for Mental Health and The National Stillbirth Study Group. The Health Education Council, 78 New Oxford Street, London WC1A 1AH.

Towards an Integrated Child Health Service (1973) Edinburgh: HMSO

Walker, C. H. M. (1977) Neonatal records and the computer. *Archives of Disease in Childhood*, 52, 452–461.

Index